A Dictionary of Neuropsychology

Diana M. Goodwin

A Dictionary
of Neuropsychology

Springer-Verlag
New York Berlin Heidelberg
London Paris Tokyo Hong Kong

Diana M. Goodwin
Pacific Graduate School of Psychology
935 East Meadow Drive
Palo Alto, CA 94303
U.S.A.

Library of Congress Cataloging-in-Publication Data
Goodwin, Diana M.
    A dictionary of neuropsychology / Diana M. Goodwin.
       p.   cm.
    ISBN 0-387-97123-8
    1. Neuropsychology—Dictionaries.   I. Title.
    [DNLM: 1. Neuropsychology—dictionaries.   WL 13 G656d]
QP360.G66   1989
612.8′03—dc20
DNLM/DLC   89-21704

Printed on acid-free paper.

Camera-ready copy supplied by the author.
Printed and bound by Edwards Brothers, Inc., Ann Arbor, Michigan.
Printed in the United States of America.

9 8 7 6 5 4 3 2 1

ISBN 0-387-97123-8 Springer-Verlag New York Berlin Heidelberg
ISBN 3-540-97123-8 Springer-Verlag Berlin Heidelberg New York

Preface

Neuropsychology is becoming a well-established specialty within the field of rehabilitation medicine. Neuropsychologists need to know many aspects of neurology, physiatry, psychiatry, and the various interpretations of the commonly used psychological tests as they relate to neuropsychology.

The emerging speciality in neuropsychology has prompted many experienced neuropsychologists to write text and reference books on the subject. Much of the test information for this book was taken from *Neuropsychological Assessment* by Murial Lezak (1983). Information on syndromes and detailed neurological functions was taken, in part, from *Fundamentals of Neuropsychology* by Kolb and Whishaw (1980), *Neurological Differential Diagnosis* by John Patton (1977), *Brain's Clinical Neurology*, 6th Ed., revised by Sir Roger Bannister (1985), and *Neuroanatomy and Neuropathology* by Reitan and Wolfson (1985).

The purpose of this book is to provide a cross-referenced, alphabetical listing of terms, common medical abbreviations, diseases, symptoms, syndromes, brain structures and locations, and test instruments used in neuropsychology and their neuropsychological interpretations. It is intended to be useful to all levels of neuropsychologists and, perhaps, others in related fields. It is what this author would have like to have had when first starting into this field and is a result of accumulated notes. Everything is alphabetized so that there is no need for an index; if multiple definitions or listings are made, each alphabetical listing of the subject is referenced to all related material.

Some historical information is included as well as current basic neuropsychological knowledge. In some cases, tests are simply described as to their diagnostic function so that if one were to need to explore deficits or assets in these certain functions, the reader would be able to use the test appropriately. Tests or test batteries may need to be administered by well-trained psychologists or speech pathologists; this fact is so stated. Most of the tests listed are published with a manual to guide the administration of the test. However, since neuropsychologists often use tests that were originally intended for uses other than neuropsychological assessment, the manuals may not always be adequate guides for neuropsychological interpretation. The intention of this book, in part, is to present any specialized administration and interpretation needed to answer the specific neuropsychological question as researched by practicing neuropsychologists.

Since it is well-known that human behavior is funneled through multiple neurological pathways, this book describes the current information of these major neurological connections and pathways and how impairments in any of these pathways will affect the behavioral outcome. Conversely, observed behavior is followed back to possible foci of function or injury.

Abbreviations and acronyms in medical notes are a fact of life. However, for the neophyte, it is not always easy to translate these abbreviations at first reading. Therefore, some more commonly used abbreviations, acronyms, and symbols found in medical notes are included in this book.

It was difficult to reach a cut-off point; there always seemed to be something more to add. However, the emerging field of neuropsychology will always have something new to add tomorrow.

D.M.G.

Sacramento, California
January, 1989

A

A: Axis.

ABASIA: inability to walk.

ABCESS (BRAIN): begins as a small focus of purulent bacteria secondary to bacterial infection elsewhere in the body that causes necrosis (death) of cells in the affected region; as the organisms multiply and destroy more brain cells, the abcess behaves as an expanding mass, frequently hollow in the center, producing increasing intracranial pressure.

ABDUCENS NERVE: sixth cranial nerve; motor nerve that supplies the lateral rectus muscle of the eye; originates in the pons, beneath the floor of the fourth ventricle, emerging from the brainstem anteriorly between the pons and medulla oblongata.

ABDUCT: to draw away from the median plane or (in the digits) from the axial line of a limb.

ABIENT: avoiding the source of stimulation; said of a response to a stimulus.

ABLATION: removal or damaging of a part or tissue, particularly by cutting.

ABREACTION: the process of working off a repressed disagreeable experience by living through it again in speech and action; the method used to bring the repressed material into consciousness is called catharsis.

ABSENCE ATTACK: see petit mal seizure.

ABSOLUTE HEMIANOPIA: blindness to light, color, and form in half of the visual field.

ABSTRACT THINKING: ability to form concepts, use categories, generalize from single instances, apply procedural rules and general principles, be aware of subtle or intrinsic aspects of a problem, be able to distinguish what is relevant, what is essential, and what is appropriate; thought by Luria (1973) to take place in the tertiary zones of the cortical sensory unit (parietal, temporal, occipital lobes); Brodmann's areas 5, 7, 21, 22, 39, & 40.

ABSTRACT WORDS TEST: (Tow, 1955) a conceptual function test; sensitive to frontal-lobe disease.

ABULIA: loss or deficiency of will power, initiative, or drive; speech: laconic with long pauses between utterances; inability to sustain monologue and narrative; also see social abulia .

ABULIA-SOCIAL: social inactivity resulting from inability to select a course of action although a wish to participate may be present.

ABULOMANIA: mental disorder characterized by weakness of the will or indecision of character.

A

A/C: anticonvulsant therapy.

ACA: anterior cerebral artery.

ACALCULIA: inability to perform simple arithmetical calculations; lesion located in left parietal-lobe in the area of the angular gyrus; see also Gerstmann's Syndrome; Brodmann's areas 39 & 40, left (Hécaen, 1969).

ACCESSORY NERVE: see spinal accessory nerve (XI).

ACETYLCHOLINE (ACh): chemical neurotransmitter; secreted in synaptic endings; plays important role in the transmission of neuronal impulses; as soon as it excites the adjoining neuron it is destroyed by acetylcholine esterase (an enzyme) which restores the resting potential in the postsynaptic neuron.

ACh: acetylcholine.

ACHROMATOPSIA: inability to distinguish different hues in the presence of normally pigmented cells in the retina; cortical color blindness, which differs from congenital color blindness in that achromatopsia affects all parts of the color spectrum; colors appear less bright, and the environment is drained of color or, in severe cases, totally lacking color; results from bilateral lesions of Brodmann's areas 18, 19, & probably 37 (Meadows, 1974b) because the cells responsible for color coding have been destroyed.

ACOPIA: inability to copy complex spatial stimuli; may be a result of a disconnection syndrome following a sectioning of the corpus collosum.

ACOUSTIC APHASIA: auditory aphasia.

ACOUSTIC NERVE TUMOR: see cerebello-pontine angle lesions.

ACROMEGALY: characterized by enlargement of the extremities of the skeleton (nose, jaws, fingers, and toes); result of hypersecretion of somatotropic hormone; in adult, condition caused by hypersecretion of the pituitary growth hormone after maturity; the converse of acromicria; also called Marie's disease.

ACROMICRIA: a condition characterized by hypoplasia of the extremities of the skeleton (the nose, jaws, fingers, and toes); the converse of acromegaly; congenital acromicria is also called Down's syndrome.

ACROPARESTHESIA: most frequent in females; intense numbness, tingling, and prickling, in fingers and hands after being asleep for a few hours; also aching, burning pains or tightness; usually bilateral.

ACTH: see adrenocorticotropic hormone; also sometimes called corticotropin.

ACTING OUT: an expressing of unconscious mental conflicts in the form of overt behavior rather than in the form of neurotic symptoms.

ACTION TREMOR: seen in delirium tremens, chronic alcoholism (morning shakes), general paresis, hyperthyroidism and other toxic states, and anxiety; becomes worse when patient is observed; may be abolished with ingestion of alcohol and becomes worse after effects of alcohol have warn off; see also delirium tremens.

ACTIVITY RATE: speed of mental and motor response; see also slowing.

AD: Alzheimer's Disease; also see SDAT.

ADAPTIVE BEHAVIOR SCALE: (Nihira et al., 1975) although primarily designed to evaluate the level of development of mentally retarded persons, it is applicable to the adaptive and cognitive deficits of the brain-injured patient; many items relate to daily living tasks and pathological behavioral symptoms such as violent and destructive behavior and social behavior; may be used for documenting changes in behavior or for treatment planning (Millham et al., 1976).

ADDUCTION: drawing toward the median plane or (in the digits) toward the axial line of a limb.

ADENOHYPOPHYSIS: the anterior (or glandular) lobe of the pituitary gland (hypophysis) as distinguished from the posterior lobe (neurohypophysis); of vital importance in growth, maturation, and reproduction; secretes growth hormone, ACTH, alpha-MSH, beta-MSH, TSH, FSH, LH, ICSH, and prolactin which regulate the proper functioning of the thyroid, gonads, adrenal cortex, and other endocrine organs.

ADENOMA: benign epithelial tumor in which the cells form recognizable glandular structures or in which the cells are clearly derived from glandular epithelium.

ADH: antidiuretic hormone; vasopressin.

ADIPSIA: loss of thirst.

ADIPOSITY: a state of being fat; obesity.

ADL: Activities of Daily Living.

ad. lib.: as much as needed; at discretion.

ADRENAL CORTEX: the outer layer of the adrenal gland; under the influence of the pituitary hormone, adrenocorticotropin, produces 40+ different hormones chemically known as steroids; has 4 functions: 1. regulates metabolism; 2. maintains blood pressure; 3. controls sexual appearance; 4. controls sexual behavior.

ADRENAL MEDULLA: central portion of the adrenal gland; secretes epinephrine and norepinephrine.

ADRENERGIC: activated by, characteristic of, or secreting epinephrine or substances with similar activity; the term is applied to those nerve fibers that liberate norepinephrine at a synapse when a nerve impulse passes, e. g., the sympathetic fibers.

ADRENOCORTICOTROPIC HORMONE: (ACTH) secreted by the anterior pituitary gland; a hormone that originates in the anterior pituitary gland and regulates the release of hormones by the adrenal cortex; increases the output of steroids from the adrenal cortex during stress.

A

AEP: average evoked potential.

AEROCELE: a tumor formed by air filling an adventitious pouch such as laryngocele and tracheocele.

AFFECT: range and appropriateness of emotional responses; the emotional complex associated with a mental state; the feeling experienced in connection with an emotion; emotional experiences evoked by particular stimuli; can be described as constricted (restricted), appropriate (broad, normal), labile (characterized by repeated, rapid and abrupt shifts that are inappropriate to the situation), blunted (a severe reduction in the intensity of affect expression), or flat (lack of signs of affective expression; the voice may be monotonous and the face immobile).

AFFECTIVE BEHAVIOR CONTROL: social affective behavior is thought to be complementarily specialized in right- and left-hemispheres where the left-hemisphere has a subordinate role, appearing to be more analytic or literal in its analysis of input while the right-hemisphere plays a major role in analyzing and producing emotionally toned stimuli and responses; function located in the amydala and portions of the anterior temporal cortex; these structures form a system that inputs to the hypothalamus (Papez, 1937).

AFFECTIVE DISORDERS: cerebral blood flow and PET scanning suggest a right frontal-lobe deficit (Buchsbaum, 1982; Golden, 1982).

AFFECTIVE STATE ABNORMALITIES: right-hemisphere lesions impair mimicry of emotional states (Tucker et al., 1977); indifference (joke telling, lack of interest) may be seen in right-hemisphere lesioned patients (Gainotti, 1972; Goldstein, 1939) reaction in left-hemisphere lesioned patients is usually associated with aphasia and may produce catastrophic or depressive reactions; tears and swearing often precipitated by repeated failures in verbal communication; correlated with the presence of contralateral neglect; frontal-lobe lesions reduce facial expressions (Kolb, 1977); left frontal-lobe lesions reduce spontaneous talking; right frontal-lobe lesions increase talking (Kolb et al., 1980).

AFFERENT: conveying toward a center, as an afferent nerve.

AFFERENT FIBERS: fibers that carry impulses to the brain via the dorsal columns of the spinal cord.

AFFERENT PARESIS: motor disorder associated with lesion(s) of the sensory afferent mechanisms.

AFFERENT PATHWAY LESION (EYE): see Marcus-Gunn pupil.

AFTERBRAIN: metencephalon.

AGCT: Army General Classification Test.

AGE DECREMENTS: visual nonverbal memory declines more rapidly than other forms of nonverbal memory in the 60 to 80 decades; auditory or tactile memory shows greater decline than visual in the decades between 40 & 60 (Riege & Williams, 1980); diminished

4

ability for abstract and complex conceptualization (Botwinick, 1977; Denney, 1974; Reitan, 1967); mental inflexibility which causes difficulty in adapting to new situations, solving novel problems, or changing mental set (Botwinick, 1977, 1978: Kramer & Jarvik, 1979; Schaie, 1958; Williams, 1970); behavioral slowing that affects perceptual (Hines & Posner, n.d.; Kramer & Jarvik, 1979), cognitive (Botwinick, 1977; Thomas et al., 1977), memory functions, and psychomotor activity (Benton 1977; Hicks & Birren, 1970; Welford, 1977); WAIS or WAIS-R scores on the Block Design, Object Assembly, & Digit Symbol subtests are usually the most affected by age decrements; Trail Making Test A & B may also show the effects of aging, particularly B.

AGENESIS OF THE CORPUS CALLOSUM: complete or partial absence of the corpus callosum; 3 types: 1. absence of the telencephalic commissures; 2. absence of corpus callosum with preserved anterior and hippocampal commissures; 3. partial absence of the posterior part of the corpus callosum.

AGEUSIA: loss of taste; loss of taste of the posterior third of tongue is controlled by the glossopharyngeal nerve (IX).

AGEUSIC APHASIA: loss of power to express words relating to the sense of taste.

AGGRESSIVE BEHAVIOR: see thalamus, Raphè Nucleus or tegmentum, hypothalamus, and amygdala.

AGITATED: a state of continued restless, purposeless activity expressive of nervous tension and anxiety.

AGNEA: a condition in which objects are not recognized.

AGNOSIA: defect in the formulation and use of symbolic concepts, including the significance of numbers and letters, the names of parts of the body or recognition, knowing, and understanding the meaning of stimuli; loss of power to recognize the importance of sensory stimuli; the varieties correspond with several senses and are distinguished as auditory, visual, olfactory, gustatory, tactile, color, finger, time, body-image, ideational, and simultaneous.

AGNOSIA - AUDITORY: a receptive aphasia characterized by inability to recognize the significance (meaning) of sounds of the spoken language in the absence of physical disability of hearing; also called cortical deafness or auditory verbal agnosia; hears, but does not recognize or understand what is heard; see also agnosia for sounds.

AGNOSIA - BODY-IMAGE: see autotopagnosia.

AGNOSIA - FINGER: loss of ability to indicate one's own or another's fingers; also see Gerstmann's Syndrome.

AGNOSIA - IDEATIONAL: (secondary somatosenory agnosia) loss of the special associations which make up the idea of an object from its component ideas; also see asymbolia, somatosensory agnosia.

AGNOSIA - PRIMARY: inability to recognize tactile qualities of an

A

object because of an inability to evoke tactile images; may be a result of lesions in either hemisphere, in the postcentral gyrus or the thalamoparietal projections (association areas); may not appreciate the size, form, consistency and weight of an object; inability to identify an object by palpatation although primary sense data (touch, pain, temperature, and vibration) are intact.

AGNOSIA FOR SOUNDS/AUDITORY AGNOSIA: inability to identify the meaning of nonverbal sounds, such as a bell ringing; sounds either may sound all alike or be confused with one another; most often amusia and word deafness are associated; may also be a result of confusion of the auditory percept because of disconnection from the verbal or memory components necessary to label the sound; thought to be bilateral temporal-lobe dysfunction (Brodmann's areas 22 & 42).

AGNOSIA - TACTILE: inability to recognize familiar objects by touch; primary agnosia; see also tactile agnosia, astereognosia.

AGNOSIA - TIME: loss of comprehension of the succession and duration of events; see also time agnosia.

AGNOSIA - VISUAL: inability to recognize familiar objects by sight; see also visual agnosia.

AGONAL: pertaining to the death agony; occurring at the moment of or just before death.

AGONIST MUSCLE: prime mover; opposed by antagonist muscle.

AGORAPHOBIA: morbid fear of being in large open spaces.

AGRAMMATISM: sharply contracted sentence structure, lacking most small grammatic words, often with faulty use of grammar in the words remaining; loss of words such as "the" and "is" as well as grammatical inflectional endings such as plurals and past tense; lesion in the frontal operculum or insula.

AGRAPHIA: an expressive aphasia characterized by the inability to express thoughts in writing, due to a lesion of the cerebral cortex. Writing requires the translation of a language item into symbols. Linguistic messages originate in the posterior language area (Wernicke's area), are translated into visual symbols in the inferior parietal area (lesion causes agraphia with alexia), and are sent to the frontal language area (Broca's) for motor processing; lesions in any of these areas or pathways will cause agraphia; all aphasics show some agraphia; not all patients with agraphia are aphasic; does not refer to poor handwriting, gross spelling errors, or paragraphias; also see Gerstmann's syndrome.

AKATHISIA: motor restlessness ranging from a feeling of inner disquiet to inability to sit, lie quietly, or sleep; repetitive tapping and fiddling with hands and feet and facial mannerisms; seen in toxic reactions to neuroleptic medication such as phenothiazines.

AKINESIA: disinclination of the patient to use an affected part of the body, to engage it freely in all the natural actions of the body; absence or poverty of movement; see cerebellar lesions.

AKINETIC: absence or poverty of movements.

AKINETIC MUTISM: a state characterized by wakefulness but lacking impulse for speech and action; uncanny appearance of awareness; also called coma vigil; if the lesion is cortical, the patient appears much more alert and awake most of the time; the eyes remain open when awake; may have violent outbursts when aroused by external stimuli; lesion(s) may be in the subthalamic region, septal area, anterior hypothalamic area, cingulate gyri, bilateral orbital-frontal area, or may be cortical; may be due to rupture of the anterior communicating artery; if there are positive Babinski signs (increased reflexes), the lesion involves the corticospinal tract; if temperature control dysfunction is present, the lesion is in the anterior hypothalamic area; if primitive reflexes (snout and grasp) are present, the lesion is in the mesial frontal-lobe area; if the patient is difficult to arouse and drifts back to sleep or looks away when awakened (apathetic akinetic mutism), lesion(s) is in midbrain subthalamic or septal region.

AKINETIC EPILEPSY: (in adults) characterized by a sudden fall to the ground without warning; unawareness of the fall; usually gets up immediately; usually affects middle-aged obese women without history of epilepsy; often associated with cervical osteoarthritis and presumed to be a result of brainstem ischemia from compression of the vertebral arteries by cervical osteophytes (Brain, 1985).

AKINETIC SEIZURE: most often seen in children; usually the child collapses suddenly and without warning; usually of few seconds duration with no postictal depression; the falls may be quite dangerous; most children who have this disease wear protective head-gear.

ALALIA: lack of ability to talk.

ALCOHOL: ETOH; ethanol.

ALCOHOLIC DEMENTIA: loss of the abstract attitude and impaired visuomotor performance distinguish this condition from Korsakoff's psychosis (Horvath, 1975; Lishman, 1978, 1981); may also display some Korsakoff's psychosis symptoms.

ALCOHOLISM: dipsomania.

ALCOHOLISM CEREBELLAR GAIT: wide-base and short steps, trunk inclined slightly forward, arms held away from body; seen in chronic alcoholism and Korsakoff's disease.

ALCOHOLISM - CHRONIC: chronic alcohol abuse affects certain aspects of intellectual functioning while leaving many intellectual activities relatively unimpaired (Parsons, 1977; Parsons & Farr, 1981; Tarter, 1975, 1976). Binge drinkers appear to be less prone to alcohol-related cognitive deficits than those with a heavy daily alcohol intake (Sanchez-Craig, 1980.). Intellectual deficits consis-

A

tently appear on tasks involving functions associate with frontal-lobe activity (Bolter & Hannon, 1980; Parson, 1977; Talland, 1965b; Tarter, 1975; Tarter & Jones, 1971); difficulties in maintaining a cognitive set, impersistence, decreased flexibility in thinking, defective visual searching behavior, deficient motor inhibition, perseveration, loss of spatial and temporal orientation, and impaired ability to organize perceptuomotor responses and synthesize spatial elements characterize the test behavior of chronic alcoholics; characteristically perform relatively poorly on speed-dependent visual scanning tasks such as the Digit Symbol subtest of the Wechsler Intelligence Scales, the Trail Making tests, tests of motor speed, and tests of visuospatial organization of which the Wechsler Block Design subtest and the Tactual Performance Test are representative examples (Kapur & Butters, 1977; Parsons & Farr, 1981; Tarter, 1975). Verbal and arithmetic skills of the Wechsler Verbal Scale subtests generally remain relatively unimpaired; impaired motor control and integration; no consistent performance decrement on perceptuomotor tasks or motor coordination tasks that require little or no synthesizing, organizing, or orienting activity (Hirschenfang et al., 1968; Tarter, 1975, Vivian et al., 1973); subtle but consistent short-term memory and learning deficits that become more evident as task difficulty increases (Ryan & Butters, 1980b, 1982; Ryan, Butters, Adinolfi, & DiDario, 1980); deficits may be a breakdown in encoding strategies (Ryan et al., 1980). Remote memory is particularly resistant to deterioration in alcoholics (M. S. Albert et al., 1980); the greatest amount of return of function takes place in the first week of abstinence and slows down rapidly thereafter, leveling off at three to six weeks (Lezak et al., 1983).

ALERT STATE: fully awake and fully aware of normal external and internal stimuli; capable of meaningful interaction with others; basic anatomical structures which control the alert state include the brainstem reticular system and the diffuse thalamic projection system (diencephalic extension of the reticular formation).

ALEXIA/DYSLEXIA: Failure to visually recognize words; word blindness; inability to read; *cortical alexia*: a form of sensory aphasia due to lesions of the left angular gyrus; *motor alexia*: the patient understands what he sees written or printed but cannot read it aloud; *optical alexia*: word blindness; *subcortical alexia*: interruption of the connection between the optic center and the angular gyrus; lesion(s) in the left angular gyrus and/or left occipital-lobe; Brodmann's areas 7 & 40, left (Hécaen & Albert, 1978).

ALEXIA AND INABILITY TO NAME COLORS WITHOUT AGRAPHIA: lesion in the left occipital-lobe and splenium of corpus callosum.

ALEXIA WITH AGRAPHIA: unable to read or write; may not be aphasic, but may have anomia; in a right-handed patient, the lesion is in the left inferior-parietal area (angular gyrus area).

ALEXIA WITHOUT AGRAPHIA: patient is able to write normally, but is not able to read his own writing; able to understand words spelled aloud; good naming; caused by a left posterior cerebral artery occlusion in right-handed patients; the infarct damages the posterior portion of the corpus callosum and left occipital-lobe; the visual information enters the right-hemisphere but cannot be transmitted to the left-hemisphere because of damage to the corpus callosum.

ALLESTHESIA: sensory dysfunction; the sensation of touch experienced at a point remote from the point actually touched.

ALLESTHESIA-VISUAL: illusory displacement of images from one side of the visual field to the other.

ALLOCENTRIC SPATIAL RELATIONS: (Semmes et al., 1963) extrapersonal orientation (map-following) as opposed to egocentric spatial relations (personal/bodily orientation).

ALLOCHIRIA: a condition in which, if one extremity is stimulated, sensation is referred to the opposite side.

ALPHA-MSH: alpha-melanocyte-stimulating hormone; secreted by the adenohypophysis; a peptide which influences the formation of deposition of melanin in the body.

ALPHA MOTOR NEURON: connects with and excites a skeletal muscle.

ALPHA RHYTHM: dominant rhythm of the posterior cortex at 8-to-12 cycles/second; generally found when a person is relaxing but awake.

alt.: alternate.

alt. hor.: every other hour.

alt. noc.: every other night.

ALTERNATING HAND MOVEMENT DEFECTS: may be either cortical (Lezak, 1983) or subcortical (Heilman, 1979); loss of sequence or perseveration suggestive of loss of ability to move from one motor movement to another and inability to shift sets; dysfunction of premotor cerebral cortex (frontal-lobe); may be tested with the fist-palm-side test adapted from Luria (1973a).

ALTERNATE HEMIPLEGIA: paralysis of one part on one side of the body and another part on the opposite side.

ALTERNATING OCULOMOTOR HEMIPLEGIA: see Weber's syndrome.

ALTITUDE ANOXIA: anoxia caused by the reduced pressure of oxygen at high altitudes.

ALTITUDINAL HEMIANOPIA: defective vision or blindness in a horizontal half of the visual field.

ALZHEIMER'S DISEASE (AD/SDAT): characterized by progressive degenerative nerve cell changes within the cerebral hemispheres with concomitant progressive global deterioration of intellect and

A

personality (Roth, 1978); before age 59/64 called AD; after age 59/64 called SDAT (senile dementia of the Alzheimer's type); also called primary degenerative dementia; neuropathological indicators are neurofibrillary tangles and senile plaques throughout the brain, but particularly in hippocampal and amygdaloid areas (Berry, 1975; Lishman, 1978; Terry, 1980); a greater amount of senile plaques are found in the parietal-lobe (Roth, 1978); thinning of the cortical mantle, enlargement of the lateral ventricles, and flattening of the surface of the cortex; may be lower tissue densities in frontal- and temporal-lobes and the anterior portion of the caudate nucleus within the corpus striatum (Bondareff et al., 1981); etiology unknown; *Early signs*: failing recent memory, depression, irritability, and sometimes seizures; early symptoms of inattentiveness, mild cognitive dulling, social withdrawal, and emotional blunting or agitation are often confused with depression; perseverations (speech); paralogisms with syntax preserved (Golper & Binder, 1981; Marin & Gordon, 1979); dysnomia; intrusions; language impairment my include loss of spontaneous speech or intrusions (Fuld et al., 1982; Lezak, 1983) and /or dysfluency such as paraphasias and articulatory errors (Golper & Binder, 1981; Obler & Albert, 1980); memory impairment and depression usually precede personality deterioration; *Late signs*: restless apathy may alternate with aggressive demands for attention and petulant irritability; *Final stages*: severe handicapping apraxias, disruption of effective speech production, disturbances of posture and gait, incontinence, totally dependency, and bedridden; *Neuropsychological Assessment*: on the WAIS the highest scores are achieved on tests of overlearned behaviors presented in a familiar format and immediate memory recall (Information, Vocabulary, Comprehension, and Similarities and Digits Forward); poor scores are achieved on Block Design, Digit Symbol, Digits Backward, and Object Assembly subtests; Object Assembly subtest score may be a little higher than scores on the Block Design and Digit Symbol subtests; Vocabulary subtest score at least twice as large as Block Design subtest score is a highly likely indicator of dementia and rarely occurs among depressed patients (Coolidge, 1982); patients may fail reasoning such as Raven's progressive matrices, unfamiliar, or timed tests such as verbal fluency tests, and both storage and retrieval components of memory learning tests (Fuld, 1978; Gainotti et al., 1980; Lezak, 1983); see also Pick's disease.

ALZHEIMER WAIS SCORES: see WAIS subtest scores, Alzheimer's.

AMAUROSIS: blindness from any cause; especially blindness occurring without apparent lesion to the eye.

AMBIDEXTERITY: the ability to perform acts requiring manual skill with either hand.

AMBIGUOUS VISUAL STIMULI TEST: Rorschach.

AMBIVALENCE: the simultaneous existence of contradictory and contrasting emotions.

AMBLYOPIA: impairment or loss of vision which is not due to an error refraction or to other diseases of the eye. *[handwritten: Lazy eye]*

AMBLYOPIA EX ANOPSIA: diminished visual acuity due to strabismus and the suppression of images in one eye; lazy eye.

AMEBIASIS: amebic dysentery; caused by an infestation of the protozoan ameba, Entomoeba histolytica, resulting in encephalitis and brain abscesses.

AMENORRHEA: absence or abnormal stoppage of the menses.

AMENTIA: congenital feeblemindedness.

AMINO ACIDS: a class of organic compounds that form the chief structure of proteins, several of which are essential for human nutrition (natural amino acids); essential amino acid is one that is essential for optimal growth in a young animal or for nitrogen equilibrium in an adult.

AMNEMONIC APHASIA: forgetfulness of words with consequent aphasia.

AMNESIA: partial or total loss of memory; loss of past memory coupled with an inability to form new memory traces or to learn; see also retrograde amnesia, anterograde amnesia, posttraumatic amnesia, PTA.

AMNESIA-ANTEROGRADE: see anterograde amnesia.

AMNESIA-RETROGRADE: see retrograde amnesia.

AMNESIC APRAXIA: loss of ability to carry out a movement on command as a result of inability to remember the command although ability to perform the movement is present.

AMNESIC THEORY ON LEARNING: (Warrington & Weiskrantz, 1978) amnesics have difficulty controlling and restraining the influence of prior learning on present performance; may be a type of response disinhibition that manifests as perseveration.

AMNESTIC-DYSNOMIC APHASIA: loss of ability to produce names on demand including nouns, adjectives, and other descriptive parts of speech; pauses in speech; groping for words; substitution of other words or phrases that conveys the meaning (circumlocution); early or isolated manifestation of disease of the nervous system; caused by lesion(s) deep in the temporal-lobe or left parietal-lobe; interrupts connections of sensory speech areas with the hippocampal/parahippocampal regions; concerned with learning and memory; usually due to mass lesions; may be involved in early Alzheimer's disease and senile dementia or in confusional states caused by metabolic, infectious, intoxicative or other acute medical illnesses.

AMOK: a psychiatric disturbance marked by a period of depression followed by violent attempts to kill people.

A

AMOSMIC APHASIA: inability to express, in words, sensations of smell.

AMPHETAMINE: a drug that causes an initial elevation in mood and energy through an increase in norepinephrine; CNS stimulant that raises blood pressure, reduces appetite, reduces nasal congestion, and may cause insomnia; abuse may lead to auditory/visual hallucinations, loss of REM sleep, agitation, paranoia, and depression following withdrawal.

AMUSIA: defective perception of music or its components (i.e., rhythm, pitch, timbre, measure, tempo, or harmonics); auditory agnosia for music; includes tone deafness, melody deafness; usually associated with temporal-lobe disease, and is more likely to occur with right-than left-sided lesions; roughly Brodmann's areas 22 and 42.

AMUSIA TESTS: the examiner can whistle or hum several simple and generally familiar melodies which the patient can identify; pitch discrimination can be tested with a pitch pipe; rhythm patterns can be evaluated by requiring the patient either to discriminate similar and different sets of rhythmic taps or to mimic patterns tapped out by the examiner; tests available in the Luria/ Christiansen battery or the Luria-Nebraska Test.

AMYELIA: total absence of spinal cord; only found in association with anencephaly.

AMYGDALA: almond shaped mass; see amygdaloid nucleus.

AMYGDALOID NUCLEUS: small mass of subcortical gray matter located within the tip of the temporal-lobe; anterior to the inferior horn of the lateral ventricle of the brain (anterior and medial part of the temporal-lobe); has direct connections with the primitive centers involving the sense of smell; has partial control over semi-automatic viseral activities concerned with feeding such as chewing, salivating, licking, gagging, and viseral components of the fear reactions; controls mediation of defensive-aggressive behavior; integrates coordinates, and directs the activity of the more primitive emotional centers of the midbrain, hypothalamus, and thalamus; plays role in positive reinforcement and goal-directed behavior; also involved in memory retrieval.

AMYGDALOID NUCLEUS ABLATION: eliminates uncontrollable rage reactions in psychotic patients.

AMYGDALOID NUCLEUS LESION: tends to produce a marked calming and taming effect; animals lose fear and aggressive tendencies and are unable to compete appropriately in social situations; may show compulsive, oral behavior and hypersexuality-like behavior; impaired ability to associate reward with environmental stimuli; irrational violence that often accompanies temporal-lobe (psychomotor) epilepsy.

AMYGDALOID NUCLEUS SEIZURES: typically cause brief olfactory or gustatory hallucinations which are usually unpleasant like rotting cabbage or burning rubber.

AMYGDALOID NUCLEUS STIMULATION: revival of complex emotional stimuli with rise in blood pressure, increased pulse rate, hyperventilation, and fear.

AMYOSTASIA: a tremor of the muscles; seen especially in locomotor ataxia.

AMYOSTATIC SYNDROME: Parkinson's syndrome.

AMYOTROPHIC LATERAL SCLEROSIS: a disease marked by progressive degeneration of the neurons that give rise to the cortico-spinal tract and of the motor cells of the brainstem and spinal cord, and resulting in a deficit of upper and lower motor neurons; usually ends fatally within two to three years; also called Charcot's syndrome.

ANALYZERS (BRAIN): left-hemisphere in right-handed persons; secondary and tertiary processes in the brain that analyze and synthesize input from various sensory channels (Luria, 1973b).

ANAPHYLACTIC REACTION: an unusual or exaggerated allergic reaction of an organism to foreign protein or other substances following a prior sensitivity.

ANARTHRIA: severe dysarthria resulting in speechlessness; see also stuttering, literalis anarthria, aphasia, speechlessness.

ANASTOMOSES: connection between parallel blood vessels that allows them to intercommunicate their blood flows; if one vessel is blocked, a given region might therefore be spared an infarct because the blood has an alternate route to the affected zone.

ANDROGEN: a hormone that controls fertility and development of secondary sexual characteristics; normal gonadal function depends upon stimulation from gonadotropic hormones of adenohypophysis (anterior pituitary gland).

ANEMIA: a reduction below normal in the number of erythrocytes per cu. mm., in the quantity of hemoglobin, or in the volume of packed red cells per 100 ml. of blood which occurs when the equilibrium between blood loss and blood production is disturbed.

ANEMIC ANOXIA: anoxia resulting from a decrease in amount of hemoglobin or number of erythrocytes in the blood; a deficiency in the oxygen-carrying power of the blood; may be caused by carbon monoxide poisoning or blood loss.

ANEMIC HYPOXIA: hypoxia due to reduction of the oxygen-carrying capacity of the blood as a result of a decrease in the total hemoglobin or an alteration of the hemoglobin constituents.

ANENCEPHALY: absence of cerebral hemispheres, diencephalon, and midbrain.

ANERGASIA: Meyer's term for a psychosis associated with a structural lesion of the central nervous system causing lack of functional activity (e.g., loss of memory and judgment, fits, contractures, palsies, etc.).

ANESTHESIA, SENSORY: loss of all forms of sensation.

ANEURYSM: a sac formed by the dilatation of the wall of an artery, a vein, or the heart; vascular dilations resulting from localized defects in the elasticity of the vessel; balloonlike expansions of vessels which are usually weak and prone to rupture; most often congenital, but may be produced by hypertension, arteriosclerosis, embolisms, or infections; if the aneurysm is in the brain, symptoms included severe headache, which may be present for years because of pressure on the dura from the aneurysm; a "berry" (subarachnoid) aneurysm is a small saccular aneurysm of a cerebral artery; occur most often in the vicinity of the anterior part of the circle of Willis, but may arise from the vertebral, basilar, and posterior cerebral arteries; usually at the bifurcation of a cerebral vessel; most common sites are the terminal portion of the internal carotid artery, the junction of the anterior cerebral and anterior communicating arteries, and the middle cerebral artery where it divides at the lateral sulcus; most frequent sites in the vertebral-basilar system: posterior inferior cerebral artery where it arises from the vertebral artery, and the division of the basilar artery into the posterior cerebral arteries (Reitan & Wolfson, 1985); mortality rate is about 60% within six months; 33% of the survivors show residual paralysis, epilepsy, headache or mental symptoms (Leech & Shuman, 1982).

ANEURYSM RUPTURE - ANTERIOR COMMUNICATING ARTERY: (behavioral sequelae) lack of spontaneity, childishness, indifference, and Korsakoff-type memory disorder; any deficits/behavioral changes associated with frontal-lobe lesions (Okawa et al., 1980).

ANGIOBLASTOMA: blood-vessel tumor of the brain.

ANGIOGRAM/ANGIOGRAPHY: an x-ray technique of imaging the brain's blood vessels after dye is injected into the vertebral or carotid artery; valuable in diagnosing and locating vascular abnormalities and some tumors.

ANGIOMAS: congenital collections of abnormal vessels, including capillary, venous, or arteriovenous malformations that result in abnormal blood flow; composed of a mass of enlarged and tortuous cortical vessels that are supplied by one or more large arteries and are drained by one or more large veins, most frequently in the field of the middle cerebral artery; may lead to stroke or to inadequate distribution of blood in the regions surrounding the vessels; arterial blood may bypass tissue and flow directly into veins; symptoms are characterized by frequent focal epileptic seizures and progressive impairment of the blood supply which may give rise to increasing hemiparesis.

ANGOR ANIMI: sense of impending death.

ANGULAR GYRUS: a convolution of the inferior-parietal lobule, arching over the posterior end of the superior-temporal sulcus and continuous with the middle temporal gyrus; *speech*: (Geschwind model, 1972) combines sensory input to house "visual patterns" of letters, words, etc., and acts in some way to convert a visual stimulus into the appropriate auditory form.

ANGULAR GYRUS LESION: (dominant side): dysnomia; nominal aphasia; inability to read; anomic aphasia; also see Gerstmann's syndrome.

ANHEDONIA: total loss of feeling of pleasure in acts that normally give pleasure.

ANION: negatively charged organic ion.

ANISEIKONIA: a rare condition in which the two optical images from each eye record themselves on the brain as similar objects but of different size and/or shape.

ANISOMETROPIA: a difference in the refractive power of each eye.

ANISOPIA: inequality of vision in the two eyes.

ANKYLOSIS: immobility and consolidation of a joint due to disease, injury, or surgical procedure.

ANNULOSPIRAL ENDINGS: stretch receptors that wrap around the nuclear bag of intrafusal muscle fibers; firing initiates the stretch reflex.

ANOMALY: marked deviation from the normal standard, especially as a result of congenital or hereditary defects.

ANOMIA: loss of power to name objects or to recognize and recall their names; see also nominal aphasia, dysnomia, and anomic aphasia.

ANOMIC APHASIA: fluent aphasia in which comprehension and repetition are both preserved; normal speech except for inability to name objects and paraphasic errors; understands both written and verbal speech; no hemiplegia; word-finding difficulty only; word-finding pauses; circumlocution often present; paraphasias when searching for specific object names; two-way dissociation of naming: can't name objects and has difficulty recognizing objects by name; also called amnesic aphasia; caused by diffuse encephalopathy, or focal space-occupying lesions in speech area; the most severe anomic aphasia is caused by temporal-lobe lesions involving the 2nd & 3rd temporal gyri including important pathways from the occipital-lobe to the limbic system; parietotemporal lesions result in severe anomia with substantial alexias with agraphia; may be caused by a lesion in the angular gyrus (not a proven theory, Kolb & Whishaw, 1980); may be tested by confrontation naming of common and uncommon items in several categories (Strub & Black, 1977).

ANOPIA: absence or rudimentary condition of the eye.

ANOPSIA: nonuse of or suppression of vision in one eye; may be caused

A

by damage to the Optic nerve (II).

ANOREXIA: lack or loss of appetite for food; may be due to a dsyfunction of the lateral hypothalamus; also called anorexia nervosa.

ANOSMIA: absence of the sense of smell; may be caused by damage to the Olfactory nerve (I).

ANOSODIAPHORIA: indifference to illness or disease.

ANOSODIAPHORIAS - UNILATERAL, LEFT SIDE: lesion of the posterior-parietal region in the right-hemisphere.

ANOSOGNOSIA: (Babinski) implicit unawareness of neurologic or bodily deficits/condition; confabulation or delusions may be present to explain bodily deficits; may be associated with left hemiparesis; caused by large lesions to the nondominant parietal-lobe.

ANOSOGNOSIA - UNILATERAL LEFT SIDE: lesion of the posterior-parietal region in the right-hemisphere.

ANOSOGNOSIA WITH AMNESIA FOR AFFECTED SIDE: lesions penetrating only to the transmission fibers from the thalamus to the parietal cortex (Gerstmann, 1942).

ANOSOGNOSIA WITH UNILATERAL NEGLECT: patient ignores unilateral paralysis; lesions of the right optic region of the thalamus (Gerstmann, 1942).

ANOXIA: absence or lack of oxygen; reduction of oxygen in body tissue below physiologic levels; severe sequelae include: clinically similar state to coma vigil; bilateral decortication with double hemiplegia and primitive reflexes (apallic state); diffuse brain-damage; types: altitude a., anemic a., anoxic a., fulminating a., histotoxic a., myocardial a., neonatorum., stagnant a., hypokinetic a.; see also hypoxia.

ANOXIC ANOXIA: anoxia resulting from interference with the source of oxygen; most often refers to diminished oxygen in the arterial blood despite normal ability to contain and carry oxygen; may result from respiratory obstruction, paralysis or other dysfunction of respiratory muscles, brainstem dysfunction, impaired lung function, ingestion of gases that produce anesthesia, or altitudinal oxygen deficiency.

ANOXIC ENCEPHALOPATHY: if oxygen consumption is reduced by more than 30%, brain-dysfunction/damage may occur; gray matter often more affected than white matter because of the difference in metabolic rate; frontal-lobes often more affected; neurons in the medulla may survive the longest; characterized by impairment of higher-level neuropsychological functions, followed by perceptual and visual difficulties, loss of consciousness, and decorticate and decerebrate motor syndromes; may proceed to respiratory failure and death; sequelae may include cognitive dysfunction, generalized rigidity with mild parkinson-like tremor, severe brain dysfunction with involuntary movements, myoclonic jerks, and decerebrate rigidity (Reitan & Wolfson, 1985).

ANS: autonomic nervous system; anterior nasal spine.

ANTABUSE: a trademark for a preparation of disulfiram; often used as a deterrent to alcohol ingestion; taken in combination with alcohol causes severe nausea.

ANTAGONIST MUSCLE: a muscle that acts in opposition to the action of another muscle, its agonist.

ANTERIOR: situated in front of or in the forward part of an organ; toward the head end of the body; ventral or belly surface of the body; opposite of posterior.

ANTERIOR CAROTID ARTERY: arises directly from the carotid artery, runs backwards along the optic tract to the area under the internal capsule, and eventually supplies the choroid plexus of the lateral ventricle; has a variable distribution that includes the optic tract and the basal ganglia.

ANTERIOR CAROTID ARTERY OCCLUSIONS: symptoms include hemiparesis, hemisensory loss, hemianopia with no flaccidity, no drowsiness, no dysphasia or dyspraxia; may mimic a cerebral tumor.

ANTERIOR CEREBRAL ARTERY: one of two major divisions of the internal carotid artery; the other division is the middle cerebral artery; irrigates the anterior and middle portions of the cortex as well as the subcortical structures of this same area; joins with the middle cerebral artery to form the anterior communicating artery.

ANTERIOR CEREBRAL ARTERY INFARCTION: rare unilateral lesions of the proximal portion of the artery may result in contra-lateral hemiplegia and sensory loss affecting the lower limb; distal portion (supplies the medial aspect of the frontal-lobe and the paracentral lobules) may result in paralysis and sensory loss of the lower limb without significant involvement of the upper limb; occlusion of the left anterior cerebral artery may produce dysphasia characterized by motor or expressive deficits (Reitan & Wolfson, 1985).

ANTERIOR CEREBRAL ARTERY OCCLUSION: causes flaccid paralysis of the entire leg, with cortical sensory loss; if a recurrent artery of Heubner is present and the blockage occurs proximal to its origin, the anterior internal capsule will also be infarcted giving rise to a typical upper motor neuron facial weakness, a spastic arm, and a useless flaccid leg; incontinence of urine; considerable intellectual deficit and memory disturbance may occur due to damage to fronto-parietal and fronto-temporal fibers in the cingulate gyrus; *Terminal branch occlusion*: both motor and sensory functions are affected; flaccid weakness of the leg; the sensory loss affects accurate touch perception and joint position sense; intellectual disturbances and bladder dysfunction may be less severe than that caused by a main trunk occlusion.

ANTERIOR CHOROIDAL ARTERY: supplies the optic tract, part of

A

the cerebral peduncle, the lateral geniculate body, part of the internal capsule, and the choroid plexis in the temporal horn of the lateral ventricle.

ANTERIOR CHOROIDAL ARTERY OCCLUSION: may produce symptoms resembling a middle cerebral artery occlusion (Reitan & Wolfson, 1985).

ANTERIOR COMMISSURE: smaller than the corpus callosum; functions to interconnect portions of the anterior temporal-lobe, the amygdala, and the paleocortex of the temporal-lobe surrounding the amygdala; with agenesis of the corpus callosum, the anterior commissure is greatly enlarged to connect far greater regions of the neocortex.

ANTERIOR PITUITARY GLAND: (adenohypophysis); secretes somatotropic (growth) hormone as well as numerous other hormones; see also adenohypophysis.

ANTERIOR SPINAL ARTERY SYNDROME: relative or absolute sparing of posterior column functions and only a loss of pain and temperature sensation below the level of the lesion; paralysis of motor function below the level of lesion.

ANTERIOR TEMPORAL LOBE: plays role in affective behavior control.

ANTERIOR TEMPORAL LOBE - BILATERAL REMOVAL: Klüver-Bucy syndrome.

ANTERIOR VISUAL CORTEX LESION: macular sparing homonymous hemianopia.

ANTEROGRADE AMNESIA: inability to remember events subsequent to the onset of amnesia.

ANTIADRENERGIC REACTION: see anticholinergic reaction.

ANTICHOLINERGIC MEDICATION: belladonna alkaloids.

ANTICHOLINERGIC REACTIONS: reaction to neuroleptics; acute dystonic reactions; akathisia; blockage of the passage of impulses through the parasympathetic nerves; see also extrapyramidal reaction, oculogyral crisis, cogwheel phenomenon; also called parasympatholytic reaction and antiadrenergic reaction.

ANTICONVULSANT: an agent that relieves or prevents convulsions/ seizures.

ANTIDEPRESSANT DRUGS: having the specific effect of elevating the mood of the patient.

ANTIDIURETIC HORMONE (ADH): acts on kidney tubules to control reabsorption of water; hyposecretion results in diabetes insipidus; secreted by the hypothalamus nuclei and stored in the posterior pituitary gland; vasopressin.

ANTIPSYCHOTIC AGENTS: (also known as major tranquilizers, neuroleptics, or phenothiazines) their action appears to be a result of their action on dopamine; reduce dopaminergic transmission thereby blocking dopamine receptors; reserpine reduces dopamine levels by destroying storage granules within the synapse.

ANTON'S SYMPTOM/SYNDROME: denial of, and usually unawareness of, one's own blindness, with resort to confabulation, as seen in cortical blindness due to bilateral infarction of the occipital-lobes.

ANXIETY: a feeling of apprehension, uncertainty, fear, tension, or uneasiness that stems from the anticipation of danger, which may be internal or external and without apparent stimulus; may be focused on an object, situation, or activity which is avoided (phobia), or may be unfocused (free-floating anxiety); may be experienced in periods of sudden onset and accompanied by physical symptoms (panic attacks; physiological changes such as tachycardia, sweating, tremors, etc.); common with brain-damage particularly with left-hemisphere lesions characterized by oversensitivity to impairments, exaggeration of disabilities, often compounded by depression (Buck, 1968); may cause distractability and poor concentration; may cause slowing, scrambled or blocked thoughts and words, and memory failure/impairment; also called catastrophic reaction.

APALLIC STATE: may be caused by anoxia, hypoglycemia, circulatory or metabolic embarrassment; clinically similar to coma vigil; bilateral decortication with double hemiplegia; primitive reflexes present; diffuse damage to the neocortex and neopallium.

APATHETIC: indifferent; undemonstrative; marked emotional blunting; may be due to bilateral frontal-lobe lesions or large right-hemisphere lesions; also seen in functional depression.

APATHETIC AKINETIC MUTISM: see akinetic mutism.

APATHY: indifference to the environment, feelings, or physical state.

APGAR SCORE: a numerical expression of the condition of a newborn infant, usually determined at 60 sec. after birth; the sum of points gained on assessment of the heart rate, respiratory effort, muscle tone, reflex irritability, and color.

APHAGIA: abstention from eating.

APHASIA: difficulties, ranging from mild to severe, in understanding spoken and written language and in using language for oral or written communication; may be accompanied by a disturbance in speech; true language disturbance in which patient produces errors of grammer and word choice; basic aphasic defect is in higher integrative language processing although articulation and praxic errors may be present; always agraphic and frequently alexic; lesion of the dominant parietal- or frontal-lobe or connections between the two; Brodmann's areas 7,& 40, left (Hécaen & Albert 1978); implies dysfunction of the middle cerebral artery territory and is often caused by disease of the internal carotid in the neck; sudden onset of aphasia with hemiparesis suggests embolus; also see speech problems, word-finding problems, dysphasia, anarthria, dysarthria,

A

aphonia, dysphonia, global aphasia, conduction aphasia, motor aphasia, abulia, akinetic mutism, Broca's aphasia, Wernicke's sensory aphasia (fluent a.), central aphasia, pure word deafness, pure word blindness, amnestic-dysnomic aphasia, developmental aphasia, jargon aphasia (gibberish a.), nominal aphasia, paraphasia, disconnection syndrome, receptive and expressive aphasia (global), elective mutism, acoustic aphasia, agrammatism, and paragrammatism; other types of aphasia include: ageusic, amosmic, associative, auditory (word deafness), combined, commissural (frontolenticular or lenticular), complete, cortical (global), expressive (Broca's a., frontocortical, verbal, ataxic), functional, graphomotor, Grashey's, Lichtheim's, mixed (global), motor (Broca's a.), nonfluent (Broca's a.), optic, parieto-occipital, psychosensory (receptive, Wernicke's a.), semantic, sensory (Wernicke's a.), subcortical, syntactical (jargon a.), tactile, temporoparietal (Wernicke's a.), transcortical, true (intellectual a.), verbal (Broca's a.), visual (word blindness).

APHASIA - BROCA'S: left Brodmann's area 44; see also Broca's aphasia.

APHASIA SCREENING TESTS: best used as supplements to a neuropsychological test battery; they do not provide the fine discriminations of the complete aphasia test batteries: Aphasia Screening Test (Halstead & Wepman, 1959) takes about 30 minutes to complete and is included in the Halstead-Reitan Neuropsychological Test Battery; a shortened version of the Aphasia Screening Test (Heimburger & Reitan, 1961) consists of four tasks: 1. Copy a square, Greek cross, and triangle without lifting the pencil from the paper; 2. Name each copied figure; 3. spell each name; 4. Repeat; "He shouted the warning"; then explain and write it; may discriminate between left- and right-hemisphere lesions; left-hemisphere lesioned patients can copy the designs but cannot write; right-hemisphere lesioned patients cannot reproduce the designs but can write; Token Test (de Renzi & Vignolo, 1962).

APHASIA TESTS: aphasia tests differ from other verbal tests in that they focus on disorders of symbol formulation and associated apraxia and agnosias (Benton, 1967b); usually designed to elicit samples of behavior in each communication modality — listening, speaking, reading, writing, and gesturing; examination of the central "linguistic processing of verbal symbols" is their common denominator (Darley, 1972; Wepman & Jones, 1967); The Boston Diagnostic Aphasia Examination (BDAE) (Goodglass & Kaplan, 1972); Communication abilities in Daily Living (CADL) (Holland, 1980); Minnesota Test for Differential Diagnosis of Aphasia - revised edition (Schuell, 1972); Multilingual Aphasia Examination (Benton & Hamsher, 1978); Neurosensory Center Comprehensive Examination for Aphasia (Spreen & Benton, 1969); Porch Index of Communicative Ability (Porch, 1967); Western Aphasia Battery (Kertesz, 1979); Functional Communicative Profile (Sarno, 1969); Wepman-Jones language modalities test for aphasia (Wepman & Jones, 1961).

APHEMIA: Broca's first name for aphasia.

APHONIA: loss of voice; total inability to adduct vocal cords and make audible sounds; may be a result of a functional conversion symptom; see also aphasia, elective mutism, dysarthria.

APHRASIA: inability to speak or to understand words arranged as phrases.

APNEA: cessation of breathing; asphyxia.

APOPLEXY: sudden neurologic impairment due to a cerebrovascular disorder; see also CVA, stroke.

APPERCEPTION: conscious perception and appreciation; the power of receiving, appreciating, and interpreting sensory impressions.

APPERCEPTIVE VISUAL AGNOSIA: able to see but cannot synthesize what is seen; cannot organize discrete parts of symbols into a perceptual whole.

APPETITE - LACK OF: aphagia.

APPETITE CONTROL: controlled by the posterior hypothalamus.

APPETITIVE MOVEMENTS: also called voluntary, instrumental, purposive, or operant movements.

APPOSITIONAL CAPACITY: right-hemispheric processing of percepts in terms of their structural similarity.

APRAXIA: difficulty or loss of ability in performing well-learned skills; failure to execute purposive movements voluntarily in the correct context while retaining the ability to carry out the individual movements upon which such acts depend; the left parietal cortex (particularly Brodmann's area 40) is the critical area for control of complex movement (Leipmann, 1908); control is mediated via the left frontal-lobe (Brodmann's area 4) which controls the right side of the body; disruption anywhere along this route in the left-hemisphere would produce apraxia of the right limbs; control over the left side proposed by Leipmann (1920) to be mediated through a series of corticocortical connections running from the left-parietal cortex to the left-frontal cortex and finally to the right-frontal cortex via the corpus callosum; Brodmann's areas 7 & 40, left (Brown 1972; Geschwind 1975); some disconnection between the "command" centers and Brodmann's area 4 (Lawrence & Kuypere, 1968); expressive function; usually associated with some specific sensory impairment and share a common pattern of localization (Hécaen, 1962); use and gesture apraxias most often due to left-sided cortical lesions (Kimura, 1979); symbolic and use apraxias often are associated with receptive language disorders (Dee et al., 1970) and gesture recognition (Ferro et al., 1980); imitating symbolic gestures is sensitive to brain-damage in general regardless of laterality of lesion. *Types of apraxia*:

A

akinetic, amnestic, constructional, cortical, ideational, ideokinetic or ideomotor (transcortical a.), motor (cortical), and sensory (ideational).

APRAXIA-CONSTRUCTIONAL: see Gerstmann's syndrome, constructional apraxia, constructional functions, constructional tasks, drawing tests/tasks, drawing agnosia, and drawing disabilities.

APRAXIA - MOTOR TESTS FOR: (Christensen, 1979; Luria, 1966, 1973); test of learned movements: tested by imitation of the examiner's movements or commands; Kimura Box test (Kimura, 1979); inability to perform the movement (providing there are no sensory deficits, motor weaknesses, or subcortical involvement of the motor system) suggests apraxia.

ARACHNOID (arachnoidea): a delicate membrane interposed between the dura mater and the pia mater, being separated from the pia mater by the subarachnoid space.

ARAS: ascending reticular activating system.

ARCHICEREBELLUM: first cerebellar structure to differentiate in the human fetus; makes up the more medial and ventral portion of the cerebellum.

ARCUATE FASCICULUS: connects Wernicke's area to Broca's area; a bundle of association fibers in the cerebrum extending from the frontal-lobe to the posterior end of the lateral sulcus and interrelating the cortex of the frontal, temporal, parietal, and occipital lobes.

ARCUATE FASCICULUS LESION: causes fluent but paraphasic speech and writing with nearly perfect comprehension of spoken or written language; repetition, reading, writing, and spelling are severely affected; conduction aphasia; also called central aphasia.

ARD: acute respiratory disease.

AREA PYRAMIDALIS: precentral gyrus, primary motor cortex; also called Betz cell area, excitomotor area, psychomotor area, and rolandic area.

AREAS OF THE BRAIN: also called zones; hierarchical layers of at least three cortical zones, built one above the other; found in the three "blocks" or functional units: primary (projection area); secondary (projection-association areas); tertiary (zones of overlapping) (Luria, 1973b).

ARGYLL-ROBERTSON PUPIL: small, irregular pupil that is fixed to light, but reacts to accommodation to a near object; classical sign of meningo-vascular syphilis; other causes are pinealomas, diabetes, brainstem encephalitis, damage in the periaqueductal area, or damage to midbrain relays of the third nerve.

ARITHMETIC CALCULATION TESTS: WAIS-R Arithmetic subtest; Wide Range Achievement Test (WRAT); Calculations subtest of the Psycho-educational Battery; Luria-type computational questions; verbal and written complex examples from Strub & Black

(1977) mental status examination.

ARITHMETIC REASONING PROBLEMS: Luria's arithmetic reasoning problems; Stanford-Binet subtests: Ingenuity I and II; Enclosed Box Problem (SA I); Induction (XIV); Reasoning I and II; Block Counting (level X); Cube Counting; Luria/Christensen's block counting; MacQuarrie Test for Mechanical Ability block-counting subtest.

ARITHMETIC SUBTEST: (WAIS-R) mediocre value as measures of general ability; reflects concentration and ideational discipline (Saunders, 1960a); not a good test of verbal ability for normal subjects; there is a tendency for scores to drop with brain-damaged patients because of the considerable memory and concentration components of oral arithmetic (Morrow & Mark, 1955; Newcombe, 1969); slight but regular tendency for left-hemisphere patients to do a little worse (Spreen & Benton, 1965; Warrington & Rabin, 1970); left-parietal lesioned patients tend to have significantly lowered Arithmetic scores (McFie, 1975); left temporal-lobe lesions produce lower scores (Long & Brown, 1979); right-hemisphere lesioned patients may have lower scores on the Arithmetic subtest than on verbal subtests which may be due to impaired ability to organize the elements of the problems, memory impairments, attention deficits, conceptual manipulation and tracking difficulties (Lezak, 1983); brain-damaged patients usually can perform the first several questions quickly and correctly (one operation), but as the questions become operationally complex the patient may lose or confuse the elements or goal of the problem; not an adequate test for testing basic arithmetic symbol recognition or spatial dyscalculia (Lezak, 1983); assesses knowledge of and ability to apply arithmetic operations only.

ARMY GENERAL CLASSIFICATION TEST (AGCT): depressed scores may follow frontal-lobe, left temporal-lobe, and left parietal-lobe injuries; largely a language and speeded test.

AROUSAL: mediated through the hypothalamus with the ARAS and nonspecific thalamic nuclei; arousal level may be affected by pressure on the midbrain from hippocampal or uncal herniation; see also midbrain, ascending reticular formation, tegmentum, subthalamic lesion, septal region lesion, apathetic akinetic mutism, coma vigil, anterior hypothalamus, cingulate gyri, bilateral orbital frontal cortex, ruptured anterior communicating artery (aneurysm), deep frontal-lobe tumor, anterior cingulate gyrus tumor, mesial frontal-lobe damage, drug intoxication, metabolic balance, sepsis brainstem lesion, reticular system in thalamus or hypothalamus, persistent vegetative state, hysteric coma-like state, locked-in syndrome.

ARRYTHMIA: any variation from the normal rhythm of the heart beat.

ARTERIAL OCCLUSION: (CVA) three locations: 1. main trunk of parent vessel; 2. important penetrating artery; 3. terminal branch.

ARTERIOSCLEROSIS: see cerebral arteriosclerosis.

A

ARTERIOSCLEROTIC DEMENTIA: see multi-infarct dementia.

ARTERIOSCLEROTIC PSYCHOSIS: see multi-infarct dementia.

ARTERIOVENOUS MALFORMATIONS: a tangle of abnormal blood vessels of various sizes; may cause primary subarachnoid hemorrhage; may be found in any part of brain or spinal cord; parietal lobe most common site; may cause epilepsy, migraine-like headaches, chronic progressive dementia, progressive gliosis, and hydrocephalus; bleeding most often venous, recurrent subarachnoid hemorrhage; symptoms may include hemiparesis, hemisensory deficits, homonymous hemianopia, and dysphasia; may show neuropsychological dysfunction of the homologous area of the non-affected cerebral hemisphere (Reitan & Wolfson, 1985).

ARTHEROMA: a mass of plaque of degenerated, thickened arterial intima occurring in atherosclerosis.

ARTHRALGIA: a pain in a joint.

ARTICULATION: contractions of the tongue, lips, pharynx, and palate which interrupt or alter the vocal sounds.

ARTICULATION, DEFECTS IN: see paretic, spastic, rigid, choreic, myoclonic, and ataxic dysarthria.

ARTICULATION DISORDERS: Speaking requires the ability to make the sounds of vowels and consonants, which will then be placed in different combinations to form words and sentences. Patients with severe deficits in articulation are unable to produce simple sounds, even by imitation. Noises may be produced, but each attempt to form a word may produce the same nonsense syllable. In milder forms, the patient may be able to articulate many sounds, especially vowel sounds, but usually will have extreme difficulty in making difficult sounds such as consonant blends; deficits in articulation may result from any of three different causes: 1. defect in peripheral speech mechanisms of the larynx, pharynx, and tongue; 2. defect in choosing the desired sound from all those available in a person's repertoire; 3. deficit in the motor system that prevents the desired sound from being properly pronounced.

ASCENDING RETICULAR ACTIVATING SYSTEM: (ARAS) mediates arousal and wakefulness; ascending fibers project diffusely to all areas of the cerebral cortex; exitation produces and maintains the conscious state; partial inhibition by pontine nuclei brings about sleep; sectioning produces coma; hallucinogenic and stimulant drugs have ARAS as an important site of action; originates in brainstem reticular formation in the medulla oblongata and extends to the cortex via the diffuse nonspecific thalamic projection system; specialized reticular neurons in the tegmentum portion of the midbrain and upper pons have the specific capacity to activate higher centers; these neurons are located in a perimedian portion of the brainstem and receive collateral input from most ascending and descending fiber systems; see also reticular activating system.

ASCENDING HEMIPLEGIA: ascending paralysis of one lateral half of the body.

ASEPTIC MENINGITIS: most common viral invasions are Coxsackie B, mumps, ECHO, and lymphocytic choriomeningitis.

ASHD: arteriosclerotic heart disease.

ASOMATOGNOSIA: the loss of knowledge/awareness about one's own body and bodily condition; see also anosognosia, anosodiaphoria, autotopognosis, asymbolia for pain.

ASPHYXIA: a condition due to lack of oxygen in respired air resulting in impending or actual cessation of apparent life; cessation of breathing; apnea.

ASSOCIATE LEARNING SUBTEST (WMS): test of verbal learning; paired word-learning task; tests recall of well-learned verbal associations and retention of new, unfamiliar verbal material; a test which may be used to expose malingering. (Gronwall, quoted in Lezak, 1983).

ASSOCIATION AREAS: overlapping zones of the cortex which are involved in integration and refinement of raw percepts or simple motor responses emanating from the primary projection zones; located peripherally to functional centers where the neuronal components of two or more different functions are interspersed; lesions produce a pattern of deficits running through related functions or as an impairment of a general capcity; lesions do not produce specific sensory or motor defects.

ASSOCIATION AREAS - PARIETAL LOBES: generally thought to mediate affect, memory, and language functions; specialized for the mediation of complex cognitive processes and cognition (the highest form of sensory integration, reasoning, thought, perception, etc).

ASSOCIATION FIBERS: two types: 1. long fiber bundles that interconnect distant neocortical areas, and 2. short subcortical U-fibers that interconnect adjacent neocortical areas. The long fiber bundles include the uncinate fasciculus, the cingulum, the inferior longitudinal fasciculus, and the inferior frontal occipital fasciculus; provides for integration of the functions mediated by the association zones.

ASSOCIATIONS: (thought processes): ideas which are connected or linked in some logical way; may be loose or clanging in schizophrenia or bipolar disorder; see also loose or clang associations and derailment.

ASSOCIATIVE APHASIA: disturbance of connection between the parts comprising the central structure.

ASSOCIATIVE VISUAL AGNOSIA: perceives the whole of what is seen but cannot recognize it.

ASTEREOGNOSIA: 2 types: 1. primary somatosensory agnosia (see

A

agnosia also - primary agnosia - tactile) and 2. secondary somatosensory agnosia or asymbolia (see also agnosia - ideational).

ASTHENIA: lack or loss of strength and energy; weakness.

ASTIGMATISM: images entering the eye focus in different planes.

ASTROCYTES: a neuroglial cell of ectodermal origin, characterized by fibrous or protoplasmic processes; collectively called astroglia.

ASTROCYTOMA: see tumor.

ASTROGLIA: neuroglial cells of ectodermal origin that give structural support to and repair neurons.

ASYMBOLIA: secondary somatosensory agnosia; tactile images are preserved but are disconnected or isolated from other sensory representations so that the full significance of the object cannot be appreciated; lesion in the posterior-parietal cortex, roughly Brodmann's areas 5 and 7.

ASYMBOLIA FOR PAIN: absence of normal reactions to pain; thought to be caused by a lesion in the left parietal-lobe, probably the secondary zones, or a disconnection from affective regions of the brain; may be one or both hemispheres.

ASYMMETRY OF BRAIN: The planum temporale, which is the cortical area just posterior to the auditory cortex (Heschl's gyrus) within the Sylvian fissure, is larger on the left in 65% of the brains and usually 1 cm. longer on the right (Geschwind & Levitsky, 1968); there are usually two Heschl's gyri on the right and only one on the left, complementary to the larger planum temporale on the left. The slope of the Sylvian fissure is different in the two sides, being gentler on the left than on the right (specialized role in integrating the spatial characteristics of sensory stimuli). The frontal operculum (Broca's area) is significantly larger (by about one-third) on the right side. Anatomical asymmetry is significantly greater in males than in females, as is functional asymmetry. The distribution of noradrenergic neurons is strongly lateralized in the thalamus, being more heavily concentrated in the pulvinar of the left-hemisphere and the ventral-lateral thalamus of the right-hemisphere. The right-hemisphere extends further anteriorly than the left, the left-hemisphere extends further posteriorly than the right, and the occipital horn of the lateral ventricles are five times more likely to be longer on the right than on the left. The total mass of the two sides are essentially identical.

ASYMMETRY OF CHEWING: damage to the trigaminial nerve (V).

ASYMMETRY OF EYE MOVEMENTS: may indicate malfunctions of the third, fourth, and sixth cranial nerves.

ASYNERGIA: lack of coordination among parts or organs normally acting in harmony such as muscle contractions; different components of an act need to follow in proper sequence, at the proper moment, and to the proper degree, so that the act is executed accurately; see also lateral and inferior cerebellar lesions.

ATAXIA: lesion of one cerebellar hemisphere, especially the anterior lobe, causes disturbances in coordination of volitional movements of the ipsilateral arm and leg; patient may overshoot the mark (passed pointing); afferent disorder; movements characterized by an inappropriate range, rate, and strength of each of the various components of a motor act and by an improper combination of those components; see also lesions of the lateral and inferior cerebellum.

ATAXIA OF BRUNS: inability to stand because of decomposition of gait and upright stance; wide base, flexed posture, and small shuffling steps.

ATAXIC APHASIA: Broca's aphasia.

ATAXIC DYSARTHRIA: imprecise enunciation; monotony; unnatural irregular separation of the syllables of words; poor coordination of speech and respiration; see also multiple sclerosis, Friedreich's ataxia, cerebellar atrophy, heat stroke slowness, cerebellar lesions.

ATAXIC INTENTION TREMOR: see intention tremor.

ATHEROSCLEROSIS: an extremely common form of arteriosclerosis in which deposits of yellowish plaques (atheromas) containing cholesterol, lipoid material, and lipophages are formed within the intima and inner media of large and medium-sized arteries.

ATHETOSIS: a derangement marked by ceaseless occurrence of slow, sinuous, writhing movements, especially severe in the hands, and performed involuntarily; may occur after hemiplegia, and then is known as posthemiplegic chorea; also called mobile spasm; characterized by an inability to sustain the fingers and toes, tongue, or any other group of muscles in one position; purposeless movements; most pronounced in the digits and the hands, but often involves the tongue, throat, and face; lesion(s) of anterior thalamus or ventricular nuclei with intact pyramidal tracts; see also dystonia.

ATHETOTIC GAIT: grotesque postures, arms awry, wrist and fingers alternately undergoing slow flexion, extension, and rotation, legs advance slowly and awkwardly; seen in congenital athetosis and Huntington's chorea; see also mobile spasm, posthemiplegic chorea, congenital athetosis, Huntington's chorea palsy, Voyt's syndrome, and Little's disease.

ATHETOID - PSEUDOBULBAR: combination of bilateral pyramidal and extrapyramidal signs.

ATRESIA: congenital absence or closure of a normal body orifice or tubular organ.

ATROPINE: dilates the pupils by paralyzing the parasympathetic nerve endings.

ATTENTION: ability to attend to a specific stimulus without being distracted by extraneous environmental stimuli; screens out irrelevant stimuli; contrasted to alertness in which the person can re-

A

spond to any stimuli; attention presupposes alertness; alertness does not imply attentiveness; complex interaction of limbic, neocortical and ascending activating functions; automatic, passive but focused, capacity for selective perception (Allison et al., 1968); impairment causes shortened attention span, distractibility, and susceptibility to confusion.

ATTENTION HEMIANOPIA: inability to see in one half field of vision with patient being unaware of the defect; see also homonymous hemianopia.

ATTENTION TO EXTERNAL CUES TESTS: Problem of Fact (Stanford-Binet subtest-age XIII); Cookie Theft Picture.

ATTENTIONAL DEFICITS: distractibility or impaired ability for focused behavior; impaired concentration and mental/conceptual tracking abilities; may be modality specific (Diller & Weinberg, 1972); visual perception, visual search and visual scanning tests require sustained, focused attention and concentration, and directed visual shifting; see also vigilance.

ATTENTIONAL DEFICITS TESTS: cancellation tests; mental tracking tests; reverse serial order; serial sevens; Paced Auditory Serial Addition test; Symbol Digit Modalities test; sequential Matching Memory task; Trail making test.

ATTENTIONAL DEFICITS - KORSAKOFF'S: characterized by indifference and perseveration; performs well on digit span but not random letters test.

ATTITUDE: a pattern of feeling or mental view determined by cumulative previous experience.

AUDITION IN THE COMMISSURED BRAIN: the auditory system has both crossed and uncrossed connections between the two hemispheres; however, in the commissured patient, direct access to the left side from the left ear does not appear to take place.

AUDITORY AGNOSIA: impaired capacity to recognize the nature of nonverbal acoustic stimuli; aphasia due to disease of the hearing center of the brain; word deafness; see agnosia - auditory.

AUDITORY COMPREHENSION DEFICITS: most common sources of defective auditory comprehension are deficiencies in auditory acuity resulting from conduction and/or sensorineural hearing losses and deficiencies in auditory processing associated with aphasia.

AUDITORY COMPREHENSION DISORDER: audition may be disturbed even though the primary auditory cortex is not damaged; sometimes particularly impaired when words are presented in isolation rather than in the context of a sentence; comprehension of individual words may be intact, but certain grammatical constructions are not discriminated properly.

AUDITORY DEFICIT TESTING: some patients may attempt to hide impaired hearing or refuse to wear a hearing aid because of embarrassment. If the patient is not aware of his hearing loss, it may be due to brain injury and/or he may have poor comprehension as a result of aphasia. Behavioral observation will usually identify a minor hearing loss; the patient will usually turn the "good" ear towards the examiner or compulsively watch the examiners mouth. To detect a mild to moderate hearing loss, the examiner can vary the volume of his voice or turn away to speak. Auditory discrimination problems can be tested by having the patient repeat sound-alike words and phrases; if an auditory deficit is suspected, the patient should be referred to an audiologist; hearing deficits may contribute to poor performance on tests and poor psychosocial adjustment; aphasia should always be suspected when the patient has a right hemiplegia or should be considered when the hearing deficit does not appear to be related to hearing loss, attention or concentration defects, or a functional thought disorder.

AUDITORY HALLUCINATIONS: see hallucinations - auditory.

AUDITORY INATTENTION: patients with lateralized lesions involving the temporal lobe or central auditory pathways tend to ignore auditory signals entering the ear opposite the side of the lesions; a simple method for testing auditory inattention can be performed without special equipment by an examiner standing behind the patient so that he can deliver stimulation to each ear simultaneously or randomly, varying single and simultaneous stimuli; dichotic listening tests may be used (Kimura, 1961, 1967; Walsh, 1978).

AUDITORY MEMORY: Brodmann's area 22.

AUDITORY MEATUS: external ear canal.

AUDITORY NUMBER AGNOSIA: receptive aphasia characterized by inability to understand the meaning, magnitude, or relationships of spoken numbers in the absence of physical disability of hearing.

AUDITORY PROCESSING TEST: dichotic words and melodies.

AUDITORY RECEPTION TEST: (subtest of ITPA) a few errors suggest inattention or carelessness; more than a few errors indicate a need for more thorough examination of auditory verbal receptive and processing functions.

AUDITORY REFLEXES: mediated through the inferior colliculi.

AUDITORY SENSATION AND PERCEPTION - DISORDERS: Brodmann's areas 41,42,22; temporal lobe.

AUDITORY SYSTEM: auditory projections from both left and right ears travel to both hemispheres; the major pathways cross from the ear and cochlear nucleus to the inferior colliculus, medial geniculate nucleus of the thalamus, and the cortex; the primary auditory region in the cortex is area 41, located in Heschl's gyrus, which is connected to the secondary auditory zones that include area 42 and 22; area 22 also receives direct connections from the medial geniculate, although it receives fewer than area 41; crossed pathways to the hemisphere contralateral to each ear have preferential access and input into the respective auditory cortical area; neurons of the auditory system are arranged hierarchically; the auditory input travels from the auditory nerve to the cochlear nuclei, superior olivary nuclei, inferior colliculi, medial geniculate nuclei, and finally the auditory cortex; see also cochlear nucleus, superior olivary nuclei, inferior colliculus, medial geniculate nuclei, auditory cortex.

AUDITORY SYSTEM - LESIONS: lesions of the auditory nerve produce deafness in the connected ear; bilateral lesion in Heschl's gyrus will produce deafness in both ears, but a unilateral lesion in either of Heschl's gyri will not produce deafness in either ear; lesions in the primary auditory projection cortex (area 41) cause an increase in the threshold for auditory sensation in the contralateral ear; left-temporal lesions will produce a deficit in the recall of dichotically presented digits in both ears which suggests some sort of deficit in selectively attending to and differentiating simultaneous speech sounds; left-temporal lesions produce a deficit in phonemic hearing so that the patient confuses oppositional phonemes such as da-ta, ba-pa, or sa-za probably as a result of damage to the posterior part of area 22 near Wernicke's area; lesions to the secondary zone of the right auditory cortex: analysis of music impaired, particularly timbre and tonal memory (Milner, 1971); impaired ability at locating the source of sounds in space (Shankweiler, 1966).

AUDITORY TESTS: Speech Sounds Perception Test, dichotic listening, auditory reception, Seashore Rhythm Test, Seashore Test of Musical Talent, Dorgeuille battery, auditory-verbal perception; more definitive auditory testing should be performed by an audiologist.

AUDITORY-VERBAL LEARNING TEST: (Rey, 1964; Taylor, 1959) measures immediate memory span, provides a learning curve, reveals learning strategies (or absence), elicits retroactive and proactive interference tendencies and tendencies to confusion or confabulation on memory tasks, and also measures retention following interference; numerous repetitions of the same words probably reflect a problem in self-monitoring and tracking associated with a learning defect; confabulations repeated in later word lists show a tendency to have difficulty in maintaining the distinction between information coming from the outside and own associations, or in distinguishing between data obtained at different times which suggests a breakdown in self-monitoring functions.

AUDITORY-VERBAL PERCEPTION TEST: when impairment in auditory processing is suspected, the examiner can couple an auditorally presented test with a similar task presented visually.

AUDITORY-VESTIBULAR NERVE (VIII): hearing.

AURA (epileptic): warning signs experienced by patient of impending seizure; may take the form of sensations such as odors, noises, etc., or may simply be a feeling that the seizure is going to occur.

AURAL: hearing; 8th cranial nerve.

AUSTIN MAZE: (Walsh, 1978) electrically activated maze developed to study self-correcting behavior as well as the ability to follow instructions; patients whose executive abilities are impaired may have difficulty learning from their mistakes, switching to alternative response pattern, or attending to the rules.

AUTISTIC THINKING: thinking dominated by unconscious trends and uncorrected by reality.

AUTOMATIC BEHAVIORS: behaves like an automaton, may get up, walk, drive, remove clothes, speak, cannot attend to others, and does not understand external stimuli; also called reflexive, consummatory, or respondent behaviors; units of stereotyped behavior linked in a sequence such as grooming, chewing, lapping, and rejection of food; present at the level of midbrain and below; present in high decerebrate animal.

AUTOMATIC LANGUAGE: emotional use of language as in swearing, overlearned expressions, serial speech, memorized sequences.

AUTOMATISMS ASSOCIATED WITH EPILEPSY: characterized by behavior of an individual who carries out a series of more or less complex acts without being aware of them and has no recollection of the acts; most often a manifestate of temporal-lobe epilepsy, but sometimes follows petit mal or grand mal attack (Brain, 1985).

AUTOMATISMS-VERBAL: patterned verbal material learned in early childhood and frequently used throughout life is usually recalled without difficulty or thought (e.g., alphabet, number series, days of the week, etc.); inability to repeat automatisms may reflect attentional deficits, reduced levels of consciousness, or diffuse cerebral damage.

AUTONOMIC NERVOUS SYSTEM: subdivision of the peripheral nervous system; contains some afferent (sensory) fibers; emphasis is on motor functions; primary function: to innervate smooth muscles and glands; also called vegetative or involuntary nervous system; controls activity of the viscera; divided into the sympathetic nervous system and the parasympathetic nervous system which work together and in opposition to control visceral reflexes and to regulate peripheral emotional responsivity.

AUTONOMIC HYPERREFLEXIA: paroxysmal hypertension, bradycardia, sweating of the forehead, severe headache, and gooseflesh due to distention of the bladder and rectum; it is associated with lesions above the outflow of the splanchnic nerves.

AUTOTOPAGNOSIA: inability to localize, name, or orient correctly different parts of the body; body image agnosia; most often a result of left frontal-lobe lesions (Teuber, 1964); aphasia often present (Diller et al., 1974; Weinstein, 1964); Personal Orientation Test;

31

B

Body Center Test; Right-Left Orientation; tests should include pointing on command, naming body parts, imitating body positions or movements and crosswise imitations.

AVERAGE EVOKED POTENTIALS(AEP): see evoked potential.

AVM: arteriovenous malformations.

AWOL: unauthorized absence; absent without leave.

AXIS: 1. a line about which a revolving body turns or about which a structure would turn if it revolved; a line around which specified parts of the body are arranged; 2. the second cervical vertebra.

AXOAXONAL: synapse between two axon.

AXODENDRITIC: synapse between axon and dendrite.

AXON: part of a neuron that sends information; the generally long and single extension of the neuron that conducts impulses away from the cell body to other neurons.

AXONAL ENDINGS: multibranching fibers at the end of axons, weaving among the dendrites, the cell bodies, and in rare cases, the axons of other neurons.

AXOSOMATIC: synapse between the axon and another nerve cell body.

B

BA: behavioral age.

BABCOCK STORY RECALL TEST: memory test (Babcock, 1930; Babcock & Levy, 1940).

BABINSKI'S LAW: law of voltaic vertigo that a normal subject inclines to the side of the positive pole; one with disease of the labyrinth falls to the side to which he tends to incline spontaneously. If the labyrinth is destroyed, there is no reaction.

BABINSKI'S REFLEX: dorsiflexion of the big toe and spreading of the other toes when the sole of the foot is stimulated; occurs in lesions of the pyramidal tract (corticospinal); indicates organic, as distinguished from hysteric, hemiplegia; also called Babinski's sign or toe sign.

BABINSKI'S SIGNS: also see Babinski's law, phenomenon, reflex, and syndrome; 1. loss or lessening of the Achilles tendon reflex in sciatica; 2. in hemiplegia, the contraction of the platysma muscle in the healthy side is more vigorous than the affected side, as seen in opening the mouth, whistling, blowing, etc.; *signs tests*: 1. patient lies on the floor, with arms crossed on chest, and makes effort to rise to a sitting position: on the paralyzed side, thigh is flexed upon the pelvis and the heel is lifted from the ground; seen in organic hemiplegia and not hysterical hemiplegia; 2. when paralyzed forearm is placed in supination, it turns over to pronation; seen only in organic paralysis; also called pronation sign.

BABINSKI-NAGEOTTE SYNDROME: a syndrome due to multiple lesions affecting the pyramidal and sensory tracts, the cerebellar peduncle, and the reticular formation; marked by contralateral hemiplegia and hemianesthesia (usually only of the pain and temperature senses), ipsilateral hemiasynergia, hemiataxia, and Horner's syndrome.

BACKGROUND INTERFERENCE PROCEDURE: (Canter, 1966, 1968) a version of the Bender-Gestalt test which is reported to be a better screening device for brain-damage; identifies senility; disrupts the performance of patients with right-hemisphere damage (Nemec, 1978).

BACTERIAL INFECTIONS: (of the brain) result from an infestation of bacteria, usually via the blood stream; most common: meningitis and brain abcess.

BACTERIUM: a loose generic name for any one-celled microorganism that has no chlorophyll and multiplies by simple division.

BALANCE: see cerebellar lesions/functions.

BALINT'S SYNDROME: cortical paralysis of visual fixation, optic ataxia, and distrubance of visual attention, with preservation of spontaneous and reflex eye movements; caused by bilateral lesions of the parieto-occipital lobes.

BALLISMUS: violent movements of the limbs resembling a forceful throwing movement which exhaust and incapacitate the patient; cause seems to be due to damage in the contralateral subthalamic nucleus, as a result of vascular disease, tumor, or infection; see also hemiballismus.

BALTHAZAR SCALES OF ADAPTIVE BEHAVIOR: (Balthazar, 1956) assesses daily living abilities in minute detail and has a manual for use in developing specific training programs from the ratings.

BASAL GANGLIA: collection of large nuclei lying mainly beneath the anterior regions of the neocortex and lateral to the thalamus; includes putamen, globus pallidus, caudate nucleus, amygdala; primarily (but not exclusively) involved with extrapyramidal regulation of motor activity; may have other functions, such as sequencing a number of complex movements into a smoothly executed response; the bundle of motor fibers which make up the the internal capsule originate in the primary motor cortex and descend through the basal ganglia; presumed to control the ability to link automatic movements to voluntary movements so that the behaviors are biologically adaptive such as moving towards food and stopping at the right time and place (Kolb & Whishaw, 1980); principal structures are the corpus striatum which consists of the caudate nucleus and the

B

lenticular nucleus which, in turn, is divided into the putamen and the globus pallidus; more concerned with slow (ramp) movements than rapid (ballistic) movements, which are controlled by the cerebellum; probable function is to recognize that certain complex movements will take place and prepare the motor system for the accomplishment of these movements (Brain, 1985).

BASAL GANGION LESION: difficulty in rapid alternating sequences of movement (clumsiness); unable to inhibit approach behavior; damage to different parts can produce changes in posture, increases or decreases in muscle tone, and abnormal movements such as twitches, jerks, and tremors; see also Parkinson's Disease, Wilson's Disease, akinesia, dystonic postures.

BASAL GANGLIONIC: choreic, athetotic, subthalamic.

BASAL GANGLIONIC LEVEL OF FUNCTIONING: (in the decorticate animal); able to link automatic movements to voluntary movements so that the behaviors are biologically adaptive; probably involves inhibition or facilitation of voluntary movements.

BASILAR AREA LESIONS: The 3rd, 4th, & 6th nerves are subject to damage by basal meningeal disease processes, e.g., tuberculous, fungal and bacterial meningitis, carcinomatous meningitis, direct neoplastic invasion from the sinuses and nasopharynx, meningovascular syphilis, sarcoid, Guillain-Barré syndrome, and Herpes Zoster; aneurysmal dilation of the upper basilar artery may cause multiple nerve palsies and, in particular, bilateral third nerve lesions; the sixth nerve may also be affected in the basal area with increased intracranial pressure from hydrocephalus which pushes the brainstem down and the sixth nerve becomes stretched over the petrous tip; the sixth nerve may also be damaged by mastoiditis or middle ear infection which causes severe ear pain and a combination of 6th, 7th, 8th and, occasionally, 5th nerve lesions (Gradenigo's syndrome); 6th nerve lesion may be caused by a cavernous sinus thrombosis usually occurring as a complication of sepsis of the skin over the upper face or in the paranasal sinuses.

BASILAR ARTERY: the cerebral artery formed by the joining of the two vertebral arteries that enter the base of the brain; after dividing into several smaller arteries, it irrigates the cerebellum; the major division forms the posterior cerebral artery, which irrigates the medial temporal-lobe and posterior occipital-lobe; the posterior cerebral artery and the middle cerebral artery join together to form the posterior communicating artery.

BASIS PEDUNCULI (PES CEREBRI): ventral-most aspect of the midbrain; contains cerebral peduncles and substantia nigra.

BBB: blood-brain barrier.

BEAD STRINGING: (Stanford-Binet subtest) suitable for severely impaired brain-damaged patients.

BECK DEPRESSION INVENTORY: (Beck et al., 1961) a self-rating depression scale that explores mood, sense of failure, indecisiveness, work inhibition, and appetite; may be denied by patient or easily manipulated to look good or bad depending upon the desire of the patient.

BEHAVIORAL RATING SCALES: some are designed to be administered by ward staff or care takers and contain many observational questions regarding orientation and behavioral functioning; Geriatric Rating Scale; Stockton Geriatric Rating Scale; Sandoz Clinical Assessment — Geriatric; Dementia Rating Scale; Developmental Scales; Longitudinal evaluation of head-trauma patients; Boyd Developmental Progress Scale; Vineland Social Maturity Scale; Gesell Developmental Schedules; Adaptive Behavior Scale; Balthazar Scales of Adaptive Behavior; Glasgow Coma Scale; Galveston Orientation and Amnesia Test; posttraumatic amnesia questionnaire; Glasgow Outcome Scale; Katz Adjustment Scale: Relative's Form; Portland Adaptability Inventory; Rappaport Disability Rating Scale; Social Status Outcome Scale; PULSES; Sickness Impact Questionnaire.

BEHAVIORAL TRIANGLE: receptors detect the stimuli; effectors respond to the stimuli, and conductors link the two.

BEHAVIORISM: the doctrine holding that only observable responses, the measurable features of overt behavior, are suitable for psychological study.

BELL'S PALSY: facial paralysis due to lesion of the facial nerve and resulting in characteristic distortion of the face; an acute seventh nerve paralysis preceded by pain in and around the ear on the day of onset; usually caused by a viral infection with damage to the swollen nerve caused by entrapment in the facial canal.

BENDER-GESTALT TEST; a copying test; interpretations; self-regulatory aspects: cards 1, 2, and 6 tend to bring out perseverative tendencies (a symptom of frontal-lobe dysfunction) and planning aspects; the page placement of designs shows awareness of space use and spatial relations (frontal-lobe function); malingering may be demonstrated by retesting several hours or days later which may show inconsistencies in altered reproductions; organicity is generally demonstrated with simplicity of design and particular distortions are usually consistant across designs; most often organicity is shown in rotations and diffi-

B

culty with card 6 (Bender, 1938; Hutt, 1977); may also be used as a projective technique for studying personality; demonstrates the tendency to organize visual stimuli into configurational wholes; drawing impairments are more likely to occur with parietal-lobe lesions (Garron & Cheifetz, 1965); right parietal-lobe lesions are most associated with the poorest performances (Diller et al., 1974; Herschenfang, 1960); patients with right-hemisphere damage are much more susceptible to errors of rotation (Billingslea, 1963), fragmentation (Belleza et al., 1979), and omissions (Diller & Weinberg, 1965); left frontal-lobe lesioned patients may not show impairment (Garron & Cheifetz, 1965).

BENEDIKT'S SYNDROME: see midbrain vascular lesions.

BENTON VISUAL RETENTION TEST: a visuospatial memory test; norms well established; (Benton, 1974) the performance of patients with frontal-lobe lesions differs with the side of injury: bilateral hemispheric lesioned patients make the most errors, right-sided damage the next most, and left-sided damage the least and comparable to normal scores (Benton, 1968); may show perseverative responses (a frontal-lobe dysfunction) (Benton, 1974); sensitive to unilateral spatial neglect; spatial organization problems may show up in the handling of size and placement relationships of the three figures; impaired immediate recall or an attention defect appears mostly as simplification, simple substitutions, or omission of the last one or two designs elements of a card; unilateral spatial neglect shows up as consistent omission of the figure on the same side as the lesion; visuospatial and constructional disabilities appear as defects in the execution or organization of the drawings; rotations and consistent design distortions generally indicate a perceptual problem; perseveration suggests a specific visuoperceptual, or an immediate memory impairment (Lezak, 1983); simplification of designs, including disregard of size and placement, may be associated with overall behavioral regression in patients with bilateral or diffuse damage; patients who improve their performance when they have a quiet delay period may be suffering attention and concentration problems rather than memory problems, or they may need more than an ordinary amount of time to consolidate new information; sensitive to left brain damage as well a right because of verbal mediation of designs; constructional component more pronounced than the memory component; useful in distinguishing patients with cerebral brain-damage from psychiatric patients (Benton, 1974; Heaton et al., 1978; Marsh & Hirsch, 1982); malingerers may make many more errors of distortion but fewer errors of omission than brain-damaged patients.

BERRY ANEURYSM: subarachnoid aneurysm.

BETA-MSH: secreted by the adenohypophysis.

BETA RHYTHM: dominant rhythm of the precentral and postcentral sensorimotor area at 20-to-25 cycles/second.

BETZ CELLS: large pyramidal ganglion cells forming one of the layers of the motor area of the gray matter of the brain; called also giant pyramids and giant pyramidal cells.

BIFURCATION: the site where a single structure divides into two.

BID: two times a day.

BICYCLE DRAWING TEST: (Taylor, 1959); a test of mechanical reasoning as well as visuographic functioning; may be used to test reasoning, comprehension of relationships, logical thinking, and practical judgment; tends to bring out the drawing distortions characteristic of lateral damage: right-hemisphere lesioned patients tend to reproduce many of the component parts of the machine, sometimes with much elaboration and care, but misplace them in relation to one another; left-hemisphere lesioned patients are more likely to preserve the overall proportions but simplify (Lebrun & Hoops, 1974; McFie & Zangwill, 1960); severely impaired patients, regardless of the site of the lesion, perform this task with great difficulty, producing incomplete and simplistic drawings (Lezak, 1983).

BILATERAL: structures that lie on both side.

BILATERAL DYSFUNCTION OF TEMPERAL LOBES: 1. Korsakoff's amnesic defect; 2. apathy and plastidity; 3. loss of sexual capacity; 4. loss of other unilateral functions; 5. Klüver-Bucy syndrome.

BILATERAL HEMIANOPIA: true hemianopia.

BILATERAL PREFRONTAL LESIONS: severe impairment in reporting the time of day and in decoding proverbs, perseveration (inflexible behavior, inability to change response sets), impaired response inhibition (impulsivity).

BINASAL HEMIANOPIA: heteronymous hemianopia in which the defects are in the nasal half of the field of vision in each eye.

BINGSWANGER'S DEMENTIA: a form of presenile dementia caused by demyelination of the subcortical white matter of the brain accompanying sclerotic changes in the blood vessels supplying it.

BINOCULAR HEMIANOPIA: true hemianopia.

BIOFEEDBACK TRAINING: a procedure for training subjects to control their internal environment (autonomic responses such as blood pressure or central nervous system responses such as brain waves) by giving reinforcement each time the desired response occurs. With repeated reinforcements, the response increases in strength.

BIPOLAR NEURON: a neuron that has one axon and one dendrite

B

issuing from its cell body.

BITEMPORAL HEMIANOPIA: loss of vision in the temporal half of the field of vision in each eye as a result of a lesion of the medial region of chiasmal compression; heteronymous hemianopia.

BLINDNESS: visual anesthesia, amaurosis.

BLINDSIGHT: (Weiskrantz et al., 1974) a phenomenon of visual perception in which patients are apparently blind but are able to grasp objects in motion and can indicate the direction of motion, even if they reported not having seen the object (Riddoch, 1917).

BLIND SPOT: the area where the optic nerve leaves the retina of each eye; an object projected here cannot be seen because there are neither rods nor cones in this area; also known as the optic disc.

BLOCK COUNTING: Stanford-Binet subtest level X; a test of reasoning ability; sensitive to right-hemisphere lesions (Newcombe, 1969; McFie & Zangwill, 1960; Warrington & Rabin, 1970) and left visuospatial inattention (Campbell & Oxbury, 1976); also called Cube Analysis (Newcombe, 1969) or Cube Counting (McFie & Zangwill, 1960).

BLOCK COUNTING SUBTEST: MacQuarrie - Test for Mechanical Ability; test of spatial reasoning; norms available.

BLOCK COUNTING TESTS: Stanford-Binet Block Counting subtest-level X; Cube Counting, Luria/Christensen's block counting, MacQuarrie Test for Mechanical Ability block counting subtest.

BLOCK DESIGN TEST (WAIS-R): two dimensional space constructional task; best measure of visuospatial organization; reflects general ability so that intellectually capable but academically or culturally limited persons frequently obtain their highest score on this test; may provide information about ability to order, plan ahead naturally and effectively, laboriouly, inconsistently, or not at all (frontal-lobe planning dysfunction); concrete-minded persons and right-hemisphere damaged patients with visuospatial deficits have particular difficulty constructing diagonal patterns; visuospatial comprehension: highest level — patient comprehends the design at a glance, does not need to refer back; average level — trial and error; *work habits*: orderliness, planning, speed vs impulsiveness; ability to perceive errors and willingness/ability to correct them; *tempermental characteristics*: cautiousness, carefulness, impulsivity, impatience, apathy, etc; self-deprecatory or self-congratulatory statements; requests for help and rejection of the task betray patient's feelings about self; *frontal-lobe damage*: patients may say they understand the task, but may confuse the designs; with less severe damage, frontal-lobe lesioned patients may fail items because of impulsivity and carelessness; a concrete perspective that prevents logical analysis of the designs may result in random approaches to solving the problem or not seeing or correcting errors; *concrete thinking*: patients will try to make the sides as well as the top of their construction match that of the model in the first item; may fail item 8 (WAIS) or 7 (WAIS-R) by laying out red and white stripes with whole blocks rather than abstracting the 3x3 format and shifting their conceptualization of the design to a solution based on diagonals; scores are usually lower in the presence of any kind of brain injury; scores are least affected when the lesion is confined to the left hemisphere, except when the left parietal-lobe is involved (McFie, 1975); scores are moderately depressed by diffuse or bilateral brain lesions such as those resulting from traumatic injuries or diffuse degenerative processes that do not primarily involve cortical tissue (Lezak, 1983); most pronounced deficits associated with posterior lesions, particularly right parietal lesions (Strub & Black, 1977; Newcombe, 1969; Smith, 1966); in split-brain lesioned patients: neither hemisphere alone can do the task (Geschwind, 1979); left-parietal lesioned patients show confusion, simplification, and concrete handling; although orderly, they usually work from left to right and usually preserve the square shape but may have trouble placing the last block (McFie, 1975); right-hemisphere lesioned patients may begin at the right of the design and work left; visuospatial deficits show up in disorientation, design distortions, misperceptions, or loss of squared or self-contained format; left-visuospatial inattention may compound these design-copying problems, resulting in two or more block solutions to the four-block designs in which the whole left half or one left quadrant of the design is omitted; there may be more errors on the side of the design contralateral to the side of the lesion; errors more at the top suggest temporal-lobe components, lower errors have parietal components.

BLOCK DESIGN SUBTEST IN DEMENTIA/ALZHEIMER'S DISEASE: often one of the lowest ranking scores of the WAIS-R along with Digit Symbol and Digits Backward; slowness in learning new response sets is typical of aging, dementing, frontal-lobe disease, or head injury and may show up with failure on the first two items while the succeeding two or three or more items are passed, each more rapidly than the last; diffuse loss of cortical neurons (Alzheimer's disease): in *early stages*, patients will understand the task and may be able to copy one or two designs. In *later stages* they may get confused between one block and another or between their constructions and the examiner's model so that they may be able to imitate the placement of only one or two blocks (constructional apraxia) (Lezak, 1983).

BLOCKING: mental condition characterized by difficulty in logical verbal expression, inability to keep track of associations, and interruption of a train of thought or idea; there may be sudden stops in midsentence or no response to a question; produced when complex material or anxiety producing material is presented; may be seen in schizophrenia, severe psychotic depression, and bipolar disorders; also called derailment or a symptom of formal thought disorder; usually the person indicates that he/she cannot recall what he/she meant to say; blocking should be judged to be present only if the person spontaneously describes losing the thought or, if upon questioning by the interviewer, the person gives that as a reason for pausing.

BLOCKS OR FUNCTIONAL UNITS: three principal functional units of the brain whose participation is necessary for any mental activity: block 1. (brainstem, reticular activating system, limbic system) regulates tonicity of cortex or waking state; block 2. (occipital, temporal, parietal lobes) a unit for obtaining, processing, and storing information arriving from the outside world; block 3. (frontal and prefrontal lobes) a unit for programming, regulating, monitoring, and verifying or evaluating mental activity (Luria, 1973b).

BLOCK-TAPPING: (Milner, 1971) Corsi's test of immediate recall span; sensitive to right-temporal lobe resections when significant amounts of the hippocampus are removed.

BLOOD-BRAIN BARRIER: (cerebral) a barrier separating the blood from the parenchyma of the central nervous system; consists of the walls of capillaries of the CNS and the surrounding glial membranes; filters, inhibits, prohibits passage of certain substances into the brain including antibodies (Reitan & Wolfson, 1985).

BLOOD PRESSURE: the pressure of the blood on the walls of the arteries, dependent on the energy of the heart action, the elasticity of the walls of the arteries, and the volume and viscosity of the blood; maximum pressure occurs near the end of the stroke output of the left ventricle of the heart and is termed maximum or systolic pressure; minimum pressure occurs late in ventricular diastole and is termed minimum or diastolic pressure; mean blood pressure is the average of the blood pressure levels; basic blood pressure is the pressure during quiet rest or basal conditions.

BLOOD CLOT: see thrombosis or embolism.

BLOOD SUPPLY OF THE BRAINSTEM: main blood supply is

derived from the paired vertebral arteries which join at the pontomedullary junction to form the basilar artery. From its medial side each vertebral artery gives rise to a branch that joins with its fellow to form the anterior spinal artery which supplies part of the central medulla and the bulk of the spinal cord down to S1. Laterally, each vertebral artery gives off a variable branch, the posterior inferior cerebellar artery which may be absent in 25% of people. When it is present it runs a tortuous course along the side of the medulla, which it supplies. The other brainstem vessels follow the same pattern of distribution; from below upwards: the anterior inferior cerebellar artery, the transverse pontine arteries, the superior cerebellar arteries, and the posterior cerebral arteries. Each gives off a long penetrating paramedial branch that supplies the central area of the brainstem to the floor of the ventricle, and a series of short branches that supply the basal area of the brainstem, while the main trunk of the vessel passes around the brainstem to supply the dorsolateral quadrant of the brainstem and part of the cerebellum. The superior cerebellar artery supplies all the deep structures of the cerebellum including the nuclei. The anterior inferior cerebellar artery usually gives off a branch called the internal auditory artery that supplies the inner ear and the vestibular apparatus.

BLOOD SUPPLY TO THE BRAIN: see cerebral vascular system, location or function.

BLUNTING/ BLUNTED AFFECT: emotional dulling; common in brain damage and schizophrenia, and may be present in depression.

BODY CENTER TEST: (Diller et al., 1974) a test of body disorientation in relation to scanning problems; poor performance is associated with severe aphasia.

BODY IMAGE: the patient's mental picture of the characteristics of his/her body.

BODY IMAGE AGNOSIA: see autotopagnosia.

BODY ORIENTATION: see autotopagnosia.

BODY PARTS - DENIAL OF: see autotopagnosia, asomatognosia.

BOSTON DIAGNOSITIC APHASIA EXAMINATION: (Goodglass & Kaplan, 1972) may take from one to four hours for administration and is reported to be an excellent tool for the description of aphasic disorders and for treatment planning; should be administered by an experienced examiner.

BOVINE COUGH: see 10th cranial nerve.

BOXER'S SYNDROME: believed to result from cumulative effects of cerebral concussion and subsequent cortical atrophy; also known as punch-drunk syndrome.

BOYD DEVELOPMENTAL PROGRESS SCALE: (Boyd, 1974)

assesses adaptive behavior in three areas: motor, communication, and self-sufficiency; appropriate for evaluations early in recovery from brain injury.

BP: blood pressure.

BRADYKINESIA: abnormal slowness of movement; sluggishness of physical and mental responses.

BRAIN ABSCESS: 30% fatal due to brain compression, usually brainstem; may be caused by infections from the middle ear, sinus, bone infections, bacteria entering through cortical venous vessels, osteomyelitis of the skull, infectious lesions of the skin of the face, or an abscess around an infected tooth, or penetrating wounds of the skull; most common sites: frontal and parietal lobes; brainstem and spinal cord abscesses are rare; may be caused by bacteria, fungi, yeasts, and other organisms; most often found deep within the hemisphere; acute symptoms may include rapidly increasing intracranial pressure, headache, vomiting, cognitive impairment, severe papilledema, seizures, abnormal EEG; residual impairments may include paralysis and seizures (Reitan & Wolfson, 1985).

BRAIN DEATH SYNDROME: irreversible coma in which for a period of 24-hours there is complete unreceptivity and unresponsitivity even to the most intensely painful stimuli, no spontaneous movement or breathing, absence of elicitable reflexes, and an isoelectric electroencephalogram.

BRAIN LESION - EFFECTS: 3 types: 1. loss of function, partial or complete; 2. release of function (disorder of an inhibitory structure that allows uninhibited behaviors to emerge), and 3. disorganization of function (bits or pieces of behavior still occur but following lesioning the behaviors occur in the incorrect order or at the wrong time and place).

BRAINSTEM: the stem-like portion of the brain connecting the cerebral hemispheres with the spinal cord and comprising the pons, medulla oblongata, and mesencephalon; the part of the brain that contains the areas between the medulla and the thalamus; the brainstem structures are arranged in layers: the ventral layer contains motor pathways; intermediate layer carries mainly sensory pathways; dorsal layer contains the nuclei of the cranial nerves; extrapyramidal, cerebellar, and vestibular connections run across all areas; see also motor pathways, corticospinal pathways, cortico-bulbar pathways, sensory pathways, dorsal column sensation, spino-thalamic sensation, trigeminal sensory system, cranial nerve nuclei, and blood supply of the brainstem.

BRAINSTEM DISORDERS: (see under the following headings) brainstem vascular syndromes, mid-brain vascular lesions, pontine vascular lesions, medullary vascular lesions, transient brainstem ischemic attacks, intracranial hemorrhage, multiple sclerosis and the brainstem, pontine glioma, posterior fossa tumors, metabolic brainstem dysfunction.

BRAINSTEM LESIONS: lesions of the medulla and lower pons cause crossed sensory disturbances (loss of pain and temperature sensation of one side of face and opposite side of body); involvement of trigeminal tract or nucleus and lateral spinothalamic tract on one side of brainstem (upper pons and midbrain where spinothalamic tracts and medial lemniscus join) cause loss of all superficial and deep sensation over the contralateral side of the body; may be associated with cranial nerve palsies; usually due to lateral medullary infarction; see also Wallenburg's syndrome.

BRIDGE SUBTEST: (Stanford-Binet) spatial construction task; sensitive to right parietal-lobe lesion.

BRIEF PSYCHIATRIC RATING SCALE: (Overall & Gorham, 1962) a widely used 16-item rating scale derived from psychiatric rating data; intended for use by psychiatrists and psychologists; rating scored with a 7-point rating scale of Severe to Not Present; assesses behavior and emotions.

BROCA'S APHASIA: expressive aphasia; a complex syndrome characterized by a failure of motor aspects of speaking and writing, with an accompanying agrammatism and a variable impairment in language comprehension; comprehension of written and verbal speech is good; repetition of single words is good although may be effortful; phrase repetition is poor; speech is slow, nonfluent, produced with great effort, and poorly articulated; total speech output is reduced and small words may be omitted; the use of mostly nouns and verbs leads to the descriptive term "telegraphic speech"; verb forms often reduced to the infinitive or participle; nouns are usually expressed in the singular; conjunctions, adjectives, adverbs, and articles are used infrequently; only key words necessary for communication are used; naming to confrontation fair to good; reading aloud poor; naming is occasionally paraphasic; auditory and reading comprehension good; spontaneous speech is poor, comprehension is intact, repetition is limited, naming limited; the basic deficit is one of switching from one sound to another; imitation of examiner's actions are better performed than execution of acts on command; self-initiated actions are often normal; may be able to hum a melody normally and to articulate curses well; caused by a large lesion involving anterosuperior sylvian operculum and insula, in the territory of the supply of the upper division of the left middle cerebral artery; may be accompanied by a weak-

B

ness and sagging of the lower part of the right face area with deviation of the tongue to the weak side, and usually weakness of right arm and leg with the hemiparesis greater in the arm than the leg; there may be lingual or pharyngeal apraxia; the patient is aware of deficits which usually cause frustration and depression; also called motor aphasia, nonfluent aphasia, expressive aphasia, ataxic aphasia, frontocortical aphasia, verbal aphasia.

BROCA'S AREA INFARCTION: lower premotor cortex adjacent to the motor cortex for the oropharynx, larynx, and respiratory apparatus; interrupts skilled movements of these muscle groups; dyspraxia in speech takes the form of impaired transitions between syllables and words, and dysprosody.

BROCA'S SPEECH AREA: dominant frontal lobe; controls motor mechanisms concerned with articulation; complex coordination of muscles for speech; lesion disrupts the articulation of speech; see Broca's aphasia.

BRODMANN'S AREAS OF THE CORTEX: *vision*: primary - area 17, secondary - areas 18 & 19, tertiary - 20 & 21; *auditory*: primary - area 41, secondary - areas 22 & 42; *body senses*: primary - areas 1, 2, & 3; secondary - areas 5 & 7; tertiary - areas 7, 21, 22, 37, 39, & 40; *motor*: primary - area 4, secondary - area 6, eye movement - area 8, speech 44, tertiary - areas 9, 10, 11, 45, 46, & 47; see also the specific area numbers below:

BRODMANN'S AREAS 1, 2, & 3: primary zones for body senses.

BRODMANN'S AREA 4: frontal lobes; primary zone: motor strip; final cortical motor command area.

BRODMANN'S AREAS 5 & 7: superior parietal; contributes to apraxias; lesion causes astereognosia.

BRODMANN'S AREAS 5, 7, & 37 lesion: tactile agnosia.

BRODMANN'S AREAS 5, 7, 9, 10, 11, 21, 22, 37, 39, 40, 45, 46, & 47: tertiary zones of the posterior part of the brain lie on the boundary of the occipital, temporal and parietal cortex; function of the tertiary zones is to integrate the excitation arriving from the different sensory systems and translate into symbolic processes and abstract thinking; lesion causes concrete thinking.

BRODMANN'S AREAS 6 & 8: premotor area; secondary zone; frontal lobes; motor programs are prepared for execution by the primary area (area 4).

BRODMANN'S AREAS 6 & 8 lesion: impairment in smooth muscle transition of separate axial, limb, and hand movements into fluid series of movements; produces subtle deficits/impairments.

BRODMANN'S AREA 7 lesion: short-term memory deficit.

BRODMANN'S AREAS 7, 40 lesion, left: right-left confusion;

right: construction apraxia; contralateral neglect.

BRODMANN'S AREAS 8 & 9: controls voluntary gaze.

BRODMANN'S AREAS 8 & 9 lesion: poor voluntary eye gaze.

BRODMANN'S AREA 9 lesion: left: impaired response inhibition (perseveration) (Milner, 1964); severe inability to shift response sets on the Wisconsin Card Sort test.

BRODMANN'S AREAS 9, 10, 11, 45, 46, & 47: tertiary zones of the frontal-lobe unit; prefrontal or granular frontal cortex; formation of intentions; integrated area of function ("the superstructure above all other parts of the cerebral cortex" - Luria, 1973b); executive functions.

BRODMANN'S AREAS 9, 10, 45, 46, & 47 lesions: alterations of personality and social activities.

BRODMANN'S AREAS 9 & 10 lesion: impaired response inhibition.

BRODMANN'S AREA 17: primary zone: projection areas of vision.

BRODMANN'S AREA 17 lesion: homonymous hemianopia or, if large, blindness.

BRODMANN'S AREAS 18 & 19: visual association area; secondary zones: projection areas of the primary visual zones; secondary zones maintain the modality of functional sensation, but have a less fixed topographic organization.

BRODMANN'S AREAS 20 & 21: visual association cortex.

BRODMANN'S AREAS 20 & 21 lesions: lesions on the right produce larger deficits in perception of complex visual forms such as faces and geometric patterns; lesions on the left produce large deficits in perception of verbally related material.

BRODMANN'S AREAS 20, 21, 37 & 38: tertiary zone; temporal lobe.

BRODMANN'S AREAS 20 & 38: inferior temporal gyrus.

BRODMANN'S AREA 21: hippocampus; long-term memory.

BRODMANN'S AREA 21 lesion: visual memory defects.

BRODMANN'S AREAS 21 & 38 lesions: amygdala; personality and affective changes.

BRODMANN'S AREAS 21, 37, & 38: middle temporal gyrus.

BRODMANN'S AREA 22: superior temporal gyrus; lesion may cause auditory illusions.

BRODMANN'S AREAS 22 & 42 lesions: thought to be the cause of agnosia for sounds including amusia.

BRODMANN'S AREA 38: anterior temporal lobe.

BRODMANN'S AREA 39: angular gyrus.

BRODMANN'S AREA 39 lesion: dyslexia, deficits in reading because letters no longer form meaningful words (defect of perception); see also Gerstmann's syndrome.

BRODMANN'S AREAS 39 & 40 lesion: acalculia.

C

BRODMANN'S AREAS 39 & 40, left: reasoning, thought, perception.

BRODMANN'S AREAS 40 & 43: inferior parietal lobe.

BRODMANN'S AREA 41: primary auditory region in Heschl's gyrus.

BRODMANN'S AREAS 41 & 42: hearing.

BRODMANN'S AREAS 42 & 22: secondary auditory zones.

BRODMANN'S AREA 43: somatosensory cortex.

BRODMANN'S AREA 44 lesion, left: Wernicke's aphasia.

BRODMANN'S MAP/NUMBERS: a cytoarchitectonic map of the brain; numbers were assigned randomly as Brodmann located them.

BROWN-SEQUARD SYNDROME: homolateral paralysis combined with a loss of vibratory and position sense on the same side and a contralateral loss of pain and temperature sense; disease of the spinal cord on one side.

BRUIT: a sound or murmur heard in auscultation, especially an abnormal one.

BUCCOFACIAL APRAXIA: oral apraxia; inability to carry out skilled movements of face and speech apparatus in presence of normal comprehension, muscle strength, and coordination.

BULIMIA: abnormal sensation of hunger; hyperphagia; see also Kleine-Levin syndrome, Pickwickian syndrome.

BUN: blood urea nitrogen.

C

c̄: with.

C: Cervical; centigrade.

C1; C2; etc.:1st cervical vertebra; 2nd cervical vertebra; etc.

CA: carcinoma; cancer; chronological age.

CALCULATIONS SUBTEST: (Psycho-Educational Battery; Woodcock, 1977) a test for spatial dyscalculia; a test of basic arithmetic including recognition of symbols, ability to calculate spatially, and calculation of adult level mathematical concepts such as fractions, decimals, squares, and algebraic functions.

CANCELLATION OF RAPIDLY RECURRING TARGET FIGURES: test of concentration and dyslexia.

CANCELLATION TESTS: Letter Cancellation task, Digit Vigilance Test, Perceptual Speed task, Cancellation of Rapidly Recurring Target Figures test.

CANNULA: a tube for insertion into a duct or cavity.

CANTER BACKGROUND INTERFERENCE PROCEDURE:

(Canter, 1966; 1976) used to enhance the usefulness of the Bender-Gestalt as a neuropsychological screening instrument; reduces the number of false-positives among psychiatric patients and the false negatives among neurological patients (Canter, 1976; Golden, 1979; Heaton et al., 1978).

CARD SORTING TEST: (Caine et al., 1977); tests ability to think and sort cards in categories.

CARDIAC ARREST: sudden cessation of cardiac function with disappearance of arterial blood pressure, connoting either ventricular fibrillation or ventricular standstill.

CAROTID SODIUM AMYTAL: (Wada, 1960) injection of sodium amytal into the carotid artery to produce a brief period of anesthesia of the ipsilateral hemisphere; results in localization of speech; test results in arrest of speech lasting up to several minutes; characterized by aphasic errors as speech returns; injection into the nonspeaking hemisphere may produce no, or only brief, speech arrest; injection into the right hemisphere affects singing, which becomes monotone, and devoid of correct pitch.

CATALYST: a substance that accelerates chemical reactions but remains unchanged when the reactions are over.

CATAPLEXY: sudden loss of muscle tone provoked by exaggerated emotion such as excessive laughter or anger. May be associated with narcolepsy (70%); head falls forward, jaw drops to open, knees buckle; usual duration from 1 to 2 minutes.

CATASTROPHIC REACTION: extreme and disruptive transient emotional disturbance; acute, disorganized anxiety, agitation, or tearfulness which disrupts the activity that provoked it; often occurs when patients are confronted with their limitations; most often displayed by left-hemisphere lesioned patients.

CATATONIC: marked motor anomalies, generally limited to disturbances in the context of a diagnosis of a non-organic psychotic disorder; see also catatonic excitement, catatonic negativism, catatonic rigidity, catatonic posturing, catatonic stupor, catatonic waxy flexibility.

CATATONIC EXCITEMENT: excited motor activity, purposeless and not influenced by external stimuli.

CATATONIC NEGATIVISM: resistance to all instructions or attempts to be moved; when passive, the person may resist any effort to be moved; when active, the person may do the opposite of what is asked.

CATATONIC POSTURING: voluntary assumption of an inappropriate or bizarre posture, usually for a long time.

CATATONIC RIGIDITY: maintenance of a rigid posture against all efforts to be moved.

CATATONIC STUPOR: marked decrease in reactivity to environment

C

with reduction in movements and activity, sometimes to the point of appearing to be unaware of one's surroundings.

CATATONIC WAXY FLEXIBILITY: limbs can be "molded" into any position, which is then maintained. When the limb is being moved, it feels to the examiner as if it were made of wax.

CATECHOLAMINES: one of a group of similar compounds having a sympathomimetic action; includes dopamine, norepinephrine, and epinephrine; formed from amino acids; excitatory neurotransmitters; action regulated by enzymes, which break them down, and by the presynaptic membrane, which reuses them.

CATEGORICAL MEMORY OR LEARNING TESTS: WAIS Information and Vocabulary Subtests.

CATEGORY TEST: (Halstead-Reitan subtest) test of abstracting ability; also has a visuospatial component (Lansdell & Donnelly, 1977).

CATHARSIS: Freud's treatment of psychoneuroses to bring about abreation, by encouraging the patient to tell everything that happens to be associated with a given train of thought, thus "purging" the mind of the repressed material that is the cause of the symptoms.

CATION: positively charged organic ion.

CAUDATE NUCLEUS: part of the basal ganglia; an elongated, arched gray mass closely related to the lateral ventricle throughout its entire extent and consisting of a head, body, and tail; along with the putamen forms a functional unit (the neostriatum) of the corpus striatum; serves an important role in motor inhibition; electrical stimulation causes stoppage of motion; destruction leads to "obstinate progression"; insufficient transmitter substance (dopamine) at the caudate synapse is responsible for the clinical syndrome of Parkinson's disease; extrapyramidal reaction (EPR)depletion of dopamine levels by neuroleptic medications; see also chorea, choreoathetosis, Sydenham's chorea, Huntington's chorea, senile chorea, tardive dyskinesia, lupus erythematosus.

CAUSALGIA: see thalamic pain, parasthesia.

CBC: complete blood count.

cc: cubic centimeter.

CENTRAL APHASIA: see conduction aphasia; global aphasia.

CENTRAL GRAY: part of tegmentum in midbrain; excitation elicits strong fear and/or rage reactions; destruction markedly impairs ability to display defensive-aggressive behavior; also known as periaqueductal gray.

CENTRAL LESION: any lesion of the central nervous system.

CENTRAL NERVOUS SYSTEM: (CNS) the neural and supportive tissue inside the brain and the spinal cord.

CENTRAL SULCUS: Fissure of Rolando; curves toward the posterior part of the brain as it moves medially across the superior surface of the cortex; divides the frontal lobes of the cerebral cortex from the parietal lobes; separates the motor projection areas from the somesthetic areas.

CEREBELLAR AGENESIS: absence or malformation portions of the cerebellum, basal ganglia, or spinal cord.

CEREBELLAR DISEASE: (bilateral) severe disturbance in all movements; patient may not be able to stand, walk, or use limbs effectively; ocular and speech disturbances such as nystagmus, dysmetria, and dysarthria.

CEREBELLAR GAIT: unsteadiness, irregularity, lateral reeling, uncertainty of steps, shuffling, may be caused by multiple sclerosis, cerebellar tumors of medulloblastoma of cerebellar vermis, paraneoplastic diseases, and cerebellar degeneration.

CEREBELLAR LESIONS: (lateral and inferior parts of cerebellum) ataxia, asynergia, dysmetria, hypotonia; midline lesions produce severe ataxia; lingula lesions extend into the superior medullary velum producing 4th nerve palsies or into the superior cerebellar peduncle producing severe tremor of the arm on the same side; lesions in the vermis cause severe ataxia; lesions in the flocculonodular region cause ataxia, vertigo, and vomiting if they extend into the floor of the 4th ventricle; tumors in midline sites tend to cause early obstruction of the aqueduct or 4th ventricle resulting in headache and papilledema; metastatic malignant disease accounts for the majority of cerebellar tumors in the adult.

CEREBELLAR SIGNS: finger-to-nose ataxia; difficulty with rapid alternating movements of the limbs; the ataxia is almost always on the same side as the lesion.

CEREBELLAR VERMIS: median lobe of the cerebellum.

CEREBELLO-PONTINE ANGLE: a shallow triangle lying between the cerebellum, the lateral pons, and the inner third of the petrous ridge. The vertical extent of the angle is from the fifth nerve above, on its course from the pons to the petrous apex, and the ninth nerve below, passing from the lateral medulla to the jugular foramen. The abducens nerve (VI) runs upwards and forwards on the medial edge of the area and the seventh and eighth cranial nerves traverse the angle to enter the internal auditory canal.

CEREBELLO-PONTINE ANGLE LESIONS: 7th & 8th cranial nerve damage: wide range of vestibular, auditory, and motor abnormalities may occur; acoustic nerve tumor (8th nerve): usually arises on the vestibular division of the nerve, but the earliest symptoms are auditory; tinnitis is followed by slowly progressive loss of hearing; vertigo may be present; facial nerve palsy is usually a late manifestation of an acoustic nerve lesion; other causes of lesions in this area: meningiomas, cholesteatomas, hemangioblastomas, and aneurysms of the basilar artery; neuromas of the 5th, 7th and 9th nerves can produce similar clinical pictures; see also Jakob-Creutzfeldt disease.

C

CEREBELLUM: a large, convoluted structure mushrooming out from the pons; regulates movement and balance on the basis of information from the somatosensory areas and the vestibular system.

CEREBELLUM FUNCTION: concerned in the coordination of movements; coordination of the reflexes, timing, and fine-tuning of ongoing skilled motor behaviors; important role in posture and balance.

CEREBELLUM LESIONS: causes akinesia, impairments of equilibrium, postural defects, and impairments of skilled motor activity; smooth movements may be broken down into sequential components, thus making movements jerky; ability to perform rapidly alternating movements may be impaired; directed movements may overshoot their mark (passed pointing); muscle tone may be abnormal so that movements are difficult to initiate.

CEREBELLUM LOCATION: dorsal-most aspect of the hindbrain overlying the brainstem; the part of the metencephalon that occupies the posterior cranial fossa behind the brainstem; a fissured mass consisting of a median lobe (vermis) and two lateral lobes (the hemispheres); connected with the brainstem by three pairs of peduncles; two basic regions: the midline structures and the cerebellar hemispheres; the midline groups including the lingula anteriorly, the vermis in the middle, and the flocculo-nodular lobe posteriorly; these lobes are divided into a small anterior lobe and a large posterior lobe; each hemisphere contains a large main nucleus, the dentate, through which the bulk of efferent cerebellar information is discharged. There are smaller roof nuclei which are mainly concerned with vestibular reflexes and ocular movements.

CEREBELLUM AND THE EXTRAPYRAMIDAL SYSTEM: The extrapyramidal system is attached to the brainstem by three major fiber pathways in which all afferent fibers pass to its cortex and all efferent fibers originate in the underlying cerebellar nuclei and then pass on to other brain structures. Movement is initiated through the direct cortico-spinal pyramidal system. The continual postural adjustments that underlie smooth and coordinated movement are initiated by the cortico-pallidal system which projects mainly into the putamen. Final volitional activity enters the cerebellum through the cortico-ponto-cerebellar projections through the middle cerebellar peduncle. Main sensory input to the system comes from the muscle, tendon, and joint position sense nerve endings, mainly via the spino-cerebellar tracts, and from the vestibular apparatus via the vestibular nuclei. Information from both sources enters the cerebellum through the inferior cerebellar peduncle. Large axon from each Purkinje cell projects to the central cerebellar nuclei, mainly to the dentate nucleus on the same side. This nucleus relays the information to the opposite ventral-lateral thalamus and cortex via the dentato-rubral, rubro-thalamic, dentato-thalamic and tha-lamo-cortical projections. Pathways leave the cerebellum in the superior cerebellar peduncle and decussate through the region of, or relay in, the red nucleus. Information reaching the thalamus is projected to the extrapyramidal cortical areas and directed to the basal ganglia, particularly to the putamen, caudate, and external globus pallidus. An important inner loop, a relay through the subthalamic nucleus, appears to have an inhibitory feed-back effect on the globus pallidus; damage to this relay loop causes hemiballis-mus. Parts receiving most of their impulses from the vestibular system help to maintain the body's equilibrium; parts receiving impulses mainly from body senses are involved with postural re-flexes and coordinating functionally related muscles. The major part of the cerebellum receives impulses from the neocortex and functions primarily to promote the efficiency of skilled movements.

CEREBELLUM & THE MOTOR SYSTEMS: the cerebellum projects to a number of nuclei that join the lateral or ventromedial systems of the spinal cord; projections from the medial and ventral portions of the cerebellum pass from its medial cerebellar nuclei to the reticular formation and the vestibular nuclei; forms part of the ventromedial projection of the spinal cord which is instrumental in controlling more proximal movements of the body, such as posture and locomotion; damage to this area disrupts upright posture and walking, but does not substantially disrupt other movements.

CEREBRAL ARTERIOSCLEROSIS: narrowing of cerebral arteries as a result of thickening and hardening of the arteries; most common cause of narrowing of the blood vessels of the brain; other causes may include vasculitis or spasm.

CEREBRAL COMPRESSION: following traumatic head injury a hematoma may develop which compresses brain substance, causing behavioral changes much like a tumor would.

CEREBRAL CONTUSION: primarily a vascular injury, resulting in bruising, edema, and hemorrhage of capillaries, most often at the poles of the frontal and temporal lobes; often a result of coup and contracoup injuries as a result of acceleration/deceleration head trauma as in automobile accidents or falls.

CEREBRAL DAMAGE IN CHILDHOOD: (Lenneberg, 1967); later-alization of function develops rapidly between ages of two or three to five, and proceeds more slowly until complete at puberty; damage to either cerebral hemisphere up to age three: recovery could be complete and rapid, because language would be acquired by undam-aged brain tissue; damage to either cerebral hemisphere at this age could produce language disturbance because the two hemispheres are equipotential for language, although the left one has a predispo-sition for development of language; between ages 3 & 10: cerebral

C

damage may produce aphasia, but recovery occurs over time because the cerebral hemispheres, particularly the right one, are still able to assume language functions; damage after age 10: produce language disorders resembling those observed in adults because the brain becomes decreasingly able to adapt and reorganize; by about age 14: the ability to reorganize appears to be lost and prognosis for recovery is poor.

CEREBRAL DOMINANCE: 90% of the population is strongly right-handed; 99% are strongly left-hemisphere dominant for language; 40% of left-handers are right-hemisphere dominant for speech; 60% of left-handers have left-hemisphere dominance for speech (Benson & Geschwind, 1968), but the degree of dominance is less strong than in right-handers; 80% of left-handers have some mixed dominance for language (Gloning & Hoff, 1969).

CEREBRAL HEMISPHERE: either of the identical halves of the forebrain connected by the corpus callosum.

CEREBRAL HEMORRHAGE: massive bleeding into the substance of the brain; most frequent cause is hypertension; other causes are congenital defects such as aneurysms or angiomas, blood disorders such as leukemia, or toxic chemicals; onset abrupt and frequently fatal; usually occurs during waking hours.

CEREBRAL LACERATION: contusions severe enough to physically breach the brain substance; most often produced by missiles or fragments of bomb penetrating the brain substance.

CEREBRAL PALSY: a persisting qualitative motor disorder appearing before age 3, due to a nonprogressive damage to the anterior thalamus, ventricular nuclei; characterized by lack of voluntary muscle control; may involve seizures, speech, language, articulation difficulties, and limitation in learning ability.

CEREBRAL PEDUNCLES: part of the basis pedunculi in the midbrain; comprised mainly of giant bundles of descending motor fibers.

CEREBRAL SPINAL FLUID: (CSF) a clear and colorless fluid that lubricates and serves as a buffer between the brain and spinal cord and the framework of the dura mater, skull, and vertebral column; generated by the choroid plexis, located within the lateral, third, and fourth ventricles; circulates from the lateral ventricles through the foramina of Monro into the third ventricle, through the cerebral aqueduct (Sylvius), and into the fourth ventricle; communicates with the subarachnoid space through the two lateral foramina of Luschka and the medial aperture in the roof of the fourth ventricle (foramen of Magendie); continues into the cisterna magna and then circulates through the subarachnoid space of the cerebellar hemispheres, through the basilar cisterns, and caudally to the spinal subarachnoid space; progresses from the base of the cisterns through the interpeduncular and prechiasmatic cisterns, the Sylvian fissures, and the cisterns of the corpus callosum to the lateral and frontal hemispheric subarachnoid space, to the medial and posterior cerebral hemispheric subarachnoid space; absorbed by the arachnoid villi of the dural sinuses (Reitan & Wolfson, 1985; Tourtellotte & Shorr, 1982).

CEREBRAL VASCULAR ACCIDENT (CVA): a blockage or rupture of the vascular system of the brain; usually produces a characteristic paralysis on one side of the body; other symptoms depend on the hemisphere of the brain affected; see also cerebral vascular disorders, CVA, stroke.

CEREBRAL VASCULAR DISEASE: vascular disease can produce reduction of both oxygen and glucose resulting in interference of cellular energy metabolism; if the interference is total for longer than 10 minutes, all cells affected will die.

CEREBRAL VASCULAR DISORDERS: stroke, CVA, cerebral vascular accident, infarct, encephalomalacia, thrombosis, embolism, cerebral arteriosclerosis, cerebral hemorrhage, angioma, aneurysm.

CEREBRAL VASCULAR SYSTEM: two internal carotid and two vertebral arteries, one of each in either side of the body, enter the the skull at the base of the brain and give off a number of smaller arteries and two major arteries: anterior cerebral artery and middle cerebral artery; vertebral arteries enter at base of brain, and join together to form the basilar artery which, again, divides into the posterior cerebral arteries; see also internal carotid artery, vertebral arteries (cerebral), anterior cerebral artery, middle cerebral artery, basilar artery, posterior cerebral arteries, anterior and posterior communicating arteries.

CEREBRAL VENTRICLES: third, fourth, and two lateral ventricles; cavities within the brain which are filled with cerebrospinal fluid.

CEREBROSPINAL FLUID: (CSF) a colorless liquid that circulates throughout the central nervous system; buffers the brain against blows to the head.

CEREBROSPINAL FLUID PUNCTURE: the only method of looking at the subarachnoid space without opening the skull; most often performed by a puncture made in the lumbar, or lower portion of the spinal column; reasons for this procedure include: removal of toxic, inflammatory, or other substances in the CSF, allow analysis of CSF for blood (indicating a CVA), introduction of therapeutic substances into the subarachnoid space, or introduction of air or opaque media for radiographic studies.

CEREBRUM: the main portion of the brain, located at the top of the brainstem; occupies the upper part of the cranial cavity; the most recently evolved and most elaborated brain structure; consists of two hemispheres which are almost mirror images; contains the basal ganglia, amygdala, white matter (association, commissural, & pro-

C

jection fibers); the two hemispheres are united by the corpus callosum; the largest part of the central nervous system in man; derived from the telencephalon of the embryo; this term is sometimes used to refer to the entire brain.

CERTIFICATION: commitment to a mental hospital on the certificates of physicians and other authorized persons.

CHARCOT-MARIE-TOOTH DISEASE/SYNDROME: peroneal muscular atrophy; also see amyostatic lateral sclerosis.

CHEMORECEPTORS: taste and smell receptors that specialize in transforming chemicals into neural impulses.

CHEWING: see fifth cranial nerve (Trigeminal nerve).

CHEWING-ASYMMETRICAL: Trigeminal nerve (V) damage.

CHEYNE-STOKES RESPIRATION: characterized by rhythmic waxing and waning of the depth of respiration, with regularly recurring periods of apnea; seen especially in coma resulting from affection of the nervous centers.

CHIASM: located above the pituitary gland; the site where the optic tract splits and decussates.

CHIASM/CHIASMA: decussation or X-shaped crossing; see also commissure, optic chiasma.

CHILDISHNESS: frontal-lobe dysfunction/damage.

CHIMERIC FIGURES TEST: (Levy, 1972) a test for split-brain functioning in which faces and other patterns have been split down the center and recombined; commissured patients choose the face seen in the left visual field and thus by their right hemisphere, demonstrating that the right hemisphere has a special role in the recognition of faces and designs.

CHOLINERGIC FIBERS: neural fibers that release acetylcholine at the synapse.

CHOLINESTERASE: enzyme which inactivates acetylcholine in nerve synapses.

CHOREA: ceaseless occurrence of involuntary, complex, arrhythmic movements of a forcible, rapid, jerky type, noted for their irregularity, variability, and relative speed; may appear to be well coordinated, but are never combined into a coordinated acts; grimacing and peculiar respiratory sounds may be present; caused by damage to putamen and striatum .

CHOREIC: see subthalamic, basal ganglionic, chorea.

CHOREIC AND MYOCLONIC DYSARTHRIA: (hiccup speech) abrupt interruption in the pronunciation of words by abnormal movements; grimacing and other characteristic motor signs must be depended upon for diagnosis.

CHOREOATHETOSIS: see Syndenham's chorea, Huntington's chorea, tardive dyskinesia, senile chorea, lupus erythematosus, putamen, striatum, caudate nucleus, basal ganglia.

C

CHOROID PLEXUS: vascular fringe-like folds in the pia mater in the third, fourth, and lateral ventricles.

CHROMATIC: pertaining to color or hue.

CHROMOSOMES: genetic material that perpetuates traits from one generation to the next; threadlike structures, consisting mainly of protein and DNA, found in the nucleus of every plant and animal cell.

CHRONIC BASAL MENINGITIS: complication of syphilis characterized by sudden onset of diplopia (third and sixth cranial nerve involvement) followed by paralysis of other cranial nerves, trigeminal neuralgia, bilateral facial palsy, eighth nerve signs of tinnitus, vertigo, and deafness, difficulty in swallowing and wasting of the tongue muscles (twelfth cranial nerve involvement) (Reitan & Wolfson, 1985).

CHRONIC BRAIN DAMAGE: most common complaints include temper outbursts, fatigue, poor memory, depression (Brooks & Aughton, 1979b; Lezak, 1978b, Lezak et al., 1980, Lishman, 1978; Munday, 1980), irritability (Bond, 1979; Brodal, 1973; Brooks, 1979; Lezak, 1978a, b; Oddy et al., 1978), and perplexity (Lezak, 1978b).

CHRONIC OBSTRUCTIVE PULMONARY DISEASE: (COPD) may cause overall cognitive impairment on neuropsychological measures and depression (McSweeney et al., 1982).

CINGULUM: an encircling structure or part; anything that circles a body.

CINGULATE CORTEX/GYRUS: a bundle of association fibers immediately above and partially encircling the the corpus callosum; interrelates the cingulate and hippocampal gyri; traverses the isthmus posteriorly and extends forward to Broca's olfactory area; involved in motor function via the extrapyramidal tract and, according to Papez (1937), in emotion via the hypothalamus.

CIRCLE OF WILLIS: location of interconnections of all cerebral arteries; see cerebral vascular system, location or function.

CIRCLE OF WILLIS LESION: mnestic impairment; see also third ventricle lesion.

CIRCUMDUCTION: the active or passive circular movement of a limb or an eye.

CIRCUMLOCUTION: describing; "talking around"; naming functions or characteristics, substitution of another word or phrase that conveys the meaning of the sought after word or name; characteristic symptom of anomic aphasia (amnesic aphasia); may be a defect/lesion of the angular gyrus.

CIRCUMSCRIBED CORTICAL ATROPHY: see Pick's disease.

CIRCUMSTANTIALITY: a term used to describe speech that is indirect and delayed in reaching the point because of unnecessary, tedious details and parenthetic remarks.

CISTERN (cisterna): a closed space serving as a reservoir for fluid

C

(lymph or other bodily fluid), especially one of the enlarged subarachnoid spaces containing cerebrospinal fluid.

Cl: chloride.

CLANGING: speech in which sounds of words are linked by similarity of sound rather than by meaning.

CLANG ASSOCIATIONS: association of disconnected ideas resulting only from the similarity of the sounds of words; also called klang associations; may be seen in bipolar and schizophrenic disorders.

CLASSICAL CONDITIONING: the pairing of a conditioned stimulus with an unconditioned stimulus until an organism learns to respond to the conditioned stimulus whether or not the unconditioned stimulus occurs; also called Pavlovian response.

CLOCK FACE TEST: may expose unilateral visual inattention (Battersby et al., 1956); right-hemisphere lesioned patients may have trouble rounding out the left side of their drawing; part of the Parietal Lobe Battery (Borod et al., 1980; Goodglass & Kaplan, 1972) and the Luria Battery.

CLONIC STAGE OF MAJOR SEIZURE DISORDER: alternating muscle spasms; loss of bladder and bowel control.

CLOSED HEAD INJURY MECHANICS: (static injuries) a blow to the head produces several kinds of damage: force of impact causes an inward molding of the skull and compensatory adjacent outbending followed by rebound effects (Gurdjian & Gurdjian, 1978) causing coup and contracoup lesions; shearing effects (Strich, 1961) are caused by the combination of translatory force and rotational acceleration of the brain within the skull which tear blood vessels and bruise brain tissue; injuries to the brain tend to be concentrated in the undersides of the frontal and temporal lobes (Grubb & Coxe, 1978; Ommaya et al., 1971); ventricular enlargement has been found in 72% of severe closed-head injuries (Levin, Meyers, Grossman, & Sarwar, 1981); enlarged ventricles are most likely to occur in patients with prolonged coma following moving vehicle accidents and are associated with poorer outcomes.

CLOSURE FACES TEST: see Mooney's Closure Test.

CLOSURE FLEXIBILITY TEST (Concealed Figures): (Thurstone & Jeffrey, 1956); multiple-choice version of the Hidden Figures Test; tests the ability to hold a closure against distraction; test of frontal-lobe dysfunction.

CLOUDING OF CONSCIOUSNESS: a mental state in which clear-mindedness is impaired and orientation partially lost.

CLUMSINESS: see cerebellar lesion.

cc: cubic centimeter.

cm: centimeter.

CNS: central nervous system.

c/o: complained of.

COCAINE: used medically as a local narcotic anesthetic applied topically to mucus membranes; when misused as a stimulant or a narcotic it dilates the pupils of the eye by preventing the reuptake of norepinephrine into the nerve endings; may become psychologically addictive.

COCHLEAR NUCLEI: ventral and dorsal chochlear nuclei: the nuclei of termination of the sensory fibers of the pars chochlearis nervi vestibulocochlearis, which enter the brain through the inferior root of the nerve. The nuclei partly encircle the inferior cerebellar peduncle at the junction between the medulla oblongata and pons. The dorsal cochlear nucleus forms an eminence (the acoustic tubercle) on the most lateral part of the floor of the fourth ventricle.

CODES TEST: AA & SA II; Stanford-Binet subtest, 1937 revision; reasoning task; sensitive to mild verbal dysfunctions that do not appear on tests involving well-practiced verbal abilities.

COGNITIVE: pertaining to the processes of learning and knowing (reasoning, memory, understanding, and judgment).

COGNITIVE DEFICITS FOLLOWING ACUTE HEAD INJURY: mental slowing, attentional deficits, decreased cognitive efficiency in high-level concept formation and complex reasoning (Deelman, 1977; Gronwall, 1980; Gronwall & Sampson, 1974; Van Zomeren & Deelman, 1978); usually reflected by complaints of inability to concentrate or to perform complex mental operations, confusion and perplexity in thinking, irritatability, fatigue, and inability to do things as well as before the accident which keep the patient from realizing premorbid goals or repeating premorbid accomplishments; some patients may not recognize their deficits and are unrealistic in their expectations for future abilities and capabilities; usually caused by a significant frontal-lobe injury.

COGNITIVE DISTORTION: characteristic of psychosis; cognitive changes are usually global, resulting in an overall decrease in cognitive ability, most often manifested as a distortion of thought processes.

COGNITIVE FUNCTIONING: pertaining to the use of symbols, concepts, reasoning, thought, perception, etc., and language; integrative function of the tertiary zones of the parietal lobe (approximately Brodmann's areas 39 & 40 of the left temporal-parietal lobe; the supramarginal and angular gyri).

COGNITIVE PERFORMANCE FOLLOWING DIFFUSE HEAD INJURY: slowed thinking and reaction times may result in significantly lowered scores on timed tests despite the capacity to perform the required task accurately; tracking tasks are particularly sensitive to diffuse effects (Eson & Bourke, 1980a; Gronwall, 1980); performance relatively poor on tasks requiring concentration and mental tracking such as oral arithmetic or sequential arithmetic and

C

reason problems that must be performed mentally (Gronwall & Wrightson, 1981); cognitive deficits associated with diffuse damage are likely to persist indefinitely when moderate and severe head injuries have been incurred.

COGWHEEL PHENOMENON: muscular rigidity during passive stretching of hypertonic muscle; resistance may be rhythmically jerky as though the resistance of the limb were controlled by a ratchet; increased simultaneous muscle tone in both extensor and flexor muscles which is particularly evident when the limbs are moved passively at a joint.

COLLET-SICARD SYNDROME: glossolayrngoscapulopharyngeal hemiplegia due to complete lesion of the 9th, 10th, 11th, and 12th cranial nerves.

COLOR AGNOSIA: inability to recognize colors; 2 types: 1. color naming and 2. color recognition; results from a variety of lesions that disconnect the color recognition areas from memory functions or from language areas.

COLOR AGNOSIA (color naming): inability to name colors and to evoke the specific colors of color-specific objects, in the absence of aphasia, due to a disconnection of visual input from the language area; also associated with alexia with agraphia; there is no damage to the language area and no other evidence of aphasia.

COLOR AGNOSIA (recognition): the inability to associate particular colors with objects or particular objects with colors; inability to select all colors of the same hue from a group of colored objects, to pick out or point to colors on command, a defect of color perception; inability to relate colors to objects in the presence of intact color vision; usually found in association with other visual agnosias — most commonly with word blindness (Gloning et al., 1969); usually associated with prosopagnosia; caused by bilateral inferior temporo-occipital lesions.

COLOR ANOMIA: inability to name colors; color aphasia; generally associate with other aphasic symptoms; lesion of the speech zones or a disconnection of the speech zones from areas 18, 19, and 37, thus isolating the regions from one another.

COLOR APHASIA: see color anomia.

COLOR ASSOCIATION TEST: (Varney, 1982) test for the correctness of color associations; test to discriminate between color agnosia and color anomia; see also color perception tests: Color Association test, Coloring of Pictures test, Color Form Sorting test.

COLOR BLINDNESS: see color agnosia, achromatopsia, color anomia.

COLOR FORM SORTING TEST: (K. Goldstein & Scheerer, 1941, 1953; Weigl, 1941); shift in concept appears to present a major problem for bilateral and left frontal-lobe patients.

COLOR PERCEPTION BATTERY: (De Renzi & Spinnler, 1967); six-test battery: color matching test, Ishihara plates, color naming, point to color, verbal memory for color, and color drawing.

COLOR PERCEPTION TESTS: used to identify persons with congenitally defective color vision (color blindness) with color agnosia and related defects; Ishihara Test (Ishihara, 1954); Dvorine Test; H-R-R Pseudoisochromatic Plates (Hardy et al., 1955); 100-hue and Dichotomous test for Color Vision (Farnsworth, 1943); Color Sorting Test (K. Goldstein & Scheerer, 1953); Color Perception Battery (De Renzi & Spinnler, 1967); Coloring of Pictures (Damasio et al., 1979); Wrongly Colored Pictures; Color Association Test (Varney, 1982).

COLOR SORTING TEST: (K. Goldstein & Scheerer, 1941, 1953) test for accuracy of color perception; measure of abstract and concrete thought; also called the Gelb-Goldstein Wool Sorting Test.

COLORING OF PICTURES TEST: (Damasio et al., 1979); test to discriminate between color agnosia and color anomia.

COMA: patient appears to be asleep but is unreceptive to stimuli; there may or may not be extensor rigidity of limbs, possible decerebration signs, respiration slow or rapid, sometimes irregular reflexes; see also midbrain, ascending reticular formation, tegmentum.

COMATOSE: a state of unconsciousness.

COMA VIGIL: bilateral decortication with double hemiplegia and only primitive reflexes; caused by damage to the cortical mantle (neocortex or neopallium) from anoxia, hypoglycemia or circulatory/metabolic dysfunction; also called apallic state or akinetic mutism.

COMBINED APHASIA: two or more forms of aphasia occurring concomitantly in the same person.

COMMISSURAL APHASIA: aphasia due to a lesion in the insula interrupting the path between the motor and sensory speech centers; also called frontolenticular and lenticular aphasia.

COMMISSURAL FIBERS: white matter of cerebral hemispheres; primary functions are to conduct neural impulses between cortical points of the two hemispheres; see also corpus callosum, anterior commissure, posterior commissure, and hippocampal commissure.

COMMISSURES: interhemispheric connections (axon projections) between homotopic areas in the brain and spinal cord.

COMMISSUROTOMY: surgical procedure for cutting the corpus callosum which makes each hemisphere independent; also known as split-brain lesioning; produces profound behavioral discontinuities in perception, comprehension, and response.

COMMUNICATION ABILITIES IN DAILY LIVING TEST: (CADL) (Holland, 1980) examines how the patient might handle daily life activities by engaging him in role-playing in a series of simulated situations complete with props.

COMPENSATION: a mental mechanism in which one unconsciously covers up an undesirable trait by calling into play and developing a

C

desirable trait.

COMPLETE APHASIA: aphasia due to lesions of all the speech centers, producing inability to communicate with others in any way.

COMPLETE HEMIANOPIA: hemianopia affecting an entire half of the visual field of each eye.

COMPLEX FIGURE TEST: (Rey, 1941) tests both perceptual organization and visual memory in brain-damaged patients; also called Rey-Osterrieth (Osterrieth, 1944); brain-damaged patients may not be able to perceive the large rectangle and parts of the main lines and details are drawn intermingled, working from top to bottom and from left to right (Visser, 1973); left-sided lesioned patients tend to display more fragmentation than right-sided lesioned patients, but right-sided lesioned patients may omit units, probably due to unilateral neglect (Binder, 1982); the fragmented or piecemeal approach to copying the complex figure, characteristic of brain-damaged persons reflects their inability to process as much information at a time as do normals; brain-damaged patients tend to deal with smaller visual units, building the figure in a piecemeal fashion; many may ultimately produce a reasonably accurate reproduction, but the piecemeal approach increases the likelihood of size and relationship errors (Messerli et al., 1979); frontal-lobe patients frequently repeat an element already copied because the patient loses track of what he had previously drawn due to a disorganized approach; a design element may be transformed into a familiar representation; there may be some perseveration in the form of additional cross-hatches or parallel lines; may have trouble programming the approach to copying the figure; tend to perseverate, confabulate, personalize, or otherwise distort the design that first appears on the initial copy or the immediate recall trial, and tend to exaggerate with repeated recall (Messerli et al., 1979; Osterrieth, 1944; Rey, 1941); poor planning may show up as a haphazard and fragmented approach to the drawing of the figure; left-hemisphere lesioned patients tend to break up the design into units that are smaller than normally perceived; on recall, tend to reproduce the basic rectangular outline and the structural elements as a configural whole, suggesting slow processing, but able to get a gestalt eventually; make more simplifications than right-sided lesioned patients (Archibald, no date); left-sided damaged patients simplify by rounding angles, drawing dashes instead of dots, or leaving the cross incomplete; right-hemisphere lesioned patients omit elements (Binder, 1981); those having had difficulty copying the figures display even greater problems with recall (Milner, 1975; L. B. Taylor, 1969); tend to lose many of the elements of the design, making increasingly impoverished reproductions of the original figures as they go from the immediate to the delayed recall trial; those who have visuospatial problems or who are subject to perceptual fragmentation will also increasingly distort and confuse the configurational elements of the design; parietal-occipital lesioned patients may have difficulty with spatial organization of the figure; psychiatric patients may add bizarre embellishments, interpret details concretely, or fill in parts of the design (Osterreith, 1944; Snow, 1979; Wood et al., 1982).

COMPLEX PARTIAL EPILEPSY:(Temporal-lobe epilepsy) disturbance of content of consciousness which may take many forms, e.g., sensory hallucinations, especially of smell or taste, or of a more elaborate kind such as a remembered visual scene or musical tune; disordered awareness of the external world involving the size or distance of objects seen, or of own body parts; déjà vu phenomenon; abnormal emotional experiences of an unpleasant kind, especially states of fear or depression; may be dazed but not usually in coma; may progress to a generalized convulsion; automatisms; aggressive behavior may be present; lesion in or near one temporal lobe (Brain, 1985).

COMPREHENSION OF SPOKEN LANGUAGE: should be assessed in a structured fashion without reliance upon the patient's ability to produce speech; testing should require a minimal verbal response from the patient in order to assess patient's understanding; two methods of testing may be used: 1. pointing commands either of single objects or increasingly complex sequences; a patient without aphasia should be able to sequence pointing to four or more objects; 2. asking the patient six or more simple and complex questions which require yes or no answers only.

COMPREHENSION SUBTEST: (WAIS-R) fair test of general ability; measures remote memory in older persons; reflects social knowledgeability and judgment; impulsivity or dependency sometimes appear in response to questions about dealing with a found letter or finding one's way out of a forest; the proverb questions test verbal abstract reasoning; holds up well as a record of the premorbid intellectual achievement of brain-damaged patients generally, except that the questions are more sensitive than other predominantly verbal subtests to left-hemisphere damage; may be used to test reasoning (logical thinking and practical judgment) (Lezak, 1983).

COMPREHENSION SUBTEST (WAIS-R) IN DEMENTIA: may be a relatively normal score; overlearned material often survives dementing process for a long time past the patient's ability to care for self; fair test of general ability; measures remote memory in older subjects; reflects social knowledgeability and judgment; tendencies to impulsivity or dependency may show up in the response to finding a letter, getting out of a forest, or discovery of a fire; sensitive to left-hemisphere damage; the quality of performance may be comparable to that on the Similarities subtest (Lezak, 1983).

C

COMPULSION: a morbid and often irresistible urge for the repetitious performance of an act which serves as a defense against anxiety.

COMPUTERIZED TRANSAXIAL TOMOGRAPHY (CT-scan): provides a three-dimensional representation of the brain; a narrow beam of x-ray is passed through the brain from one side of the head and the amount of radiation not absorbed by the intervening tissue is absorbed by radiation detectors. The x-ray tube is moved laterally across the patient's head and the amount of radiation detected is recorded at 160 equally spaced positions. These data are stored in a computer. The x-ray beam is then rotated one degree and the procedure is repeated. In all, the beam is rotated through 180 degrees. When all the projections are completed, the resulting x-ray sums (160 X 180) are processed by the computer. A reconstruction of the patient's head in cross-section is then printed out by the computer (usually about 8).

CONCEALED FIGURES TEST: see Closure Flexibility Test.

CONCENTRATION: voluntary ability to sustain attention over an extended period of time as a result of an effortful, usually deliberate, heightened, and focused state of attention (Lezak, 1983); the cortical structures used are the frontal lobes plus the limbic system; emotional importance to the object of attention may be a critical factor in screening out extraneous stimuli; see also vigilance.

CONCENTRATION DEFICITS: inability to maintain purposeful attention; visual perception tests require visual attention and concentration; visual search and visual scanning tests require sustained, focused concentration, and directed visual shifting; impairment may result in shortened attention span, distractibility, confusion, and unpredictable performance; see delirium tremens, dementia, pre-senile dementia, post-head injury cognitive deficits, frontal-lobe disorders, Korsakoff's syndrome.

CONCENTRATION TESTS: WISC-R/WAIS-R Digit Span and Arithmetic subtests, Coding, Mazes subtests; cancellation of Rapidly Recurring Target Figures; Random letters with target letter (Strub & Black, 1981); serial 7s.

CONCEPT FORMATION TESTS: proverbs; word usage tests; Gorham's Proverbs Test; Abstract Words Test; Luria's methods; Stanford-Binet subtests: Similarities subtests (Two Things; Three Things; Essential Similarities); Difference subtests (Differences; Differences between Abstract Words; Essential Differences); Similarities and Differences subtests (Pictorial Similarities and Differences I and II; Similarities and Differences); three levels of Abstract Word subtests; Opposite Analogies; The Halstead Reitan Category Test; Symbol Pattern Tests (Thurstone Reasoning Tests in the Primary Mental Abilities battery and American Council on Education Psychological Test; The Kasanin-Hanfmann Concept Formation Test;

C

Card Sorting); Sort and Shift Tests (The Color Form Sorting Test; The Object Classification Test; modified Weigl's Test; The Object Sorting Test; Free and serial classification; The Wisconsin Card Sorting Test; Modified Card Sorting Test; Sequential Concept Formation).

CONCEPTUAL FUNCTIONS: sensitive to the effects of brain injury regardless of site (Luria, 1966; Yacorzynski, 1965); concrete thinking is usually the common sign of impaired conceptual functions; requires an intact system for organizing perceptions, a retrievable store of remembered material, the integrity of the cortical and subcortical interconnections and interaction patterns that underlie "thought," the capacity to process two or more mental events at a time, a response modality sufficiently integrated with central cortical activity to transform conceptual experience into manifest behavior, and a well-functioning response feedback system for continuous monitoring and modulation of output (Lezak, 1983).

CONCEPTUAL PRODUCTIVITY TESTS: (test of cognitive flexibility); tests of frontal-lobe functioning; see self-regulatory tests; planning .test; purposive behavior test; executive function tests.

CONCEPTUAL TRACKING - COMPLEX: ability to entertain two or more ideas or stimulus patterns simultaneously and sequentially without confusing or losing them; necessary to solve problems requiring chained associations (Reitan & Kløve, 1959); a frontal-lobe function.

CONCEPTUAL/ MENTAL TRACKING DEFICITS: usually due to attentional and concentration deficits; see frontal-lobe dysfunction.

CONCRETE RESPONSES: difficulty with the diagonal patterns of the Block Design subtest; difficulties with proverbs; different and strange answers to the Picture Completion subtest; difficulty giving categorical responses to the Similarities subtest.

CONCRETE THINKING: absence of abstract attitude; characteristic of persons whose general intellectual functioning tends to be low in the average or below average range, of certain kinds of psychiatric patients (R. W. Payne, 1970), and of brain-damaged patients; most common signs of impaired conceptual functions: difficulty forming concepts, using categories, generalizing from a single instance, applying procedural rules and general principles; preference for obvious, superficial solutions; unawareness of or inability to identify intrinsic aspects of a problem; unable to distinguish what is relevant, what is essential, and what is appropriate; each event is dealt with as if it were novel, an isolated experience with a unique set of rules; conceptual inflexibility can be present without concreteness particularly in frontal-lobe damage (Zangwill, 1966); lowered scores on Similarities and Picture Completion subtests of the WAIS-R; failures or one-point answers on the three proverb items of the

63

C

Comprehension subtest when responses to the other Comprehension items are of good quality; an inability to conceptualize the squared format of the Block Designs or appreciate the size relationships of the blocks relative to the pictured designs; *brain-damaged patients*: concrete thinking associated with brain damage may be distinguished from the normal thinking of persons of lower intellectual ability when the examiner finds one or more scores or responses reflecting a higher level of intellectual capability than the patient's present inability to abstract would warrant; lowered scores on subtests sensitive to memory defect, distractibility, and motor slowing; distinguishable from psychiatric patient's responses by consistency of deficits regardless of the emotional meaningfulness of the stimulus; a bright person who has had a mild brain-injury may have relatively depressed Similarities score, with perhaps some lowering of Comprehension, Block Design, or Picture Completion scores; prefrontal-lobe lesioned patients may be quite impaired in their capacity to handle abstractions or to take the abstract attitude and yet not show pronouned deficits on the close-ended, well-structured Wechsler test questions.

CONCRETE THINKING (LURIA'S THEORY): lesion(s) of the tertiary zones of the sensory cortical unit; Brodmann's areas 5, 7, 21, 22, 39, 40.

CONCUSSION: a condition of widespread paralysis of the functions of the brain which comes on as an immediate consequence of a blow on the head; frequent spontaneous recovery; not necessarily associated with any gross organic damage in the brain substance (Bannister, 1977); believed to produce permanent microscopic morphological changes in brain cells; may produce loss of consciousness and loss of memory of events just preceding it; severe or repeated concussion may produce diffuse cerebral atrophy; may be diagnosed from an increase in ventricle size (boxer's syndrome or punch-drunk syndrome); mild concussion: transient loss of consciousness with possible impairment of the higher mental functions, such as retrograde amnesia and emotional lability; severe concussion: prolonged unconsciousness with impairment of the functions of the brainstem, such as transient loss of respiratory reflex, vasomotor activity, and dilatation of the pupils of the eyes.

CONDITIONED RESPONSE: a response elicited by a conditioned stimulus after that stimulus has been paired with an unconditioned stimulus.

CONDITIONED STIMULUS: the stimulus that elicits a conditioned response after training.

CONDUCTORS: cells or groups of cells that specialize in the transmission of information, generally from receptors to effectors, but often to other conductors; neurons and blood cells are both conductors.

C

CONDUCTION APHASIA: (fluent aphasia) fluent but paraphasic speech with nearly perfect comprehension of spoken or written language; resembles Wernicke's aphasia; paraphasia in self-initiated speech which may not make sense in repeating what is heard and in reading aloud; no difficulty comprehending words that are heard or seen; no dysarthria or dysposody; repetition is severely affected; writing errors in spelling, word choice, and syntax; penmanship preserved; also called central aphasia or disconnection syndrome; lesion located in the arcuate fasciculus and/or connecting fibers which connect Wernicke's area with Broca's area; in the upper bank of the sylvian fissure, involving the supramarginal gyrus of the inferior-parietal lobe and occasionally the posterior part of the superior-temporal region; fiber systems in the insula are interrupted; impairment caused by disconnection of auditory input from motor output (Geschwind, 1965); hemiparesis, if present, is usually mild; may be caused by an embolus in the ascending parietal or posterior-temporal branch of middle cerebral artery.

CONDUCTIVE DEAFNESS: disease of the middle ear, such as otosclerosis, chronic otitis, or occlusion of the external auditory canal or eustachian tube.

CONFABULATION: dislocation of events in time and the fabrication of stories to fill in forgotten sequences; made up stories about past events rather than admission of memory loss; often based on past experiences and may sound plausible; differs from lying in that the individual is not consciously attempting to deceive; symptom of Korsakoff-Wernicke's disease as a result of chronic alcoholism; frontal-lobe dysfunction.

CONFABULATION IN HEMIPLEGIA: elaborate excuses of fatigue when asked to perform with paralyzed limb.

CONFABULATION QUESTIONNAIRE: (Mercer et al., 1977); a mental status exam to evaluate Korsakoff's psychosis; distinguishes mild from severe confabulators and characterizes each group in terms of memory deficits, response latencies, self-corrections, and the use of cues.

CONFIGURAL MEMORY TESTS: Configural Tests of Visual Memory Functions: Recurring Figures Test, Visual Retention Test (Metric Figures), Object and Picture Memory Span, Non-language Paired Associate Learning Test; Design Reproduction tests: Visual Reproduction subtest of the Wechsler Memory Scale, Complex Figure Test, Benton Visual Retention Test, Memory for Designs Test; Sequence Recall tests: Block-tapping, Knox Cube Imitation Test, Learning Logical and Sequential Order Test, and Learning a Code Test.

CONFUSION: inability to think with customary speed and coherence; distractible; unaware of much of the environment, disoriented to time and space; poor memory (inadequate registration and fixation).

C

CONFUSION TESTING: memory, abstract reasoning, and writing will be poor; orientation most likely poor; rule out severe anxiety/panic, agitated depression, and mania.

CONFUSIONAL STATES - ACUTE: acute onset; inattentive; incoherent conversation (tangential); recent event memory inconsistancy; fluctuations in level of consciousness; visual hallucinations and delusions; agitation; may shout incoherently; may require restraints; confusional state may wax and wane; nocturnal accentuation due to reduced environmental stimuli; may be present in any of the following: toxic confusional states, temporal-lobe automatisms, dementia, psychosis, auditory hallucinations, hypothalamic lesions, delirium tremens, alcohol hallucinosis, uremia, liver failure, meningitis, subarachnoid hemorrhage, hypoglycemia, hypoxic states, congestive cardiac failure, temporal-lobe epilepsy, migraine headache, dysphasia, toxic encephalopathy, acute brain syndrome, organic brain syndrome with psychosis; metabolic imbalance; sepsis; rising intracranial pressure; withdrawal reactions; early cardiac, pulmonary, or hepatic failure; usually a reflection of widespread cortical and subcortical neuronal dysfunction; cortical dysfunction causes alteration in content of consciousness while the ascending activating system dysfunction leads to disturbance of basic arousal.

CONGENITAL ATHETOSIS: bilateral athetosis due to birth trauma; may occur in association with spastic paraplegia, as in Vogt's syndrome and Little's disease.

CONGENITAL FEEBLEMINDEDNESS: amentia.

CONGRUOUS HEMIANOPIA: homonymous hemianopia in which the defects in the field of vision in each eye are symmetrical in position and similar in all other respects.

CONJUGATE EYE MOVEMENTS: eyes have central connections that function like the steering linkage on a car, allowing the eyes to move together (e.g., conjugate movements); mechanisms develop in the first few months of life unless the baby is blind; in blindness from birth, wild, roving eye movements exist; three basic control mechanisms are: 1. eyes flick (saccadic movements) in a scanning fashion until they locate a point of interest; with each saccadic movement a still picture is registered; frontal lobes control these voluntary eye movements; 2. the object is held on the same point of the retina despite any movement it may make (pursuit movements); controlled by the parieto-occipital area in close liaison with the visual cortex; 3. eyes are held in a straight ahead position by the continual adjustment of the eye position in relation to the head position and is maintained by vestibular activity and proprioceptive information from the neck muscles integrated at the brainstem level.

CONJUGATE GAZE: see frontal-lobe lesion; conjugate eye movements.

C

CONNECTIONS OF NEOCORTEX: three major types: 1. projection fibers; 2. commissural fibers; and 3. association fibers.

CONSCIOUSNESS: active state of awareness of environment; responsiveness to psychological stimuli.

CONSCIOUSNESS - BASIC LEVELS: 1. alertness: aware of normal internal and external stimuli; 2. lethargy/somnolence: not fully alert, may drift to sleep; 3. stupor/semicoma: responds only to vigorous and persistent stimuli; 4. coma: completely unarousable (Strub & Black, 1977).

CONSOLIDATION OF MEMORIES: progressive strengthening of the memory traces in order to become permanent; two subprocesses: 1. transfer of material into LTM storage, and 2. consolidation in the storage area; transfer refers to movement of material either from STM into LTM or movement to LTM storage directly from sensory input guided by STM.

CONSONANT TRIGRAMS: (Milner, 1970, 1972) sensitive to left-hippocampal damage (left-temporal lobe).

CONSTRUCTION APRAXIA: damage to Brodmann's areas 7 and 40 (Piercy et al., 1960).

CONSTRUCTION TASKS: Block Design and Object Assembly subtests from the WAIS-R; Kohs Blocks; Stick Construction; Cube Construction; Test of Three-Dimensional Constructional Praxis, Paper Folding; Benton Visual Retention Test.

CONSTRUCTIONAL APRAXIA: discontinuity between intent and outcome; typically based on accurate perceptions and action; reflects the breakdown in the program of an activity that is central to the concept of apraxia; e.g., block design with Alzheimer's and frontal-lobe patients who cannot make the blocks do what they want them to do; disturbances in formulative activities such as assembling, building, and drawing, in which the spatial form of the product proves to be unsuccessful without there being an apraxia of single movements (Benton, 1969a); often associated with right-hemisphere lesions; may accompany defects of spatial perception.

CONSTRUCTIONAL FUNCTIONS: combines perceptual activity with motor response and always has a spatial component; constructional disturbances can occur without any concomitant impairment of visuoperceptual functions (Lezak, 1983); careful observation is needed to distinguish between perceptual failures, apraxias, spatial confusion, or attentional or motivational problems; right-hemishpere damaged patients tend to take a piecemeal, fragmented approach, losing the overall gestalt of the construction task; may neglect the left side of construction or pile up items on the left (Hécaen & Albert, 1978; Mack & Levine, 1981; Walsh, 1978); do not benefit by having a model (Hécaen & Albert, 1970) or practice (Warrington et al., 1966); site of lesion along the anterior-posterior

C

axis also affects expression of constructional tasks (Smith, 1979; Walsh, 1978): right posterior-lesioned patients will, in general, be most likely to have impaired constructional functions, right anterior-lesioned patients are least likely to experience constructional deficits; differences between right- and left-hemisphere lesioned patients constructional functioning: right-hemisphere lesioned patients do not improve with practice; poor estimation of diagonal distances between dots; position horizontal dots ok; produce less right angles than there are in a cube; underestimate angles of a star; more symmetry errors than left-hemisphere lesioned patients; more visual inattention errors on the side opposite the lesion; more likely to draw from right to left (Warrington et al., 1966); right parietal lobe lesioned patients: lose basic outline of design on the WAIS-R Block Design subtest drawings; lose ability to assess spatial relations and orientation; construction ability impaired, but verbal ability well maintained; parietal-lobe tumor and vascular accident patients may show constructional impairment in presence of normal standard neurologic examination; left-hemisphere lesioned patients: may get the overall proportions and the overall idea of the construction correct, but tend to lose details (Gainotti & Tiacci, 1970; Hècaen & Assal, 1970); improve with practice; better than right-hemisphere lesioned patients in estimating diagonal distances between dots; position horizontal dots ok; produce more right angles than there are in a cube, overestimate angles of a star; show fewer symmetry errors than right-hemisphere lesioned patients; left-parietal lobe lesioned patients maintain external configuration with loss of internal detail on the WAIS-R Block Design subtest; drawings characterized by simplification of model (lacking detail) but with preserved spatial relationships (Warrington et al., 1966).

CONSTRUCTIONAL TASK CORTICAL PATHWAYS: parietal lobes are the principle cortical areas involved in visual integration; occipital lobes and motor areas of the frontal lobes are required for completion of tests; the association cortex of the parietal lobes are responsible for the complex integration hypothesis of function; functional pathways: the visual stimuli spread from the primary sensory area (Brodmann's area 17) to the secondary association areas (Brodmann's areas 18 & 19) where perception is elaborated and compared to prior experience; spread to the tertiary association area of the inferior-parietal lobule (Brodmann's areas 39 & 40); associations made between the visual, auditory & kinesthetic images are translated into motor patterns in the perirolandic cortex.

CONSUMMATORY BEHAVIORS: also called automatic, reflexive, or respondent behaviors.

CONTRALATERAL: opposite side.

CONTRALATERAL INATTENTION: (to double simultaneous stimulation); lesion to the parietal lobe of either hemisphere.

CONTRALATERAL NEGLECT: lesion to Brodmann's areas 7 & 40, right-hemisphere (Heilman & Watson, 1977).

CONTRECOUP EFFECT: injury to an organ due to its rebound from a direct blow to the side of the organ opposite to the contrecoup lesion (Smith, 1974).

CONTROL FUNCTIONS DEFICITS: starting, stopping, speeding up, slowing down, inhibiting and exciting, modifying and regulating, and self-correcting activities are almost always adversely affected by brain damage (Lezak, 1983); emotional lability, excitability, impulsivity, erratic carelessness, rigidity, difficulty in making shifts in attention, behavior deterioration in personal grooming and cleanliness, and decreased tolerance for alcohol are often present following diffuse head-injury (Diller, 1968; Luria, 1965; Milner, 1964).

CONVERGENT THINKING: mental search for the right or logical solution; obvious, conventional, inflexible responses (lack of creativity) to a particular stimulus which may be indicative of frontal-lobe dysfunction.

CONVERSION SYMPTOMS: a loss or change of physical functioning that suggests a physical disorder but is actually due to a psychological conflict or need (such as a hysterical paralysis).

CONVULSIVE DISORDER: sudden, excessive, disorderly discharge of neurons in cortex which results in almost instantaneous disturbance of sensation, loss of consciousness, and convulsive movements.

CONVULSION-GENERALIZED: (other than grand mal) immediate loss of consciousness, with stiffening, followed by clonic rhythmic jerking of limbs or only the latter.

CONVULSION-GRAND MAL: recurrent generalized seizure; sudden loss of consciousness with a cry and a fall to the ground; tonic-clonic movements of cranium and limb muscles, sphincteric incontenence and other autonomic disorders; followed by coma of minutes to 1/2 hour, followed by mental confusion, drowsiness, and headache.

COOKIE THEFT PICTURE TEST: (Boston Diagnostic Aphasia Examination; Goodglass & Kaplan, 1972) tests the ability to infer a story from a picture using situational cues and integration of these cues; sensitive to frontal-lobe lesions.

COORDINATING SYSTEMS OF CIRCULATORY SYSTEMS: hormones conduct chemical signals via ducts or blood systems; hormones are chemical substances produced and released by effector cells called glands; there are two types of glands: 1. exocrine glands which secrete hormones that are transported through the body via ducts, and 2. endocrine glands which secrete hormones that are transported by the blood system.

COORDINATING SYSTEMS OF NERVOUS SYSTEM: neurons

C

coordinate stimulus-response with electrochemical signals.

COPD: Chronic obstructive pulmonary disease.

COPROLALIA: compulsive utterance of vile words; see Gilles de la Tourette's disease.

COPYING CROSSES/CUBES, STARS, ETC.: tests for screening of visuographic disabilities.

COPYING/DRAWING TESTS: see Drawing/ copying tests.

COROLLARY DISCHARGE: (Teuber, 1959) voluntary movements involve two sets of signals: 1. the movement command, through the motor system, to effect the movements; 2. a simultaneous signal (corollary discharge) from the frontal lobe to the parietal and temporal association areas that presets the sensory system to anticipate the motor act; the sensory system is able to interpret changes in the external world in light of information about the person's movement; a frontal-lobe lesion can disturb the production of a movement and also interfere with the message to the rest of the brain that a movement is taking place.

CORPUS CALLOSUM: an arched mass of white matter, found in the depths of the longitudinal fissure, composed of transverse fibers connecting the cerebral hemispheres and consisting, from the anterior to the posterior, of rostrum, genu, trunk, and splenium.

CORPUS LUTEUM: a yellow glandular mass in the ovary formed by an ovarian follicle that has matured and discharged its ovum; secretes progesterone hormone.

CORPUS GENICULATUM LATERALE: the lateral geniculate body; an eminence of the metathalamus produced by the underlying lateral geniculate nucleus, just lateral to the medial geniculate body; relays visual impulses from the optic tract to the calcarine cortex.

CORPUS GENICULATUM MEDIALE: the medial geniculate body; an eminence of the metathalamus produced by the underlying medical geniculate nucleus, just lateral to the superior colliculus; relays auditory impulses from the lateral lemniscus to the auditory cortex.

CORPUS STRIATUM: (striped body) largest nuclear masses in the basal ganglia consisting of several complex motor correlation centers; modulates both voluntary movements and autonomic reactions; located in front of and lateral to the thalamus in each cerebral hemisphere; gray substance is arranged in two principal masses, the caudate nucleus and lentiform nucleus which is divided into the putamen and the globus pallidus; the striate appearance on section of the area is produced by connecting bands of gray substance passing from one of these nuclei to the other through the white substance of the internal capsule; lesions may result in movement disorders; the globus pallidus lies on the medial side of the putamen and is separated from the optic thalamus and the caudate nucleus by

70

the internal capsule. On the medial side of the internal capsule and in the upper part of the midbrain lie three nuclear masses: red nucleus, substantia nigra, and subthalamic nucleus (corpus Luysi); pathways connect the subthalamic nucleus and substantia nigra with the globus pallidus; connections are to the ventral part of the optic thalamus, the cerebral cortex and the reticular formation of the brainstem (Brain, 1985).

CORTEX: convoluted outer layer of gray matter composed of nerve cell bodies and their synaptic connections; the highest and most complexly organized correlation center of the brain.

CORTEX-ORGANIZATION OF: see cortical organization, Luria's functional units, hierarchical structure, cortical zones, cytoarchitecture, Brodmann's numbering system.

CORTICAL APHASIA: global aphasia.

CORTICAL APRAXIA: motor apraxia; loss of ability to make proper use of an object, although its proper nature is recognized.

CORTICAL FUNCTION: sensory input enters the primary sensory zones, elaborated in the secondary zones, and integrated in the tertiary zones of the posterior unit; for an action to be executed, activity from the posterior tertiary sensory zones is sent to the tertiary zone of the frontal unit, then to its secondary zone, and then to the primary zone, where execution is initiated; the basic function of the cortex is to modulate input-output signals and impose voluntary control (Luria, 1973b).

CORTICAL FUNCTIONAL UNITS: see Luria's Functional Units, sensory cortical unit, motor cortical unit, lateralization.

CORTICAL HIERARCHICAL FUNCTION: to construct sequences or patterns of voluntary movements in response to external and internal cues, and to discriminate pattern in sensory input; organizes subsets of voluntary movements into patterns of movements that are appropriate to the patterns of internal or external cues (Sherrington, 1906); all components of normal behavior are produced by subcortical systems, but the cortex exerts control.

CORTICAL INATTENTION: see extinction, inattention, parietal-lobe lesions.

CORTICAL MOTOR PATHWAYS: projections from the digit area of the motor cortex connect directly to motor neurons in the contralateral, dorsolateral portion of the ventral zone of the spinal cord grey matter, decussate at the junction of the medulla and spinal cord, forming protuberances on the ventral aspect of the brainstem that are called the pyramids; these fibers are a part of the pyramidal tract; originate in the Betz cells; the digit, hand, and limb area of the motor cortex project to the interneurons in the dorsolateral portion of the intermediate zone in the contralateral spinal cord following the course of the pyramidal tract and are responsible for producing

C

relatively independent hand and arm movements. Cells in the body area of the motor cortex project bilaterally to the interneurons of the ventromedial portion of the intermediate zone both ipsilaterally and contralaterally; part of this projection follows the pyramidal tract and part remains uncrossed to form the ventral corticospinal tract; controls movements of the body and proximal limbs for such activities as walking (Kolb & Whishaw, 1980).

CORTICAL ORGANIZATION: 1. primary sensory and motor areas; 2. secondary sensory and motor areas; 3. tertiary or association areas.

CORTICAL SENSORY AREA LESIONS: animals with visual cortex lesions are unable to discriminate between two objects that differ in pattern, but are able to respond to lights in different locations of different brightness (Klüver, 1957); the superior colliculus and other midbrain visual centers are adequate for discriminating place and intensity, but the neocortex is required for pattern discrimination (Bauer & Cooper, 1964; Goodale & Cooper, 1965).

CORTICOSPINAL MOTOR NEURON PARALYSIS: lesion(s) in the cerebral cortex, subcortical white matter, internal capsule, brainstem, or spinal cord.

CORTICO-BULBAR PATHWAYS: pass via the genu of the internal capsule to the most medial part of the cerebral peduncle with the rotation of the motor tract; innervate the cranial nerve nuclei on the opposite side of the brainstem; the motor nucleus of the 5th nerve which controls the muscles of mastication derives half of its innervation from the opposite hemisphere; a unilateral lesion of the supranuclear pathway rarely leads to detectable deficit in these muscles; the supranuclear innervation of the 7th nerve controls the muscles of the facial expression; supply ratio to the forehead muscles is 50:50 so that a unilateral supranuclear lesion will not affect the forehead muscles; lower face is strongly innervated by decussating fibers with little ipsilateral control; a unilateral supranuclear lesion produces marked weakness of the lower face; supranuclear control of the nucleus ambiguous (the motor nucleus of cranial nerves IX, X, XI) is variable; most people have a 50:50 innervation ratio to these and the XII nucleus; supernuclear control of the XI nerve nucleus (spinal part): the sternomastoid muscle on the same side and the upper fibers of the trapezius muscle on the opposite side.

CORTICOSPINAL LESIONS: impaired ability to fully use movements of the hand, such as releasing objects, or to use relatively independent movements of the fingers to grasp or manipulate objects; greater loss of strength in flexion than in extension and weaker flexion at the wrist than at the elbow or shoulder.

CORTICOSPINAL PATHWAYS: *of the brainstem*: as the corticospinal fibers descend into the midbrain they rotate into the medial part of the cerebral peduncle, fibers carrying information to the leg lying laterally and fibers to the arm lying medially; *pontine levels*: the pathways are broken up into a series of bundles by the transverse pontine fibers which cross to the cerebellar hemispheres; *lower third of the pons*: the fibers come together again as a preliminary to their decussation in the medullary pyramid; the majority of the corticospinal fibers cross in the pyramid, the rest decussate in the anterior commissure at the cervical level.

CORTICOSPINAL TRACT: provides speed, strength, and agility to limb movements; provides capacity to make discrete movements of the extremities, in particular to make relatively independent movements of the fingers.

CORTICOTROPIN: see adrenocorticotropic hormone.

CORTIN: individual hormones produced by the adrenal cortex; regulate sodium and potassium metabolism; stimulate liver glycogen formation, and increases carbohydrate metabolism; mimics male sex hormones.

COUNTING DOTS TEST: (McFie et al., 1950) test of visual scanning behavior; errors may be due to visual inattention to one side, to difficulty in maintaining an orderly approach to the task, or to problems in tracking.

COUP CONTUSIONS: brain contusions at the point of impact.

COWBOY STORY: (Talland, 1965a; Talland & Ekdahl, 1959); memory test.

COXSACKIEVIRAL DISEASE: one of a heterogeneous group of enteroviruses producing a disease resembling poliomyelitis, but without paralysis.

CP: cerebral palsy.

CRANIAL NERVES: the twelve pairs of nerves that enter the brain directly, as opposed to the 31 pairs of spinal nerves that enter the central nervous system below the neck; I olfactory; II optic; III oculomotor; IV trochlear; V trigeminal; VI abducens; VII facial; VIII auditory-vestibular; IX glossopharyngeal; X vagus; XI spinal accessory; XII hypoglossal.

CRANIAL NERVES III, IV, & VI: control the upper eyelid, eye movements and pupils, and have long intracranial courses; subject to damage by a wide range of disease processes at various sites; damage to one or another of these nerves produces diplopia.

CRANIAL NERVE PATHWAYS: the first cranial nerve consists of 20 bundles which arise in the olfactory epithelium and pass through the cribriform plate of the ethmoid bone to the olfactory bulb; the second consists primarily of axons and central processes of cells of the ganglionic layer of the retina, which leave the orbit throught the optic canal, join the optic chiasm and continue as the optic tract; the third originates in the brainstem, emerging medial to cerebral peduncles and running forward in the cavernous sinus; the fascicles of the III, VI, and XII nerves traverse the entire depth of the brainstem and exit just lateral to the midline on the ventral surface; the IV nerve exits from the dorsal aspect of the brainstem after decussating in the superior medullary velum and then passes forwards around the cerebral peduncles; the V nerve passes laterally to exit from the lateral surface of the pons; the VII nerve fasciculus heads first towards the floor of the fourth ventricle, passing around the VI nerve nucleus and then turning back on itself to cross the entire depth of the brainstem in the opposite direction to exit from the ventral surface; both the 6th and 7th nerves are usually damaged together; the main motor nuclei of nerves IX, X, XI are in the nucleus ambiguous; the main parasympathetic motor nuclei (to the lacrimal and salivary glands) are the inferior salivatory nucleus to the IXth nerve, and its anatomical continuation, the dorsal efferent nucleus to the Xth nerve; gustatory reflex activity and taste sensation are relayed through the nucleus of the tractus solitarious; the vestibular nuclei occupy almost the entire lower pons with ramifications over the entire brainstem from the midbrain down to the cervical spinal cord.

CRAWLING SKIN SENSATION: see formication.

CREATIVITY TEST: Uses of Objects Test (Getzels & Jackson, 1962); test to identify creativity in bright children or for evaluating mental inflexibility.

CREPITATION: a sound like that made by rubbing the hair between the fingers, or like that made by throwing fine salt into a fire; the noise made by rubbing together the ends of a fractured bone.

CRETINISM: chronic condition caused by insufficient amounts of thyroxine during fetal development; marked by arrested physical and mental development, dystrophy of the bones and soft parts, and lowered basal metabolism. It is the congenital form of this deficiency, while myxedema is the acquired form; see also thyroid disease.

CREUTZFELDT-JAKOB SYNDROME: a rare, usually fatal, transmissible spongiform viral encephalopathy, occurring in middle life in which there is partial degeneration of the pyramidal and extrapyramidal systems accompanied by progressive dementias and sometimes wasting of the muscles, tremor, athetosis, and spastic dysarthria; called also Creutzfeldt-Jakob disease, Jakob's disease, Jakob-Creutzfeld disease, and spastic pseudoparalysis; sometimes erroneously diagnosed as Alzheimer's disease (Wells, 1978).

CROSS OR CIRCLE ON A LINE TEST: (Milner, 1972, 1974) nonverbal task sensitive to lesions of right or bilateral hippocampus; sensitive to the adverse memory effects of electroconvulsive shock therapy (Squire & Slater, 1978).

CROSS-MODAL MATCHING: Sequin-Goddard formboard test (Teuber & Weinstein, 1954).

CROSS-MODAL MATCHING DYSFUNCTION: lesions of Brodmann's areas 37 & 40 (Butters & Brody 1968).

CROSSED NERVE FIBERS: decussation, commissure, chiasm.

CROSSED PARALYSIS: common in brainstem diseases; caused by lesions of the lowermost part of the brainstem, i.e., in the medulla; affect the tongue and sometimes the pharynx and larynx on one side, and arm and leg on the other side.

CROSSED SENSORY LOSS: see trigeminal sensory system lesion; typical symptoms of a dorsolateral brainstem lesion, between mid-pontine level and C2.

CSF: cerebrospinal fluid.

CT-SCAN: see computerized transaxial tomography.

CUBE ANALYSIS: see block counting.

CUBE CONSTRUCTION TEST: a three-dimensional construction task; includes the Tower and Bridge subtests from the Stanford-Binet; sensitive to right parietal-lobe lesions.

CUBE COUNTING: see block counting.

CUBE ILLUSION TEST: see Necker Cube Test.

CUING WORD RECALL: if after 5 minutes with interference, a patient does not recall three or four words, category cuing may assist him; if the recall improves with cuing, then a retrieval rather than a storage problem is implicated.

CURARE: a poison which causes paralysis by blocking neuromuscular transmission; competes for sites on muscle-fiber membranes with acetylcholine.

CUSHING'S SYNDROME: 1. a condition more commonly seen in females due to hyperadrenocorticism resulting from neoplasms of the adrenal cortex or anterior lobe of the pituitary; symptoms include rapidly developing adiposity of the face, neck, and trunk, kyphosis caused by softening of the spine, amenorrhea, hypertrichosis (excessive growth of hair in females), impotence (in males), dusky complexion with purple markings, hypertension, polycythemia, pain in the abdomen and back, and muscular weakness; 2. in tumors of the cerebellopontine angle and acoustic tumors: subjective noises, impairment of hearing, ipsilateral cerebellar ataxia and eventually ipsilateral impairment of the sixth and seventh nerve function and elevated intracranial pressure.

CUSSING (COMPULSIVE): see coprolalia, Gilles de la Tourette's Disease.

CUTTING SCORES: the test score that separates the normal and abnormal ends of a continuum of test scores (Lezak, 1976).

CVA: cerebral vascular accident; stroke.

CVA SYMPTOMS: see under the various cerebral artery occlusions: anterior, middle, posterior, anterior choroidal.

D

CVA TYPES: arterial occlusions; hemorrhagic; intracerebral; subarachnoid; hemorrhage into tumors.

CVD: cardiovascular disease.

CYSTICERCOSIS: the condition of being infested with cysticercus which is a larval form of a tapeworm.

CYTOMEGALIC INCLUSION DISEASE: a disease, particularly of the neonatal period, characterized by hepatosplenomegaly and often microcephaly and mental or motor retardation; due to infection with cytomegalovirus which is a highly host-specific herpes viruses that produce unique, large cells bearing intranuclear inclusions; also called salivary gland virus.

D

DA: dopamine.

DANDY-WALKER SYNDROME: congenital hydrocephalus due to obstruction of the foramina of Magendie and Luschka by a posterior fossa cyst and hypoplasia of the cerebellar vermis.

D/C; DC: discontinue.

DD: developmentally disabled.

DEAFNESS: see auditory-vestibular nerve (VIII), sensorineural deafness, conductive deafness, auditory agnosia, facial nerve (VII), acoustic nerve (VIII), Meniere's disease, multiple sclerosis, cerebello-pontine angle lesions, eighth cranial nerve.

DEAFNESS IN BOTH EARS: bilateral lesion in Heschl's gyrus; Brodmann's area 41.

DEBRIDEMENT: surgical cleansing of a wound.

DECEREBRATE FUNCTIONING - HIGH: intact midbrain containing, in the tectum, the coordinating centers for vision (superior colliculus) and audition (inferior colliculus), and in the tegmentum, a number of motor nuclei; patient responds to simple features of visual and auditory stimulation; performs automatic behaviors such as grooming; performs subsets of voluntary movements (standing, walking, turning, jumping, climbing, etc.) when stimulated; all components of voluntary locomotion are present at the level of the midbrain.

DECEREBRATE FUNCTIONING - LOW: (hindbrain intact) performs units of movement (hissing, biting, growling, chewing, lapping, licking, etc) when stimulated; shows exaggerated standing, postural reflexes, and elements of sleep-waking behavior; inactive when undisturbed; no effective thermoregulatory ability; swallows food placed on tongue; decerebrate rigidity; righting reflex intact;

reflexes carried out over cranial nerves V (trigeminal) and X (vagus), primarily, as well as VIII (vestibular); also see hindbrain functioning.

DECEREBRATE RIGIDITY: (intact hindbrain and spinal cord in animals) excessive muscle tone, particularly in the antigravity muscles of the body, which are the strongest muscles; when placed in an upright position the animals limbs extend and its head flexes upward, called exaggerated standing (Sherrington, 1906); a number of postural reflexes can be elicited by changes in head position; when head of standing animal is pushed down, the front limbs flex and the hind limbs extend; when head is pushed up, the hind legs flex and the front legs extend; head turned to side elicits extension of the limbs on the same side and flexion of the limbs on the opposite side; when animal is placed on its side, lower limbs are extended and upper limbs are semiflexed; probably the result of unchecked activity in the vestibular system; humans with brainstem damage of the type that separates the lower brainstem from the rest of the brain may alternate between states of consciousness resembling sleeping and waking, make eye movements to follow moving stimuli, cough, smile, swallow food, display decerebrate rigidity, and display postural adjustments when moved (Barrett, Merritt, & Wolf, 1967); jaw clenched, neck retracted, arms and legs stiffly extended and internally rotated; cervical and thoracolumbar spine dorsifexed; caused by diencephalic-midbrain compression.

DECEREBRATION: transection of the brainstem between the anterior colliculi and the vestibular nuclei or ligation of the common carotid arteries and the basilar artery at the center of the pons.

DECORTICATE RIGIDITY: arm or arms in flexion and adduction; caused by lesions in cerebral white matter, internal capsules, and thalamus.

DECORTICATION: removal of the neocortex (either alone or with the limbic system) leaving the basal ganglia and brainstem intact.

DECUB.: decubitus ulcer.

DECUBITUS ULCER: an ulceration caused by prolonged pressure in a patient allowed to lie too still in bed for a long period of time; called and auditory stimulation; performs automatic behaviors such as grooming; performs subsets of voluntary movements (standing, walking, turning, jumping, climbing, etc.) when stimulated; all components of voluntary locomotion are present at the level of the midbrain.

DECEREBRATE FUNCTIONING - LOW: (hindbrain intact) performs units of movement (hissing, biting, growling, chewing, lapping, licking, etc) when stimulated; shows exaggerated standing, postural reflexes, and elements of sleep-waking behavior; inactive when undisturbed; no effective thermoregulatory ability; swallows

D

food placed on tongue; decerebrate rigidity; righting reflex intact; reflexes carried out over cranial nerves V (trigeminal) and X (vagus), primarily, as well as VIII (vestibular); also see hindbrain functioning.

DECEREBRATE RIGIDITY: (intact hindbrain and spinal cord in animals) excessive muscle tone, particularly in the antigravity muscles of the body, which are the strongest muscles; when placed in an upright position the animals limbs extend and its head flexes upward, called exaggerated standing (Sherrington, 1906); a number of postural reflexes can be elicited by changes in head position; when head of standing animal is pushed down, the front limbs flex and the hind limbs extend; when head is pushed up, the hind legs flex and the front legs extend; head turned to side elicits extension of the limbs on the same side and flexion of the limbs on the opposite side; when animal is placed on its side, lower limbs are extended and upper limbs are semiflexed; probably the result of unchecked activity in the vestibular system; humans with brainstem damage of the type that separates the lower brainstem from the rest of the brain may alternate between states of consciousness resembling sleeping and waking, make eye movements to follow moving stimuli, cough, smile, swallow food, display decerebrate rigidity, and display postural adjustments when moved (Barrett, Merritt, & Wolf, 1967); jaw clenched, neck retracted, arms and legs stiffly extended and internally rotated; cervical and thoracolumbar spine dorsifexed; caused by diencephalic-midbrain compression.

DECEREBRATION: transection of the brainstem between the anterior colliculi and the vestibular nuclei or ligation of the common carotid arteries and the basilar artery at the center of the pons.

DECORTICATE RIGIDITY: arm or arms in flexion and adduction; caused by lesions in cerebral white matter, internal capsules, and thalamus.

DECORTICATION: removal of the neocortex (either alone or with the limbic system) leaving the basal ganglia and brainstem intact.

DECUB.: decubitus ulcer.

DECUBITUS ULCER: an ulceration caused by prolonged pressure in a patient allowed to lie too still in bed for a long period of time; called also decubitus, bed sore, and pressure sore.

DECUSSATE: nerve fibers crossing to the opposite side.

DECUSSATION: crossing over or intersection of sensory and motor fibers to the contralateral side of the brain in the form of the letter X; see also chiasm, commissure.

DEFENSIVE-AGGRESSIVE BEHAVIOR: see Raphè Nucleus, hypothalamus, thalamus, amydala.

DEGENERATIVE DISORDERS: Alzheimer's disease (AD/SDAT), Pick's disease, multi-infarct dementia, arteriosclerotic dementia, arteriosclerotic psychosis, subcortical dementia, Parkinson's disease, Huntington's disease, normal pressure hydrocephalus, multiple sclerosis, Korsakoff's psychosis, and alcoholic dementia.

DEGENERATIVE DISORDERS (EARLY SYMPTOMS): psychosocial regression, inattentiveness, inability to concentrate or track mentally, distractibility, apathy with impaired capacity to initiate, plan, or execute complex activities, and memory impairment.

Déjà vu PHENOMENON: strange objects or persons may seem familiar; symptom of psychomotor epilepsy; right temporal-lobe/hippocampal dysfunction.

DEJERINE-ROUSSY SYNDROME: disturbances in cortical sensory discrimination (astereognosis), judgment of intensity, and recognition of differences; radiculitis: distribution of pain, motor and sensory defects in the region of the radicular (nerve root); disturbance of the nerve roots rather than along the course of the peripheral nerve; resembles tabes dorsalis; deep sensibility depressed but tactile sense normal; *bulbar lesions*: upper bulb: produce paralysis of the twelfth nerve on the side of the lesion and hemiplegia on the opposite side; lower bulb: paralysis of the larynx and soft palate; also see thalamic syndrome.

DELAYED CEREBRAL HEMORRHAGE: Spat-apoplexie; rare CVA some days or weeks after a head injury; patients are usually children with slight head injuries.

DELAYED RESPONSE TEST: (Stanford-Binet subtest) recall test of visual memory; suitable for severely impaired brain-damaged patients.

DELIRIUM: mental disturbance marked by inability to sleep because of cerebral excitement and physical restlessness, incoherence, vivid hallucinations, illusions, short unsystematized delusions, agitation, tremulousness, and tendency to convulse; usually reflects a toxic state and has a comparatively short course.

DELIRIUM TREMENS: difficulty in concentration, irritability, tremulousness, insomnia, poor appetite, and disorientation; auditory, visual, tactile and/or olfactory hallucinations; elevated pulse, temperature, and blood pressure; caused by alcohol withdrawal; see also action tremors.

DELUSIONS: characteristic of psychosis; beliefs that are opposed to reality, but are held firmly in spite of evidence to the contrary; false beliefs often centering on persecution.

DEMENTIA: a mental disorder without clouding of consciousness or disturbance of perception in an otherwise healthy person characterized by some or all of the following: cognitive dysfunction, disorders of mood and affect, behavior disorders, memory deficit, failing judgment, difficulty in abstract thought, rumination on the past, confusion for time and place, failure to identify relatives, persevera-

D

tion, confabulation, anxiety, short-tempered, depression, visual hallucinations, disinhibition, intellectual decline, paranoia; presenile (onset before age 65); senile (onset after age 65).

DEMENTIA ASSOCIATED DISEASES: see Alzheimer's disease, Pick's disease, Huntington's chorea, Schilder's disease, myoclonic epilepsy, Jacob-Creutzfeldt disease, Hallervorden-Spatz disease, Parkinson's disease, hypothyroidism, Marchiafava-Bignami disease, low-pressure hydrocephalus, Cushing's disease, pellagra, Wernicke-Korsakoff syndrome, neurosyphilis, hepatolenticular degeneration, bromidism, cerebrocerebellar degeneration, cerebral-basal ganglionic degenerations, spastic paraplegia, lipofuscinosis, basal ganglia calcification, cerebral arteriosclerosis, Steele-Richardson-Olzewski syndrome, Wallenberg's disease, atrophy, head injury, hypoglycemia, renal or hepatic failure, hypercalcemia, neurosyphilis, tuberculous meningitis, fungal meningitis, drugs, chemicals (particularly bromides), alcohol, hydrocephalus.

DEMENTIA CONFUSION: loss of insight into condition; may develop obsessional behavior patterns to avoid embarrassment; depression frequent; may become paranoid — often about the closest relatives.

DEMENTIA RATING SCALE: (Hachinsky et al., 1975); a short, structured, scorable, behavioral observation scale of primary degenerative dementia or multi-infarct dementia which covers five crucial areas: attention, initiation and perseveration, construction, concepts, and memory; can be administered in 30-45 minutes; designed to assess the patient's ability to cope with daily living activities; may be further differentiated with the addition of an Ischemic Score (see Lezak, 1983, pg. 586).

DEMENTIA SYNDROME OF DEPRESSION: seen in elderly depressives showing a mental status that simulates a dementing process; estimated to be found in 15% of elderly persons presenting with dementia (Roth, 1976).

DEMENTIA TESTS: Dementia Scale (Blessed, Tomlinson, & Roth, 1968); Mini-Mental Status Examination (Folstein, Folstein, & McHugh, 1975); Dementia Rating Scale (Hachinsky et al., 1975).

DEMYELINATING DISEASE: acquired allergic or infectious disease in which there is a breakdown or deterioration of myelin; multiple sclerosis; leukodystrophies; lipid storage diseases (Reitan & Wolfson, 1985).

DENDRITE: part of a neuron that receives information; one of the threadlike extensions of the cytoplasm of a neuron; in unipolar and bipolar neurons, they resemble axons structurally, but typically they branch into treelike processes; dendrites comprise most of the receptive surface of a neuron.

DENIAL: a mental mechanism without conscious awareness and employed to resolve emotional conflict and allay anxiety by denying a problem.

DENIAL & NEGLECT SYNDROMES: result of brain lesion, CVA, frontal-lobe disease, and/ or confusional states; range from explicit denial of illness to mild suppression of stimulation on one side of the body during bilateral simultaneous stimulation (inattention or extinction); denial most frequently seen during acute CVA; usually accompanies confusion; also see Anton's syndrome; lesion is usually vascular in the nondominant parietal hemisphere with subcortical/ cortical structures involved.

DENIAL OF BODY AND BODILY CONDITION: see asomatognosia.

DENDATE: see cerebellum location.

DEOXYRIBONUCLEIC ACID: DNA.

DEPERSONALIZATION: changes in the sense of one's self, of one's body, or of the reality of others.

DEPOLARIZATION: condition of excitability; permeability of axon membrane is temporarily changed such that sodium ions rush in and potassium ions rush out; movement of ions excite adjacent areas of axon to fire (nerve impulse); the state a neuron enters once the action potential has taken place and the neuron has fired, thereby losing its polarization; a refractory period follows.

DEPOLARIZATION OF AXON: basis of nerve impulse; reduced resting level by a stimulus.

DEPRESSION: a psychiatric syndrome consisting of dejected mood, psychomotor retardation, insomnia, and weight loss, sometimes as-sociated with irrational guilt feelings and somatic preoccupations, often of delusional proportions; may be due to neurotransmitter insufficiency or imbalance: either noradrenaline or serotonin or both; also see pseudodementia; may be a result of frontal/temporal-lobe tumors, hydrocephalus, cortical atrophy; primary depression may resemble dementia with impaired memory, poor abstract rea-soning and concentration; agitated depression may cause reduced attention and poor performance on a formal mental status examina-tion; depression in right-hemisphere injuries takes longer to develop than with left-hemisphere injuries but after it develops, a right-hemisphere depression may be more chronic, debilitating and resis-tive to intervention; common behavioral problem in brain damage; causes disinterest and reduced arousal which may look like inatten-tion; sometimes treated with antidepressants, MOAI, ECT, and/or psychotherapy; right-hemisphere dysfunction may be shown by neuropsychological test performance (Flor-Henry, 1976; Flor-Henry & Yeudall, 1979; Goldstein, Filskov, Weaver, & Ives, 1977; Kronfol, Hamsher, Digre, & Warizi, 1978; Taylor, Greenspan, & Abrams, 1979); clinical signs of depression: diurnal mood variations (feeling worse in the morning); early morning awakening; delusional guilt; psychomotor retardation; agitation with hand-wringing; appetite

D

loss or increase with weight changes; omega sign.

DEPRESSION ADJECTIVE CHECK LIST: (Lubin, 1965) contains 32 adjectives relating to mood and state.

DEPRESSION TESTS (SELF-RATING): Beck Depression Inventory; Zung Self-rating Depression Scale; Depression Adjective Check List; social adjustment rating scales; Life Satisfaction Index.

DEPRESSION TESTS/SCALES: dexamethazone suppression test, MMPI Zung Self-rating Depression Scale; Back Depression Inventory.

DERAILMENT: see loose associations; blocking.

DEREALIZATION: a mental state characterized by a peculiar change in awareness of the external world, creating a feeling of unreality.

DERIVED SCORES: elaborations of the z-score; provide the same information as do z-scores; T-Scores.

DERMATOME: segments of the skin and musculature of the body which encircle the body in a ring formation; each dermatome corresponds to a specific spinal cord segment.

DESIGN AND FIGURE RECOGNITION TESTS: perceptual recognition of meaningless designs is usually tested by having the patient draw them from models or memory; the WAIS-R Picture Completion subtest, picture vocabulary tests, such as the Peabody Picture Vocabulary Test or the Picture Vocabulary subtest of the Stanford-Binet Scales can be used to show that the subject can recognize meaningful pictures; patients with verbal comprehension problems can be examined by the picture-matching tests of the Leiter or ITPA; Discrimination of Forms subtest from the Stanford Binet; Raven's Progressive Matrices Test (first 12 items) (Lezak, 1983).

DESIGN FLUENCY TEST: (Jones-Gotman & Milner, 1977) may be used to examine conceptual productivity vs perseveration as might be present in patients with right frontal and/or central frontal-lobe lesions (Lezak, 1983).

DESIGN REPRODUCTION TESTS: Visual Reproduction subtest of the Wechsler Memory Scale, Complex Figure Test, Benton Visual Retention Test, Memory for Designs Test.

DETAILS - IMPAIRED ABILITY TO APPRECIATE: left-hemisphere damage; low scores on Block Design; rely on the overall contours of the puzzle pieces but disregard such details as internal features or relative sizes of the pieces (Lezak, 1983).

DEVELOPMENTAL APHASIA: specific delay in language acquisition disproportionate to general cognitive development.

DEVELOPMENTAL SCALES: Although developmental scales are intended to assess infant and child development, they may be used to assess the behavioral functional level of severely brain-injured patients; Boyd Developmental Progress Scale; Vineland Social Maturity Scale; Gesell Developmental Schedules; Adaptive Behavior Scale; Balthazar Scales of Adaptive Behavior; Longitudinal evaluation of head-trauma victims (Lezak, 1983).

DEXTERITY: see manual dexterity.

DIABETES INSIPIDUS: hyposecretion of ADH; disorder marked by loss of water through excessive urination, accompanied by an increase in thirst and drinking behavior.

DIABETES MELLITUS: hyperglycemia; disease marked by the inability of the pancreas to secrete insulin.

DIAGNOSTIC SCREENING PROCEDURE: for the diagnosis of developmental dyslexia (Boder, 1973).

DIASCHISIS: (von Monakow [1914], 1969) depression of relatively discrete or circumscribed clusters of related functions that takes place in areas of the brain outside the immediate site of damage (distance effects) usually in association with acute focal brain lesions (Keminsky, 1958); transient neural dysfunction that dissipates and allows the depressed functions to improve spontaneously (Gazzaniga, 1974; Laurence & Stein, 1978).

DICHOTIC LISTENING: both hemispheres receive projections from each ear; the connections from the contralateral ear appear to have preferred access to the hemisphere; sounds projected to the right ear are primarily processed by the left hemisphere; when words or musical notes are simultaneously presented to the two ears through stereophonic earphones, verbal material is more easily analyzed if presented through the right ear, so that it gets to the left hemisphere, whereas musical material is more easily analyzed if presented to the left ear, so that it gets to the right hemisphere. It is inferred that the left hemisphere specializes in language analysis and the right hemisphere in music analysis (Kimura, 1961, 1967); auditory capacity of each ear is tested separately but simultaneously; if stimulus to only one ear is heard or understood, a contralaterally located lesion of the auditory system can be suspected (Walsh, 1978).

DIENCEPHALIC FUNCTIONING: (hypothalamus and thalamus intact in decorticate animal); voluntary movements occur spontaneously and excessively but are aimless; shows well-integrated, but poorly directed affective behavior; thermoregulates effectively.

DIENCEPHALIC-MIDBRAIN COMPRESSION: by temporal-lobe pressure cone: decerebrate rigidity.

DIENCEPHALON: gross morphological area located rostral to the midbrain and situated deep within the cerebral hemispheres between the two halves of the telencephalon; the posterior portion of the forebrain; consists of three thalamic structures (thalamus, epithalamus, & hypothalamus); dictates all behavior or psychological functions except higher order cognitive processes; also called forebrain, "tween brain," interbrain.

D

DIENCEPHALON FUNCTIONING: intact olfactory system, enabling the animal to smell odorous objects located at a distance; intact hypothalamus and pituitary; sham rage or quasi-emotional phenomena; excessive and inappropriate behavior; constant activity (hyperactivity).

DIFF.: differential cell count.

DIFFERENCES BETWEEN ABSTRACT WORDS: Stanford-Binet subtest, age level AA; test of conceptual functioning.

DIFFERENCES TEST: Stanford-Binet Similarities subtests, age level VI; test of conceptual functioning.

DIGIT SEQUENCE LEARNING TEST: (Benton et al., 1983; Hamsher et al., 1980) sensitive to the mental changes that accompany normal aging of persons over 65 and bilateral brain damage.

DIGIT SPAN BACKWARD: See Digit Span subtest.

DIGIT SPAN FORWARD: see Digit Span subtest.

DIGIT SPAN MEMORY TEST: repetition of digits. The number of digits that can be recalled is termed the memory span. The maximum memory span is about eight in short-term memory after which the memories are lost. Repeated sets of digits are learned over time because they are gradually stored in long-term memory (Hebb, 1949).

DIGIT SPAN SUBTEST: (WAIS-R) failure on one of the two trials of the WAIS-R may be due to distraction, noncooperation, inattentiveness, or lack of concentration; normal range forward is six plus or minus one (Spitz et al., 1972); normal range backwards is four to five; normal span decreases about 1 point after age 70; primarily measures the efficiency of attention (Spitz et al., 1972); anxiety tends to reduce the number of digits recalled (Mueller, 1979; Pyke & Agnew, 1963); normal raw score difference between Digits Forward and Digits Backward tends to range around 1.0 (Costa, 1975); *Digits forward*: more vulnerable to left hemisphere involvement than to either right or diffuse damage (Newcombe, 1969; Weinberg et al., 1972); declines with age, a little in the late sixties to early seventies, more sharply after that (Hulicka, 1966; Kramer & Jarvik, 1979); when patient recalls more digits reversed than forward, probably reflects the patient's lack of effort on a simple task and is more a measure of efficiency of attention rather than memory (Spitz et al., 1972); in the first months following head trauma or psychosurgery, the digit span forward is likely to be subnormal, but is also likely to show returns to normal levels during the subsequent years (Goodwin, 1983a; Lezak, 1979b; Scherer et al., 1957); repetition of less than five digits forward by a non-retarded adult without obvious aphasia indicates defective attention; *Digits Backwards*: uses working memory; involves mental double-tracking in that both the memory and the reversing operations must proceed simultaneously;

may depend upon internal visual scanning (Weinberg et al., 1972); patients with left-hemisphere damage, dementia. and visual field defects have shorter backwards spans than forwards (Newcombe, 1969; Weinberg et al., 1972); may not be affected in Korsakoff's psychosis; may show little improvement over time following trauma (Lezak, 1979b) or psychosurgery (Scherer et al., 1957); *Digits in general brain disease*: 1. perseveration, 2. reverse span of less than three digits or a difference score between forwards and backwards of more than three, 3. intrusions; *Digits in dysphasia*: transpositions, omissions, intrusions of new digits; *Digits in dementia*: digits forward may be a relatively normal score; forward digits are overlearned material which often survives dementing processes for a long time past the patient's ability to care for self; digit backwards is often one of the lowest ranking scores in dementia along with Block Design and Digit Symbol (Lezak, 1983).

DIGIT SYMBOL: test of psychomotor performance that is relatively unaffected by intellectual prowess, memory, or learning (Erber et al., 1981; Glosser et al., 1977; Murstein & Leipold, 1961); right-hemisphere damaged patients are most likely to make orientation errors, usually reversals; motor persistence, sustained attention, response speed, and visuomotor coordination play important roles in a normal person's performance; more sensitive to any kind or location of brain-damage than any other WAIS-R battery subtests (Goodwin, 1983a; Murstein & Leipold, 1961; Reitan, 1966); score is most likely to be depressed even when damage is minimal (Hirschenfang, 1960); particularly affected by right-hemisphere lesions; Korsakoff's psychosis causes not only psychomotor slowing but also visuoperceptual deficits (Butters & Cermak, 1976; Glosser, Butters, & Kaplan, 1977); *in dementia*: often one of the lowest ranking scores of the WAIS-R along with Block Design and Digits Backward; difficult for low-skilled manual workers or elderly subjects; visual perception or orientation defects may show up as rotations, simplifications, or distortions; aphasics often do poorly because of slowing even though their performance may be error-free (Tissot et al., 1963).

DIGIT VIGILANCE TEST: (Lewis & Kupke, 1977) a paper and pencil cancellation task of vigilance and conceptual slowing; a subtest of the Lafayette Clinic Repeatable Neuropsychological Test Battery.

DIGITAL SUBTRACTION ANGIOGRAPHY: an alternative type of angiography that may replace arteriography.

DIPLEGIA: the perception of two images of a single object; called also ambiopia, double vision, and binocular polyopia.

DIPLOPIA: double vision; caused by weakness of the superior oblique muscle Oculomotor nerve (III), Trochlear nerve (IV), or Abducens (VI).

D

DIPSOMANIA: alcoholism.

DIRECTIONAL ORIENTATION: see right-left orientation.

DISCONJUGATE EYE MOVEMENTS: divergent squint: paralysis of both medial recti muscles; eyes may also be skewed in which one eye looks up and out and the other looks down and out — usually caused by a pontine lesion in the cerebellar peduncles; may be see-saw nystagmus in which the eyes jerk up and down alternately; classical internuclear ophthalmoplegia: medial longitudinal fasciculus is damaged and the medial recti fail to move synchronously with the lateral recti on attempted lateral gaze to either side; seen most often in multiple sclerosis; unilateral internuclear ophthalmoplegia caused by a vascular lesion of the paramedian area of the brainstem and nystagmus of the laterally moving eye; neither eye abducts completely while adduction is complete; relay to the 6th nerve impaired on both sides; reading is often impaired.

DISCONNECTION SYNDROME: corpus callosum, (anterior four-fifths): speech and perceptual areas of the left hemisphere are isolated from those of the right hemisphere; failure of the left hand to obey commands, the right one performing perfectly (left-handed apraxia.); left hand can imitate the the examiner's movements; cannot match an object seen in the right half of the visual field with one in the left half; blindfolded persons are unable to match an object held in one hand with that in the other hand, can name objects in the right hand but not the left; *splenium lesion* (posterior fifth of corpus callosum): only the visual part of the disconnection syndrome occurs; may be caused by occlusion of the left posterior cerebral artery; infarction of left occipital-lobe; causes a right homonymous hemianopia, all information needed for activating the speech areas of the left hemisphere must come from the right occipital-lobe and cross the splenium; if splenium lesioned, cannot read or name colors because the visual information cannot reach the left angular gyrus; no difficulty in copying words, but cannot read them; matching of colors without naming them is done without error (intrahemispheric); see also conduction aphasia, sympathetic apraxia in Broca's aphasia, pure word deafness, alexia and inability to name colors without agraphia, corpus callosum, anterior cerebral artery occlusion (anterior four-fifths), splenium lesions.

DISEASE OF CRANIAL NERVES 8, 9, 10, 11, and 12: loss of strength or hoarsness of the voice, nasal speech, difficulty in swallowing with nasal regurgitation of fluids or aspiration of food particles with attacks of choking.

DISEQUILIBRIUM: a disturbed state of equilibrium; see auditory-vestibular nerve (VIII)

DISORIENTATION: confusion about the date or time of day, where one is (place), or who one is (identity).

D

DISORIENTATION - RIGHT/LEFT: see Gerstmann's syndrome.

DISORDERS OF ARTICULATION AND PHONATION: see inarticulate, phonation, paretic dysarthria, spastic and rigid dysarthria, choreic, myoclonic and ataxic dysarthria.

DISORIENTATION IN SPACE: see auditory-vestibular nerve (VIII).

DISPLACEMENT: the transfer of feeling from a certain idea or object to a more acceptable idea or object.

DISPLACEMENT OF IMAGES: see visual allesthesia.

DISSOCIATIVE SPEECH SYNDROME: see conduction aphasia, pure word blindness, deafness, dyslexia with dysgraphia.

DISTAL: far away from something; opposite of proximal.

DISTANCE ESTIMATION TASKS: spatial disorientation (Benton, 1969b) and scanning defects (Diller et al., 1974); may be implicated in inability to judge distances; sensitive to left posterior/occipital lesions.

DISTORTED REALITY CONTACT: characteristic of psychosis; unable to separate events or things that are actually happening from those that are imagined.

DISTRACTIBILITY: unable to sustain attention because attention is drawn too frequently to unimportant or irrelevant external stimuli such as trivial noises or events; etiology: 1. diffuse brain dysfunction due to metabolic disturbance, drug intoxication, post-surgical states, systemic infection; 2. extensive bilateral cortical damage, atrophy, multiple infarcts, encephalitis, head trauma; tests: digit repetition; random letter test.

DIVERGENT THINKING: ability to generate many different and often unique and daring ideas without evident concern for satisfying preconceived notions of what is correct or logical; inability to think divergently may suggest frontal-lobe dysfunction (Zangwill, 1966).

DNA: (deoxyribonucleic acid) a chemical in the nucleus of cells that is involved in transmitting hereditary characteristics; consists of four paired bases (guanine, cytosine, adenine, and thymine) arranged along strands in the form of a double helix; carrier of genetic information for all organisms except RNA viruses.

DOMINANCE - CEREBRAL: cerebral dominance or handedness.

DOMINANT (LEFT) FRONTAL-LOBE LESIONS: impaired verbal fluency; see also Broca's aphasia, right hemiplegia, frontal-lobe lesion deficits.

DOPAMINE (DA): a biochemical neurotransmitter that occurs in reduced levels in Parkinson's disease and heightened levels in certain types of schizophrenia; concentrated in more circumscribed areas than norepinephrine; found primarily in brain structures that play an important role in muscle control, among them, the substantia nigra, the caudate nucleus, and the putamen; depletion of dopamine in the substantia nigra causes Parkinson's disease.

D

DOPPLER IMAGING: a computerized technique for screening for extra-cerebral stenotic vascular lesions.

DORSAL: toward the top of the brain or the back of an animal; opposite of ventral; same as posterior in human anatomy.

DORSAL COLUMN SENSATION: fibers from the dorsal columns of the spinal cord ascend to the gracile (leg) and cuneate (arm) nuclei in the dorsal medulla. The leg fibers lie medially in the dorsal column, but as the fibers decussate in the medulla through the internal arcuate fibers, the leg fibers come to lie laterally, to parallel the motor fiber arrangement. The new tract that is formed by the decussation (the medial lemniscus) is at first vertically disposed and then flattens, spreads, and merges finally with the spino-thalamic tract in the midbrain, just below the thalamus; controls touch, two point discrimination sense and joint position sense.

DORSAL ROOT: the area of the spinal cord where sensory neurons enter.

DORSAL THALAMUS: composed of a number of nuclei, each of which projects to a specific area of the neocortex which receive input from the different body sensory systems or from other brain areas; see also lateral geniculate body, medial geniculate body, ventral lateral posterior nuclei, pulvinar, dorsomedial nucleus.

DORSIFLEXED: flexed or bent backwards.

DORSOLATERAL: pertaining to the back and to the side.

DORSOLATERAL FRONTAL LOBE LESIONS: poor recency/order memory, reduced corollary discharge, poor movement programming; reduced interest in sexual behavior, although still able to perform the necessary motor acts and can perform sexually if led through the activity step by step.

DORSOMEDIAL NUCLEUS OF THE THALAMUS: three divisions; each division projects to a distinct region of the prefrontal cortex; each division is functionally and anatomically distinct; part of the "mood" or "feeling" system (Barr & Kiernan, 1983).

DORSOMEDIAL THALAMUS - LESION: memory loss; elimination of chronic pain.

DOT COUNTING: (Lezak, 1983, pp.619-620; Rey, 1941); a test which may expose malingering.

DOTTING A TARGET CIRCLE TEST: (Vernea, 1977); spatial inattention/ unilateral visuospatial inattention test.

DOUBLE SIMULTANEOUS STIMULATION TEST: see tactile inattention tests.

DOUBLE VISION: diplopia.

DOWN'S SYNDROME: a condition characterized by a small, antero-posteriorly flattened skull, short flat-bridged nose, epicanthal fold, short phalanges, and widened space between the first and second digits of hands and feet, with moderate to severe mental retardation, and associated with a chromosomal abnormality, usually trisomy of chromosome 21; also called mongolism and trisomy 21 syndrome, congenital acromicria.

DOWNWARD GAZE DEFECT: trochlear nerve (IV) lesion.

DRAW-A-HOUSE TEST: difficulties with perspective common among intellectually deteriorated patients; the alert, bright patient who struggles with a roof line or flattens the corner between the front and side of the house is more likely to have right than left hemisphere involvement; patients who complain of difficulties in finding their way, getting lost even in familiar places, can be asked to reproduce a ground plan of their home or their ward (Lezak, 1983).

DRAWING/COPYING TESTS: Bender-Gestalt, Background Interference Procedure, Minnesota Percepto-Diagnostic Test, Complex Figure Test, Benton Visual Retention Test, Copying Crosses, Human Figure Drawings, Bicycle Drawing Test, Draw-a-House, Clock.

DRAWING AGNOSIA: see visual agnosia for drawing.

DRAWING DISABILITIES: copying and/or drawing tasks are sensitive to many different kinds of organic disabilities such as perceptual deficits, praxic disabilities, and certain cognitive and motor organization disabilities (Lezak, 1983); unilateral inattention tends to be reflected in the omission of details on the side of the drawing opposite the lesion (Colombo et al., 1976) or positioning drawings on the same side of the page as the lesion (Burton, 1978; Gur et al., 1977); drawings of patients with right-hemisphere damage tend to be larger than those done by patients with left-sided lesions (Larrabee, Kane, Morrow, & Goldstein, 1982); drawings to command tend to elicit evidence of inattention more readily than does coping from a model (Frederiks, 1963).

DRAWING DYSFUNCTION: Brodmann's area 40 (Warrington et al., 1966).

DRINKING: see hypothalamus.

DRIVENESS - ORGANIC: hyperactivity and distractability; may be due to lesions in the reticular substance of the pons and medulla.

DRIVE STATES: impetus located in hypothalamus which mediates the medial forebrain bundle.

DROMEDARY GAIT: exaggerated lordosis, hips partly flexed with a tilting forward of pelvis, and knees flexed.

DROP ATTACKS: see akinetic epilepsy.

DROP-FOOT GAIT: foot lifted abnormally high to clear ground; slapping noise as foot strikes the floor; may be unilateral or bilateral; caused by paralysis of pretibial and peroneal muscles and diseases that affect peripheral nerves or motor neurons in spinal cord such as poliomyelitis, progressive muscular atrophy; see also Charcot-Marie-Tooth disease.

DRY MOUTH-PARTIAL: see glossopharyngeal nerve (IX).

D

DUCHENNE'S DISEASE: late syphilis, tabes dorsalis.

DSM III/DSM III-R: Diagnositic Statistical Manual III (R); differential listing of psychiatric disorders.

DUCT GLANDS: see exocrine glands.

DUCTLESS GLANDS: see endocrine glands.

DURA MATER: the outermost, toughest, and most fibrous of the three membranes (meninges) covering the brain and spinal cord; also called pachymeninx.

DURET'S LESION: effusion of blood in the region of the fourth ventricle of the cerebrum as a result of slight injury.

DVORINE TEST: color perception test, particularly for color blindness.

DWARFISM: result of hyposecretion of somatotropic hormone in child-

DYNAMICS: the sequence and relationship of the psychological factors that influence behavior disturbance, personality disorders, and mental illness.

DYNAMIC APHASIA: speech appears normal by surface impression without appreciable articulatory or grammatical errors. On careful listening, patient is unable to complete a series or give a coherent account of an event; responds to clues and questions given by another person.

DYSARTHRIA: poor phonation, usually due to muscle weakness; see Hallervorden-Spatz syndrome, stuttering, anarthria, Heidenhaim's syndrome, cerebellar disease.

DYSARTHRIA - SIMPLE: understands what is heard, read, and can write ok; may be unable to utter a single intelligible word; disorder of articulation in which basic language grammar, word choice, comprehension is intact; produces distorted speech sound that cannot be accurately transcribed by a listener; dysfunction in the rapid movement of the muscles of speech — sometimes including paralysis of those muscles; lesions may be in any area controlling muscles of articulation: Broca's area; basal ganglia; bulbar neurons; supramarginal gyrus.

DYSARTHRIA - SPASTIC/RIGID: pseudobulbar palsy; corticobulbar tract lesion.

DYSDIPSIA: difficulty drinking.

DYSEIDETIC DYSLEXIA: (Boder, 1973) writes phonetically; cannot read phonetically.

DYSERGIA: motor incoordination due to defect of efferent nerve impulse.

DYSESTHESIA: painful and persistent sensation induced by a gentle touch to the skin.

DYSFLUENCY: difficulty in generating words; stuttering or stammering; not aphasia, apraxia nor dysarthria; etiology unknown; may include paraphasias and articulatory errors.

D

DYSGRAPHIA: impairment in the ability to write; may be a part of a language disorder caused by a disturbance of the parietal lobe or of the motor system.

DYSLEXIA: specific developmental learning disorder of children who have normal intelligence but experience unusual difficulty in learning to read; often involves reversal of letters or words.

DYSLEXIA TEST: Cancellation of Rapidly Recurring Target Figures; Stroop color/ word test.

DYSLEXIA WITH DYSGRAPHIA: language disturbance most evident in reading and writing; auditory comprehension better than visual comprehension; visual form of Wernicke's aphasia; often a late sequel of Wernicke's aphasia; parieto-occipital region lesion.

DYSLISI: leg movements involved in restless legs syndrome.

DYSMETRIA: an afferent disorder in which there is improper measuring of distance in muscular acts; disturbance in the power to control the range of movement in muscular action; hypermetria: voluntary muscular movement over-reaches the intended goal (past-pointing); hypometria: voluntary muscular movement falls short of the intended goal; see lesions of the lateral and inferior cerebellum or cerebellar disease.

DYSNOMIA: see anomia, anomic aphasia; nominal aphasia.

DYSPHAGIA: difficulty in swallowing.

DYSPHASIA: impairment of speech, consisting of lack of coordination and failure to arrange words in their proper order; due to a central lesion; defect of symbol formulation; see also aphasia.

DYSPHASIC CONFUSION: a communication problem; may be due to receptive or expressive aphasia or combinations of both.

DYSPHONIA: any impairment of voice; difficulty in speaking.

DYSPHONIC DYSLEXIA: (Boder, 1973) capacity for recognition and fluent reading of sight vocabulary; cannot read or spell phonetically, but can spell words from their sight vocabulary.

DYSPNEA: labored breathing; abnormal, uncomfortable awareness of breathing.

DYSPRAXIA: see apraxia.

DYSPROSODY: disruption of the melodic intonation, inflection, rhythm, and phrases of speech; usually due to Broca's area infarction; monotonal, halting speech, and may mimic a foreign accent; verbal apraxia.

DYSTONIA: same as athetosis; afferent disorder; any fixed posture which may be the end result of a disease of the motor system; inability to sustain the fingers and toes, tongue, or any other group of muscles in one position; lesion of the anterior thalamus or ventricular nuclei with intact pyramidal tracts; see also Wilson's Disease, dyskinesia, Hallervorden-Spatz disease, torsion spasm, athetosis.

E

DYSTONIA MUSCULORUM DEFORMANS: one leg rigidly extended or one shoulder elevated, exaggerated lordosis, hips partly flexed with a tilting forward of pelvis, knees flexed; dromedary gait.

Dx; DX: diagnosis.

E

EARLY MORNING AWAKENING: awakening 2-3 hours before usual time of awakening with inability to return to sleep; may be symptom of depression.

EATING REFLEXES: see ventromedial hypothalamus.

ECHOLALIA: repetition (echoing) of the words or phrases of others.

ECHO VIRUS: Enteric Cytopathic Human Orphan + virus; an enteric orphan RNA virus isolated from man; separable into many serotypes; associated with human disease, especially aseptic meningitis.

ECHOPRAXIA: an involuntary and spasmodic imitation of the movements of another.

ECS/ECT: see electroconvulsive shock therapy.

ECG/EKG: electrocardiogram; a graphic tracing of the electric current produced by the excitation of the heart muscle.

EDEMA: the presence of an abnormal amount of fluid in the intercellular tissue spaces of the body; usually applied to demonstrable accumulation of excessive fluid in the subcutaneous tissues.

EEG: electroencephalogram or electroencephalograph; a recording of the potentials on the skull generated by currents emanating spontaneously from nerve cells in the brain.

EFFECTORS: cells, groups of cells, or components of single-celled organisms that respond to stimuli e.g., muscles.

EFFERENT: leaving the center; pertaining to neurons carrying impulses away from the central nervous system.

EGOCENTRIC SPATIAL RELATIONS: (Semmes et al., 1963) personal/bodily orientation as apposed to allocentric spatial relations (extrapersonal orientation).

EGO-DYSTONIC: a symptoms or personality trait that is recognized by the individual as unacceptable and undesirable; experienced as alien.

EGO-SYNTONIC: personality traits that are acceptable and desired by the patient.

EIGHTH CRANIAL NERVE: (Auditory-Vestibular nerve) relates to hearing; carries information from the vestibular apparatus and the organ of Corti which both lie deep in the temporal bone; suspended in the bone in perilymph which is basically CSF and is in continuity with the subarachnoid space; a highly specialized fluid with a high protein content, known as endolymph, fills the semicircular canals and the scala media of the cochlear; activity in the semi-circular canals is transmitted to the vestibular nucleus on the same side of the brainstem and then to the eye muscle nuclei.

EIGHTH CRANIAL NERVE LESION: tumors usually are on the vestibular division of the nerve. Early symptoms are auditory; tinnitis is followed by slowly progressive loss of hearing; vertigo is unusual in the early stages; damage to the 7th nerve is usually a late manifestation of an eighth nerve lesion; most consistent early physical signs of eighth nerve lesion is depression or absence of the corneal reflex; later, numbness over the face; occasional face pain; as the tumor extends medially, and distorts the brainstem and cerebellum, virtigo, ataxia of gait, and mild spastic paraparesis may occur; the ataxia is usually more severe on the side of the tumor; with further distortion of the brainstem the cerebral aqueduct may become blocked with subsequent hydrocephalus, headache, and papilledema.

EKG/ECG: electrocardiogram.

ELECTIVE MUTISM: refusal to speak; may be limited to mouthing words, whispering, or slow, labored, halting speech with no motor deficits apparent.

ELECTRICAL BRAIN INJURIES: brain damage may range from minor to severe; may cause death due to respiratory arrest; neuronal dysfunction may produce generalized seizures, coma, temporary confusion, dysphasia, hemiparesis, organic dementia, parkinsonian symptoms, or choreoathetosis (Reitan & Wolfson, 1985).

ELECTOCONVULSIVE SHOCK THERAPY (ECT/ECS): massive electric shock applied across the brain; may be beneficial in depression if drug therapy fails; effect on psychological functioning: 1. total amnesia for the period of unconsiousness during treatment and for the period of confusion immediately following; 2. retrograde amnesia for events just prior to treatment which decreases over time; and 3. anterograde amnesia for stimuli after ECT, such as names of people, the contents of books, etc., which may persist for as long as two to three weeks following the ECT; usually returns to normal within four weeks.

ELECTROENCEPHALOGRAM: sampling of the electrical activity of the cortex through electrodes posted in specific areas of the skull; amplified electrical activity recorded from the scalp; sum of all neural activity, action potentials, graded potentials, etc.; mostly the measure of the graded potentials of dendrites; records alpha and beta rhythm; large-amplitude spike-and-wave activity may indicate the presence of epilepsy; slow waves in a behaviorally alert individual may indicate brain damage; valuable tool for studying problems

E

such as sleep-walking, for monitoring depth of anesthesia, and for diagnosing epilepsy and brain damage.

ELECTROLYTIC BALANCE ABNORMALITIES: (causing adverse brain functioning); hyponatremia, hypernatremia, hypokalemia, hyper- and hypomagnesemia.

ELECTROMYOGRAPHY (EMG): analysis of the electrical activity of muscles by inserting a needle electrode into the muscle to be tested; useful for diagnosing the presence of damage or abnormalities in nerves.

ELECTRON: a negatively charged atomic particle.

ELEVENTH CRANIAL NERVE: spinal accessory nerve; motor supply to the sternomastoid and upper part of the trapezius muscle; damage to the nerve results in wasting and weakness of the sternomastoid and upper trapezius.

EMBOLI: plural of embolus; see embolism.

EMBOLISM: a clot or plug brought through the blood from another vessel and forced into a smaller one, where it obstructs circulation; can be a blood clot, a bubble of air, a deposit of oil or fat, or a small mass of cells detached from a tumor; most often affects the middle cerebral artery of the left side of the brain.

EMBOLOPHRASIA: see embololalia.

EMBOLOLALIA: the interpolation of meaningless words or phrases into speech; also called embolophrasia.

EMG: see electromyography.

EMOTION: a mental state involving a distinctive feeling tone.

EMOTIONS: mediated through the hypothalamus.

EMOTIONAL CENTER: (primitive) amygdala.

EMOTIONAL DISTORTION: characteristic of psychosis; blunted affect (flattened affect) or emotional lability.

EMOTIONAL ILLUSIONS: unreal fears, loneliness, sorrow; may be the result of lesions in either temporal lobe.

EMOTIONAL LABILITY: a tendency to show alternating states of gaiety and somberness which may be a result of concussion, head-injury, delirium, dementia, or cognitive distortion as a result of psychosis.

EMPLOYABILITY AFTER HEAD INJURY: frontotemporal injuries significantly reduce the employability of brain-injured patients; few ever resume their studies or return to gainful employment (Bond, 1975; Eson & Bourke, 1980b; Najenson, 1980) at the same level as before the injury (Lezak et al., 1980: Vigoroux et al., 1971; Weddell et al., 1980); combinations of impaired initiative and apathy, lack of critical capacity, defective social judgment, childishness and egocentricity, inability to plan or sustain activity, impulsivity, irritability, and low frustration tolerance usually render the post-head-injured unemployable or only marginally employable (Lezak, 1983).

E

ENCEPHALITIS: inflammation or abscess of the central nervous system caused by infection from virus, bacteria, fungi (mycotic), or parasitic infestations.

ENCEPHALITIS LETHARGICA: see hypersomnia.

ENCEPHALIZATION: ontogenetic development of behavior in the individual as successively higher levels of function mature; the gradual increase in forebrain size relative to the midbrain and the hindbrain. In general, the tendency of anterior areas of the brain to increase in size.

ENCEPHALOMALACIAS: vascular disorders that produce a softening of the brain resulting from inadequate blood flow; decreases in blood flow can have any of three causes: 1. a thrombosis; 2. an embolism; 3. reduction in blood flow such that not enough oxygen and glucose are supplied — most commonly due to cerebral arteriosclerosis; except from embolisms, onset is usually slow (hours or days); may be episodic (cerebral vascular insufficiency or transient ischemic attacks).

ENCEPHALOPATHY: inflammation of the central nervous system caused by chemicals, allegies, toxic subtances, and/or physical trauma.

ENCLOSED BOX PROBLEM TEST: (Stanford-Binet subtest, SA I level) a serial reasoning task; logical thinking; comprehension of relationships; practical judgment.

ENDOCRINE ABNORMALITIES: may produce signs and symptoms of neurological deficit; includes diabetes mellitus, hypoglycemia, hyperglycemia, hypothyroidism, hyperthyroidism, hypoparathyroidism, hyperparathyroidism, and disorders of liver and pancreatic functioning, and hormonal abnormalities of the hypothalamic-hypophyseal relationship (Reitan & Wolfson, 1985).

ENDOCRINE ACTIVITY REGULATION: mediated through the hypothalamus via the pituitary gland.

ENDOCRINE GLANDS: internal organs such as the pancreas and the pituitary gland, that produce and release hormones into the blood stream which delivers them to target organs in remote parts of the body; these hormones speed up or slow down chemical processes; also known as ductless glands.

ENDOGENOUS: developing or originating within the organism, or arising from causes within the organism rather than from external causes.

ENDORPHINS: endogenous, natural, opiate like substances in the brain.

ENGRAM: the structural change that theoretically takes place in the nervous system during learning.

ENTERAMINE: see serotonin.

ENZYME: a protein capable of accelerating or producing by catalytic action some change in a substrate for which it is often specific;

E

chemical which regulates all functions of the cell and channels energy to the appropriate areas of the cell; brings molecules together in the appropriate order; differentiates among molecules on the basis of shape; main groups: oxidoreductases, transferases, hydrolases, lyases, isomerases, and ligases; allows chemical reactions to occur at lower temperatures than would otherwise be possible and constitutes the basic control mechanism for chemical reactions in cells.

EPENDYMAL CELLS: produce central nervous system fluid and insulate the brain's ventricles.

EPICANTHAL FOLD: a vertical fold of skin on either side of the nose, sometimes covering the inner canthus; present as a normal characteristic in persons of certain races and sometimes occurs as a congenital anomaly in others; see also Down's syndrome.

EPIDERMIS: the outermost layer of skin.

EPIDURAL ABSCESS: a collection of pus that may have extended from an adjacent infection such as chronic sinusitis, acute or chronic mastoiditis, or osteomyelitis of the skull; symptoms of large abscesses may include headache, contralateral focal motor seizures, hemiparesis, drowsiness, stupor, and papilledema; fifth and sixth cranial nerve involvement may be present (Reitan & Wolfson, 1985).

EPILEPSIA PARTIALIS CONTINUA: rare form of focal convulsion; persistent clonic movements confined to a limited part of body, often the face; movements continue for days and months; result of focal lesion involving the corresponding area of the opposite motor cortex; form of myoclonic epilepsy (Brain, 1985).

EPILEPSY: condition characterized by recurrent electrographic seizures of various types that are associated with a disturbance of consciousness; may be symptomatic (identified with a specific cause such as infection, trauma, tumor, vascular malformation, toxic chemicals, very high fever, and other neurological disorders) or idiopathic (appear to arise spontaneously and in the absence of other diseases of the CNS); symptoms most often include 1. aura, 2. loss of consciousness with amnesia which may take the form of complete collapse or simply staring off into space, and 3. movement disorders during the seizure which may be shaking or automatic movements; seizures most often occur when the patient is relatively inactive; also see focal seizures, Jacksonian march, partial seizures, generalized seizures, pre-ictal, inter-ictal, post-ictal, aura, absence attack, akinetic seizures, grand mal, petit mal, clonic stage, tonic stage, automatisms, epileptogenic state; possible causes: in infancy: birth injury, cerebral anoxia, hypoglycemia, hypocalcemia, metabolic disturbances, febrile illness, prenatal toxoplasmosis, cytomegalic inclusion disease, hydrocephalus, congenital diplegia, hemiplegia, anaphylactic reaction, amaurotic family idiocy; *in childhood*: congenital or acquired lesions as listed above, constitutional or idio-pathic epilepsy, lesions of one temporal lobe, diffuse sclerosis, and subacute inclusion encephalitis; *in adult*: intracranial tumour, cere-bral atherosclerosis, Stokes-Adams attacks, spontaneous hypogly-cemia due to a tumor of the islet cells of Langerhans of the pancrease, neurosyphilis, head-injury, alcohol withdrawal, cysticercosis (Brain, 1985).

EPILEPSY EVALUATION SCALES: Brief Psychiatric Rating Scale; Psychosocial Rating Scale; Washington Psychosocial Seizure Inven-tory; Neuropsychological Battery for Epilepsy.

EPILEPSY-TEST BATTERY: see Neuropsychological battery for epilepsy.

EPILEPSY-TYPES: Generalized: absence (petit mal); atonic-myoclonic, tonic or myoclonic. Partial Complex: with temporal lobe and psycho-motor features (special sensory, autonomic, psychic, and memory disturbances); partial seizures secondarily becoming generalized; simple motor (Jacksonian); simple sensory. Special: automatisms; Epilepsy partialis continua; reflex and self-induced (Brain, 1985).

EPILEPSY-UNCINATE: dreamy state, olfactory or gustatory halluci-nations, and masticatory movements.

EPILEPTIC PSYCHOSIS: interictal behavior and symptomatology that may bear some resemblance to what is often seen in schizo-phrenic patients (Stevens, 1966).

EPILEPTOGENIC STATE: relatively inactive brain state just prior to an epileptic seizure; a consistent feature of the brain functioning in epilepsy.

EPINEPHRINE: hormone secreted by the adrenal medulla along with norepinephrine; triggers ACTH release; stimulates liver to convert glycogen to glucose; formed from norepinephrine by a chemical process known as transmethylation; also formed to a lesser extent, in the postganglionic fibers in the SNS; involved in the activity of that system, but appears to play no role in neurotransmission in the brain; arouses the body (raising blood pressure and glucose levels) in emergencies, thus mimicking the role of the SNS; found at the postganglionic nerve endings; also called adrenaline.

EPIPHYSIS CEREBRI: see pineal gland.

EPITHALAMUS: one of three parts of the diencephalon; contains the pineal body; no known function in humans.

EPRs: see extrapyramidal reaction.

EQUILATERAL HEMIANOPIA: homonymous hemianopia.

EQUILIBRIUM DISTURBANCE (SEVERE): midline tumor of cere-bellum such as medulloblastoma, or hemorrhage; symptoms may in-clude swaying, staggering, and reeling.

EQUINE GAIT: a walk accomplished mainly be flexing the hip joint; seen in crossed-leg palsy.

E

EQUIPOTENTIALITY HYPOTHESIS (CORTICAL FUNCTION): the hypothesis that states that intact areas of the brain have the capacity to assume the function of damaged areas and that each portion of a given area is able to encode or produce the behavior normally controlled by the entire area.

ESOPHORIA: tendency for the eyes to turn inward.

ESSENTIAL DIFFERENCES TEST: Stanford-Binet subtest, age levels AA and SA II; test of conceptual functioning.

ESSENTIAL SIMILARITIES TEST: Similarities subtests; Stanford-Binet, age level SA I; requires a high level of abstraction.

ESTIMATE QUESTIONS: (Shallice & Evans, 1978); evaluation of practical judgment; sensitive to anterior lesions.

ESTIMATION TESTS: WAIS-R Information subtest, Cognitive Estimate. Questions; test ability to apply knowledge, to compare, to make mental projections, and to evaluate conclusions.

ESTROGEN: controls fertility and development of secondary sexual characteristics; normal gonadal function depends upon stimulation from gonadotropic hormones of adenohypophysis (anterior pituitary gland).

et: and.

ETHANOL: ethanol, ETOH, alcohol in beverages.

ETOH: alcohol; ethanol.

EUTHYMIC: normal functioning of the thymus; used to describe normal mood states.

EUPHORIA: abnormal sense of well-being.

EVOKED POTENTIALS: (EP) consist of a short train of large slow waves recorded from the scalp and largely reflect the activities of the dendrites; usually several EPs are averaged together (AEP) to obtain an accurate estimate of the EP.

EXACERBATION: increase in severity of disease or any of its symptoms.

EXAM: examination.

EXCITOMOTOR AREA: precentral gyrus.

EXECUTIVE FUNCTIONS: four components: 1. goal formulation; 2. planning; 3. carrying out goal-directed plans; and 4. effective performance; necessary for appropriate, socially responsible, and effectively adult conduct; located in the frontal lobe particularly in the prefrontal regions in the orbital or medial structures (Damsio, 1979; Hécaen & Albert, 1978; Luria, 1966, 1973b; Seron, 1978); sensitive to damage in other parts of the brain such as subcortical lesions; other causes besides traumatic brain injury include anozia, Korsakoff's psychosis, and Parkinson's disease.

EXECUTIVE FUNCTIONS TESTS: attention to external/situational cues tests: Problem of Fact (Stanford-Binet), Cookie Theft picture from the Boston Diagnostic Aphasia Examination; planning tests:

Bender-Gestalt, Thematic Apperception Test, WAIS-R Block Design, Sentence Building (Stanford-Binet SA I, 1960 Revision), Complex Figure Test, Porteus Maze Test, goal formulation; purposive behavior tests: Tinkertoy Test; Self-regulation tests: (flexibility and the capacity to shift), Bender-Gestalt Test, Luria-type tests, Line Tracing Task, Tracing, Tapping, and Dotting (subtests of MacQuarrie Test for Mechanical Ability), Stroop Color/Word Test, motor impersistence Tests, and self-correction tests.

EXHIBITIONISM: may be caused by dorsolateral frontal-lobe dysfunction.

EXOCRINE GLANDS: duct glands whose hormones do not enter the bloodstream, but are carried to the target organs by ducts.

EXODEVIATION: see exophoria.

EXOGENOUS: arising from factors outside of the individual.

EXOPHORIA: a form of heterophoria in which there is deviation of the visual axis of one eye away from that of the other eye in the absence of visual fusional stimuli; also called exodeviation.

EXOPHTHALAMOS: abnormal protrusion of the eyeball.

EXPRESSIVE APHASIA: difficulty in producing language; see also Broca's a., ataxic a., motor a., frontocortical a., verbal a.

EXPRESSIVE DEFICIT TESTS: provide information about how effectively the subject perceives and integrates the elements of a picture (Lezak, 1982b) and about such aspects of verbal ability as word choice, vocabulary level, grammar and syntax, and richness and complexity of statements. Story Telling; Cookie Jar Theft picture from the Boston Aphasia Exam (Goodglass & Kaplan, 1972); Smashed Window picture (Wells & Ruesch, 1969); Birthday Party picture from the Stanford-Binet Scales (Terman & Merrill, 1973).

EXPRESSIVE FUNCTIONS: speaking, drawing, or writing, manipulation, physical gestures, facial expressions or movements that make up the sum of observable behavior; disturbances of expressive functions are called apraxias.

EXPRESSIVE-RECEPTIVE APHASIA: global aphasia.

ext.: external; extract.

EXTENSOR MUSCLES: any muscle that extends a joint.

EXTERNAL CUES TESTS: see attention to external cues tests.

EXTEROCEPTIVE SENSATION: superficial, cutaneous sensation.

EXTEROCEPTIVE STIMULI: stimuli originating outside the body and sensed by receptors located on or near the body surface; distinguished from interoceptive stimuli, which originate in the viscera.

EXTINCTION: see cortical inattention or inattention; suppression of stimuli from one side of the body; may be polymodality or single modality neglect; most often caused by parietal-lobe lesions; also a procedure by which learned behavior is eliminated through the omission of reinforcement.

E

EXTINCTION TESTS: visual: patient fixes eyes upon examiner's face while examiner moves fingers in both right and left peripheral fields; asked to report which fingers are moving; auditory: examiner stands behind the patient and snaps fingers or some other stimulus of equal intensity.

EXTORTION OF EYE: tilting of the upper part of the vertical meridian of the eye away from the midline of the face; lesion of the 4th nerve.

EXTRADURAL: outside the dura mater.

EXTRAFUSAL FIBERS: fibers that, along with intrafusal fibers, make up skeletal mucles; reciprocal action of the two kinds of fibers produces muscle tension, which is regulated by the stretch reflex.

EXTRA-OCCULAR MUSCLES: the medial rectus muscle of one eye and the lateral rectus muscle of the other work as a pair to produce lateral eye movements; the vertical acting rectus muscles are most effective when the eye is abducted; the oblique muscles are maximally effective when the eye is adducted.

EXTRAPYRAMIDAL DISORDER: kinesia; difficulty in rapid alternating sequences of movement; see also extrapyramidal reaction, Parkinson's disease.

EXTRAPYRAMIDAL LESION SIGNS TEST: finger-to-nose test or rapidly and repeatedly touching index finger with thumb.

EXTRAPYRAMIDAL REACTION: (EPR) body flexion, rigidity, immobility, paucity of automatic movements, head rigid, arms held stiffly in front of body, facial expression unblinking and masklike, trunk bent forward, short steps, and shuffle; usually caused by neuroleptic medication; see also oculargyral crisis.

EXTRAPYRAMIDAL SYNDROMES: disorders which result from lesions involving those parts of the brain other than the corticospinal pathways which are concerned with movement; parkinsonian syndrome, Wilson's disease, chorea (Sydenham's chorea, Huntington's chorea, hemiballismus, progressive supranuclear palsy, i.e., Richardson-Steele-Olszewski syndrome), athetosis, spasmodic torticollis, tardive dyskinesia (Brain, 1985).

EXTRAPYRAMIDAL SYSTEM: pathways in the extrapyramidal system originate in the cortex but synapse and gather information from a number of areas before they reach the spinal cord; synapse with a group of structures surrounding the thalamus, the caudate, putamen, and globus pallidus, collectively known as the basal ganglia which are thought to be involved in control of spontaneous motor activity; collect information from the reticular formation, the cerebellum, and the vestibular system, all involved to different degrees in sensing the position and balance of the body; in the medulla, it gives rise to two major tracts: the reticulospinal and the vestibulospinal, both of which continue down the cord and end in the central gray matter in the cord; the vestibulospinal tract conveys the information originally gathered by the receptors in the vestibular system (sense position of the head); both tracts synapse directly or indirectly with motor neurons in the spinal cord; two types of motor neurons involved: alpha motor neurons which synapse with the extrafusal fibers and the gamma motor neurons of the gamma efferents which are issued from the ventral part of the spinal cord and synapse with the intrafusal fibers; gamma efferents are the ultimate reason that muscle tone varies depending on the posture and position of the body; governs the information that allows muscles to assume the background condition (tension and position) necessary to movement; governs the discrete muscular movements; changes in body position sensed by the proprioceptor senses (kinesthetic) which then convey information to the cerebellum; changes in position sensed by the exteroreceptors which convey information to the sensory cortex.

EX VACUO: wasting of white matter.

EX VACUO HYDROCEPHALUS: compensatory replacement by cerebrospinal fluid of the volume of tissue lost in atrophy of the brain.

EYE DEVIATION INWARD: abducens nerve (VI).

EYE DEVIATION OUTWARD: oculomotor nerve (III).

EYE FIELD DEFECTS: right homonymous hemianopia: lesion of left optic tract or internal capsule; right macular sparing hemianopia: lesions of the left occipital cortex; bitemporal hemianopia: chiasmal compression; right upper quadrantic hemianopia: lesion of the left anterior temporal lobe.

EYE GAZE - VOLUNTARY - IMPAIRMENT: Brodmann's areas 8 & 9 (Teuber, 1964; Tyler, 1969).

EYE MUSCLE NERVES (EXTRINSIC): oculomotor, trochlear, and abducens.

F

F: Fahrenheit.

FACE-HAND SENSORY TEST: (Smith, 1980) subtest in the Michigan Neuropsychological Test Battery.

FACE-HAND TEST: (Bender et al., 1951) a test for tactile inattention/ extinction.

FACIAL HEMIPLEGIA: paralysis of one side of the face, the body being unaffected.

FACIAL NERVE (VII): controls facial movements and expression; originates in the inferior border of the pons, between the olive and inferior cerebellar peduncle; purely motor except for the chorda

F

tympani which conveys taste sensation from the anterior 2/3 of the tongue; joins the 7th nerve in the middle ear; supplies the forehead muscle (frontalis), all the muscles of facial expression, and the neck muscle (platysma); supplies the tensor tympani; a complete lesion affects auditory acuity on the affected side.

FACIAL NERVE PALSY: see Cerebello-Pontine angle lesions.

FACIAL PAIN: see trigeminal nerve (V).

FACIAL PARALYSIS: lesion of the facial nerve (VII); see also Bell's Palsy.

FACIAL RECOGNITION OF WELL-KNOWN PERSONS TEST: (Warrington & James, 1967b; Milner, 1968); has a memory component; sensitive to right-hemisphere damage.

FACIAL RECOGNITION WITHOUT MEMORY COMPONENT: (Benton & Van Allen, 1968; Benton et al., 1983); matching of pictures of faces; sensitive to right parietal-lobe lesions; sensitive to aphasic conditions (Hamsher et al., 1979).

FACIAL SENSATION: trigeminal Nerve (V).

FACICULUS CUNEATUS: an ascending spinal tract that collects pressure information from the upper part of the body and synapses in the medulla.

FACICULUS GRACILIS: an ascending tract that collects pressure information from the lower part of the body and synapses in the medulla.

FACIOBRACHIAL HEMIPLEGIA: paralysis of one half of the face and of the arm on the same side.

FACIOLINGUAL HEMIPLEGIA: paralysis of one side of the face and tongue.

FAINTNESS: lack of strength, with sensation of impending loss of consciousness.

FANTASY: an imaginary sequence of events or mental images often used to resolve emotional conflict.

FAS TEST: (Benton, 1968) a word generator test; sensitive indicator of brain dysfunction particularly frontal-lobe lesions regardless of side; left-sided lesions depress scores one-third more than right-sided lesions (Benton, 1968; Miceli et al., 1981; Perret, 1974; Ramier & Hécaen, 1970); bilateral lesions tend to lower verbal production more than one-third (Benton, 1968); Alzheimer's-type dementia reduces word generation (Miller & Hague, 1975); no depression of word generation with depression that mimics organic deterioration (Kronfol et al., 1978).

FASCICLES: the parts of a nerve that course through the substance of the brainstem.

FBS: fasting blood sugar.

FEAR/RAGE REACTIONS: see central gray, tegmentum, periaqueductal gray; hypothalamus; amydala.

FEEBLEMINDEDNESS: congenital amentia.

FEEDING REFLEXES: ventromedial hypothalamus.

FEELING TONE: state of one's emotional feelings.

FESTINATING GAIT: an involuntary tendency to take short, accelerating steps in walking; see also paralysis agitans, Parkinson's disease.

FESTINATION: involuntary increase or hastening of gait.

F. Hx: Family history.

FIBRILLATION: small, local involuntary contraction of muscle, invisible under the skin, resulting from spontaneous activation of single muscle cells or muscle fibers; *atrial f.*: atrial arrhythmia characterized by rapid randomized contractions of the atrial myocardium, causing a totally irregular, often rapid ventricular rate; *ventricular f.*: arrhythmia characterized by fibrillary contractions of the ventricular muscle due to rapid repetitive excitation of myocardial fibers without coordinated contraction of the ventricle; an expression of randomized circus movement or of an ectopic focus with a very rapid cycle.

FIELD DEFECTS: areas of blindness within the visual field of one or both eyes depending upon whether the lesion involves the visual pathways before or after the chiasma; see also scotoma.

FIFTH CRANIAL NERVE: trigeminal nerve; emerges from the lateral surface of the pons as a motor and a sensory root, together with some intermediate fibers; sensory root expands into the trigeminal ganglion, which contains the cells of origin of most of the sensory fibers, and from which the three divisions of the nerve arise (mandibularis, maxillaris, and ophthalmicus); sensory in supplying the face, teeth, mouth, and nasal cavity; motor in supplying the muscles of mastication.

FIGURE AND DESIGN RECOGNITION TESTS: Perceptual recognition of meaningless designs is usually tested by having the patient draw them from models or memory; the WAIS-R Picture Completion subtest, picture vocabulary tests, such as the Peabody Picture Vocabulary Test or the Picture Vocabulary subtest of the Stanford-Binet Scales can be used to show that the subject can recognize meaningful pictures; patients with verbal comprehension problems can be examined by the picture-matching tests of the Leiter or ITPA; or the Forms subtest from the Stanford Binet; Raven's Progressive Matrices Test (first 12 items) (Lezak, 1983).

FINAL COMMON PATHWAY: the alpha motor neuron is the final link between the central nervous system and the skeletal muscles; impulses affecting a skeletal muscle travel in an alpha motor neuron, regardless of where they originate.

FINE MOTOR REGULATION TESTS: see Line Tracing Task (Lezak, 1983); MacQuarrie Test for Mechanical Ability, Tracing, Tapping,

F

and Dotting subtests.

FINGER AGNOSIA: inability to identify fingers; may occur with lesions in either hemisphere (Benton, 1979; Boll, 1974; Kinsbourne & Warrington, 1962); also see Gerstmann's syndrome.

FINGER AGNOSIA TESTS: (Benton, 1959, 1979; Benton et al., 1983; Gainotti et al., 1972); tactile finger recognition test.

FINGER TAPPING TEST: (Reitan & Davison, 1974; Russell et al., 1970) manual dexterity test in the Halstead-Reitan battery; anxiety tends to depress score of women; slowing occurs with age; slowing of finger tapping usually is sensitive to brain damage and contralateral lesions (Finlayson & Reiten, 1980; Haaland & Delaney, 1981); sensitive to Dilantin levels (Dodrill, 1975).

FINGER-TO-NOSE TEST: to test for extrapyramidal lesion signs. the patient touches examiner's fingertip and then the tip of his own nose repeatedly.

FINGERTIP NUMBER-WRITING PERCEPTION TESTS: test for tactile-perceptual defects. (Goldstein & Shelley, 1974; Reitan & Davison, 1974); also called Fingertip Writing (Russell et al., 1970).

FISSURE OF NEOCORTEX: cleft in neocortex (sulcus) that extends deeply enough into the brain to indent the ventricles; see Sylvian and Rolandic fissures; divide the frontal lobes from the parietal lobes and the temporal lobes from the frontal and parietal lobes.

FISTULA: an abnormal passage or communication, usually between two internal organs, or leading from an internal organ to the surface of the body.

FIVE (5)-hydroxytryptamine: (5-HT): chemical neuro-transmitter, serotonin.

FIXATION: an arrest of the development of part of the personality at some point in the maturing process.

FIXED PUPILS: the pupils do not accommodate to light (constrict); see Parinaud syndrome, Argyll-Robertson pupil.

FLACCID HEMIPLEGIA: paralysis on one side with loss of tone of the muscles of the paralyzed part and absence of tendon reflexes.

FLATTENED AFFECT: see blunted affect.

FLEXED POSTURE: see Ataxia of Bruns.

FLEXOR ACTIVITY: first major reflexes to return following spinal section/lesion; consists of such movements as dorsiflexion of the big toe and fanning of the toe, dorsiflexion of the foot, and flexion of the leg and thigh.

FLEXOR MUSCLES: flexes and adducts; bends.

FLIGHT OF IDEAS: a nearly continuous flow of accelerated speech which reflect thoughts that move nimbly and abruptly from one idea to another before the first topic is concluded; associations are numerous and loosely linked although the associations are usually understandable; the ideas may be prompted by distracting stimuli, or plays on words; when severe, the speech may be incoherent; common in hypomania and manic states and sometimes occurs in acute reactions to stress, organic mental disorders, or schizophrenia.

FLOCCULONODULAR LOBE: see cerebellar location.

FLUENCY OF SPEECH: measured by the quantity of words produced or by word-naming tests, usually within a restricted category or to a stimulus, and usually within a time limit; also involves short-term memory in keeping track of what words have already been said (Estes, 1974); demonstrates how well thinking is organized; dominent frontal-lobe function.

FLUENT APHASIA: speech is well articulated and grammatically correct but lacking in content; see Wernicke's aphasia; lesion in the dominent parietal lobe.

FLUID BALANCE: see hypothalamus.

FOCAL SEIZURES: epilepic seizures that begin locally and then spread as in Jacksonian seizures: begins with jerks of single parts of the body, such as a finger, a toe, or the mouth, and then spreads to adjacent parts (Jacksonian march).

FOCI: locations of brain lesions.

FOLLICLE STIMULATING HORMONE (FSH): brings about follicular maturation (ova development in ovarian follicles) in females; acts on the seminiferous tubules to stimulate sperm production in males.

FORAMINA OF LUSCHKA: an opening at the end of each lateral recess of the fourth ventricle by which the ventricular cavity communicates with the subarachnoid space.

FORAMAN OF MAGENDIE: a deficiency in the lower portion of the roof of the fourth ventricle through which the ventricular cavity communicates with the subarachnoid space.

FOREBRAIN: forward most part of the brain; includes the telencephalon and the thalamus of the diencephalon; divided into six anatomical areas: neocortex, basal ganglia, limbic system, thalamus, olfactory bulbs and tract, and lateral ventricles; one of three major subdivisions of the brain; also called the prosencephalon.

FOREBRAIN (FRONTAL LOBE) LESION: impairment of the ability to use objects correctly because of impaired sequencing ability to organize appropriate units of voluntary movements to manipulate the object; apraxia; may also cause sexual dysfunction because of inability to voluntarily sequence actions.

FORGETTING CURVES: require reexamination over time; provide an indirect means of measuring the amount of material retained after it has been learned; poor performance may be due to the patient's lack of drive or motivation; caused by either frontal-lobe dysfunction or depression.

FORMAL THOUGHT DISORDER: this is not used as a specific

F

descriptive term in DSM III-R; see loose associations, incoherence, poverty of speech, neologisms, blocking, echolalia, and clanging.

FORMICATION: sensation as of small insects crawling over the skin.

FOSSA: a general term for a hole or depressed area.

FOURTH NERVE: (trochlear nerve) motor nerve: controls extrinsic eye muscles (superior oblique muscle); governs asymmetry of eye movements; nucleus lies in the dorsum of the brainstem and the fibers decussate in the substance of the superior medullary velum so that the right nerve originates in the left trochlear nucleus and vice versa; emerges from the back of the brainstem below the corresponding inferior colliculus; runs a very long course; leaves the posterior fossa and encircles the brainstem to enter the cavernous sinus; traverses the roof of the orbital fissure, and crosses the third nerve in order to do so.

FOURTH NERVE LESION: causes extorsion of the eye and weakness of downward gaze; most marked when the eye is turned inward; the patient has special difficulty going downstairs; head tilts to opposite shoulder to compensate for diplopia.

FOURTH NERVE PALSY: weakness of the superior oblique muscle with subtle diplopia when looking straight ahead which the patient may compensate for by tilting his head slightly away from the side of the affected eye to line up the image from the normal eye; frank diplopia occurs when the patient looks down and away from the side of the affected eye which may lead to trouble going downstairs.

FRAGMENTED VISUAL STIMULI TESTS: Hooper Visual Organization Test; Minnesota Paper Form Board Test.

FREE AND SERIAL CLASSIFICATION TEST: (Krauss, 1978) test of conceptual functioning in older persons.

FREE ASSOCIATIONS: ideas that are allowed to arise spontaneously without conscious restraint or selective criticism.

FRIEDREICH'S ATAXIA: an inherited disease, usually beginning in childhood, with sclerosis of the dorsal and lateral columns of the spinal cord; symptoms include ataxia, speech impairment, lateral curvature of the spinal column, and peculiar swaying especially of the lower limbs.

FRÖHLICH'S SYNDROME: a condition of obesity and genital atrophy; damage in the ventromedial hypothalamus.

FRONTAL LOBES: anatomically fixed boundaries; bounded posteriorly by the central sulcus, inferiorly by the lateral fissure, and medially by the cingulate sulcus just above the corpus callosum; four major gyri: superior, middle, inferior, and the precentral (in front of the central sulcus); includes the motor strip (area 4), supplementary motor area (area 6), the frontal eye fields (area 8), the cortical center for micturition (the medial surface of the frontal lobe); connections with the temporal lobe, parietal lobe, basal ganglia, hypothalamus, and cerebellum; olfactory bulb and tract, and the optic nerves lie under the lobe; play a major role in personality, particularly in respect to acquired social behavior.

FRONTAL-LOBE ATAXIA: small shuffling, hesitant steps; turning accomplished by a series of tiny, uncertain steps made with one foot, the other acting as a pivot; dementia usually present; loss of integration at the cortical and basal ganglionic level of the essential elements of stance and locomotion; Babinski's signs may or may not be present.

FRONTAL-LOBE LESION: lesions cause spastic paralysis of the contralateral face, arm, and leg; *eyes*: paralysis of contralateral gaze; eyes turn towards the side of the lesion; if bilateral, unable to turn the eyes in any direction, but retains fixation and following movements.

FRONTAL LOBE LESION DEFICITS: *left-hemisphere lesion*: reduced spontaneous verbal fluency, to a lessor degree, verbal learning; impaired block construction, memory for verbal recency/order of presentation, design copying, and proverb interpretation; *right-hemisphere lesion*: impaired memory for nonverbal or pictorial recency/ order of presentation, block construction, design copying; to a lessor degree, verbal fluency (excessive talking), verbal learning; impaired interpretation of proverbs; *bilateral lesions*: severe deficits in verbal learning, verbal fluency, interpretation of proverbs, time orientation, design copying, block construction, ability to initiate spontaneously a desired or an automatic task; loss of drive, apathy, concern for personal appearance, personal hygiene, work, etc.; dysinhibition may be present; severe decline in intellect coupled with memory impairment, perseveration, inability to perform double simultaneous tracking, poor sequencing ability; activities of daily living may be carried out at any time or place, without regard for the social consequences (Hécaen & Albert, 1975); pseudodepression/loss of interest in environment; deficits in ability to serially order complex chains of behavior in relation to varying stimuli.

FRONTAL-LOBE SYNDROME: specific personality changes; may be no cognitive deficits; apathy; unconstructive euphoria; short-lived irritability; social inappropriateness; lost interest in environmental and social activities; failure in job performance; poor family relationships; sometimes poor personal cleanliness; may not usually lower IQ.

FRONTAL-LOBE TESTS: Wisconsin card-sort; Stroop color-word test; Semmes body-placing test; left-right differentiation test; Thurstone word fluency test; motor function tests such as hand dynamometer, finger tapping speed, and movement sequencing; Token test for quick aphasia screening; spelling test; phonetic differentiation test; clinical evaluation of pseudodepression or pseu-

F

dopsychopathology.

FRONTAL-LOBE LESIONS & MEMORY DEFICITS: (Corsi, 1972; Prisko, 1963) deficit in the memory of the temporal ordering of events; asymmetry in the function of the left frontal lobe (recency memory defect for verbal material) and right frontal lobe (recency memory defect for nonverbal material).

FRONTALIS MUSCLE: forehead.

FRONTAL OPERCULUM: the part of the inferior frontal gyrus between the anterior and ascending branches of the lateral sulcus, covering over a part of the insula; lesion causes agrammatism.

FRONTOCORTICAL APHASIA: Broca's aphasia, ataxic a., motor a., and verbal a.

FRONTOLENTICULAR APHASIA: see commissural aphasia.

FSH: follicle stimulating hormone; secreted by the anterior pituitary gland.

FULD OBJECT-MEMORY EVALUATION: (Fuld, 1977) a test designed to assess several aspects of learning and retrieval in elderly persons and also provide information about tactile recognition, right-left discrimination, and verbal fluency.

FULMINATING: occurring suddenly and with great intensity.

FULMINATING ANOXIA: a rapid fall in the oxygen content of the blood.

FUNCTIONAL APHASIA: aphasia resulting from hysteria or severe hysterical disorder.

FUNCTIONAL LEVELS - SELF RATING: (Heaton, Chelune, & Lehman, 1981) Patient's Assessment of Own Functioning Inventory; an 8-category test that assesses how well the patient is aware of his own condition.

FUNCTIONAL UNITS IMPORTANT IN NEUROPSYCHOLOGICAL EVALUATION: general intelligence, visuoperceptual abilities, memory, spatial discrimination, somatosensory function, language, hippocampal function, frontal-lobe function, and motor function.

FUNGAL INFECTIONS OF CNS: include aspergillosis, cryptococcosis, histoplasmosis, actinomycosis, mucormycosis, cerebral nocardiosis, coccidioidomycosis, blastomycosis, candidiasis, and clodosporiosis [see Reitan & Wolfson (1985) for more detail].

FUNGUS: any members of a large group of lower plants that lack chlorophyll and subsist on living or dead organic matter; the fungi include yeast, molds, and mushrooms.

G

GABA: gamma-aminobutyric acid; inhibitory transmitter; hyperpolarizes the postsynaptic membrane by changing its permeability to postive potassium ions and negative chlorine ions.

GAIN, PRIMARY: the gain to the patient from the emotional illness itself; the dynamic "reason" for the illness.

GAIN, SECONDARY: the gain to the patient from outside sources (monitary settlements, attention from others, etc.) from the continued or exacerbated symptoms of the illness.

GAIT DISORDERS: may be caused by lesions to the cerebellum, peripheral nerves, posterior roots, posterior columns of spinal cord, medial lemnisci, and sometimes both parietal lobes; see cerebellar gait, alcoholism (chronic), multiple sclerosis, proprioception disorder, festinating, spastic, ataxia, sensory ataxia, marche à petits pas, extrapyramidal, athetotic, dystonic, choreic, equine, waddling, staggering, hysterical, frontal-lobe ataxia, and senile, hemiplegic, and paraplegic gaits.

GAIT, SHORT, ACCELERATING: festinating gait.

GAG REFLEX: see glossopharyngeal nerve IX.

GALLOPS: a disordered rhythm of the heart; an auscultatory finding of three or four heart sounds, the extra sound(s) by convention, being in diastole and related either to atrial contraction, to early rapid filling of a ventricle with an altered ventricular compliance, or to concurrence of atrial contraction and ventricular early rapid filling.

GALVESTON ORIENTATION AND AMNESIA TEST (GOAT): (Levin, O'Donnel, & Grossman, 1979); a short mental status exam devised to assess the extent and duration of posttraumatic amnesia and confusion; may be repeated as often as desired; error score is 0 - 100; Levin suggests that formal neuropsychological testing should not begin before the patient has achieved a GOAT score of 75 or less.

GAMMA-AMINOBUTYRIC ACID: GABA.

GAMMA EFFERENT SYSTEM: the system by which the brain controls muscle tone via the extrapyramidal system and the intrafusal fibers.

GANGLION: a general term for a group of cell bodies located outside of the CNS; occasionally applied to certain nuclear groups within the brain or spinal cord; groups of neural cell bodies and dendrites outside the brain and the spinal cord; ganglia in the autonomic nervous system include the sympathetic ganglia, which are located immediately outside the spinal cord and form the sympathetic cord, and parasympathetic ganglia, found near their target organs.

GATES-MACGINITIE READING TESTS: measure different aspects

G

of reading separately (Gates & MacGinitie, 1965, 1969).

GAZE (LATERAL): controlled by the medial longitudinal fasciculus which connects one abducens nucleus with the opposite oculomotor nucleus.

GAZE (VERTICAL): controlled by the pretectal areas and paramedian zones of midbrain tegmentum.

GAZE - VOLUNTARY - DEFICITS IN: frontal-lobe lesions (Teuber, 1964).

GELB-GOLDSTEIN WOOL SORTING TEST: see color sorting test.

GENERAL PARESIS: progressive deterioration of the brain due to syphilitic infection; symptoms include progressive mental deterioration leading to dementia, impairment of judgment, changes in personality, irritability, emotional lability, manic episodes, deterioration of personal grooming, apathy, and mental obtundity, and eventual disorientation with paranoid delusions or hallucinations (Reitan & Wolfson, 1985).

GENERALIZED SEIZURES: (grand mal) bilaterally symmetrical seizures without local onset; often preceded by an aura; characterized by loss of consciousness and sterotyped motor stages: 1. tonic stage, in which the body stiffens and breathing stops; 2. clonic stage, in which there is rhythmic shaking; and 3. post-seizure (post-ictal) depression, in which the patient is confused.

GENICULATE BODY: the part of the facial nerve at the lateral end of the internal acoustic meatus, where the fibers turn sharply postero-inferiorly, and where the geniculate ganglion is found; see also corpus geniculatum laterale, corpus geniculatum mediale.

GENICULOSTRIATE SYSTEM: projections received along the optic nerve from the retina of the eye go to the lateral geniculate nucleus of the thalamus, then to the neocortex in Brodmann's areas 17, 18, and 19, and finally 20 and 21; involved in the perception and analysis of forms, colors, and patterns; combines with the tectopulvinar system in areas 20 and 21 where the geniculostriate system analyzes the form and content which the tectopulvinar system has located.

GERIATRIC INTERPERSONAL RATING SCALE: (Plutchick et al., 1971); a check list which covers the most pertinent areas of mental status: personal orientation, attention, mental tracking, verbal abstraction, language usage, recent and remote memory, digits forward and backwards, simple math, humor, card sorting, and matching.

GERIATRIC RATING SCALE: (Plutchick et al., 1970) adapted from the Stockton Geriatric Rating Scale; 31 questions designed to be answered regarding the behavior of inpatient geriatric patients to assess social abilities such as eating, toileting, self-direction, and sociability; evaluates withdrawal/ apathy, antisocial disruptive behavior, and deficits in activities of daily living.

G

GERIATRIC INTERPERSONAL RATING SCALE: (Plutchick et al., 1971); a check list which covers the most pertinent areas of mental status: personal orientation, attention, mental tracking, verbal abstraction, language usage, recent and remote memory, digits forward and backwards, simple math, humor, card sorting, and matching.

GERIATRIC RATING SCALE: (Plutchick et al., 1970) adapted from the Stockton Geriatric Rating Scale; 31 questions designed to be answered regarding the behavior of inpatient geriatric patients to assess social abilities such as eating, toileting, self-direction, and sociability; evaluates withdrawal/ apathy, antisocial disruptive behavior, and deficits in activities of daily living.

GENU: a general term used to designate any anatomical structure bent like the knee; *capsulae internae genu of internal capsule*: the blunt angle formed by the union of the two limbs of the internal capsule, situated posterior to the caudate nucleus, anterior to the thalamus, and medial to the lentiform nucleus; *genu of the corpus callosum*: the sharp ventral curve at the anterior end of the trunk of the corpus callosum; plural: genua.

GERSTMANN'S SYNDROME: inability to write (agraphia), inability to calculate (acalulia), failure to distinguish right from left, loss of recognition of various fingers and toes, and constructional apraxia; true agnosia; lesion in the dominant angular gyrus (parietal lobe).

GESELL DEVELOPMENTAL SCHEDULES: (Gesell, 1940; Gesell et al., 1949) assesses developmental behavior from four weeks to six years that can be compared with normative data for motor, language, adaptive, and personal-social behavior; may be used for assessment of severely brain-damaged patients.

GESTALT COMPLETION TEST: see Street Completion Test.

GIANTISM: result of hypersecretion of somatotropic hormone in childhood.

GIBBERISH APHASIA: jargon aphasia; Wernicke's aphasia.

GIDDINESS: swaying type of dizziness.

GILLES DE LA TOURETTE SYNDROME: movement disorder; begins with single or multiple tics in early childhood or adolescence between age 3 and 14; initial symptoms: involuntary movements; tics of the face, arms, limbs, and trunk which are frequent, repetitive, and rapid; most common is facial tic (eye blink, nose twitch, grimmace), replaced by or added to by other tics of the neck, trunk, and limbs; other tics: kicking, stamping, touching, repetitive thoughts, and movements, and compulsions; verbal tics include grunting, throat clearing, shouting, barking, coprolalia, etc.; symptoms wax and wane; new symptoms may be added or replace old ones; symptoms may remit for a while; caused by a biochemical dysfunction in the basal ganglia; may be genetically transmitted; often treated with

G

Haloperidol (Tourette Syndrome Association).

GLAND: an organ that manufactures and secretes hormones that affect the activity of other organs; two types are endocrine glands and exocrine glands.

GLASGOW COMA SCALE: (Teasdale & Jennett, 1974) can be used to assess any posttraumatic, altered consciousness level; total scores range from 3 (most impaired) and 13 (normal); may be used by nurses or doctors although Teasdale (1974) has stated that "only physicians" are qualified to use it; accepted in many circles as a standard measure for determining severity of injury; said to be predictive of outcome (Jennett et al., 1975; Levin, Grossman et al., 1979; Plum & Caronna, 1975).

GLASGOW OUTCOME SCALE: (Jennett & Bond, 1975; Bond, 1979) a "goodness of outcome" test that has five levels: Death to Good Recovery; however, the scale does not evaluate the obvious levels of impairment within their "good recovery" category.

GLIOBLASTOMA: see tumor.

GLIA: supporting cells.

GLIOMA: a tumor composed of tissue which represents neuroglia in any one of its stages of development; term sometimes extended to include all the primary intrinsic neoplasms of the brain and spinal cord, including astrocytomas, ependymomas, neurocytomas, etc.

GLOBAL AMNESIA - TRANSIENT: see Transient Global Amnesia.

GLOBAL APHASIA: inability either to speak or comprehend; hemiparesis present; may be able to say only a few words; cannot read or write; understands only a few words and phrases; often accompanied by right hemiplegia, right hemianesthesia, and homonymous hemianopia; consciousness level varies; due to a lesion that destroys a large part of the speech areas of the major cerebral hemisphere; usually due to occlusion of the left internal carotid or middle cerebral artery at its origin.

GLOBUS PALLIDUS: part of the basal ganglia; involved in spontaneous movement and food intake; lies on the medial side of the putamen and is separated from the optic thalamus and the caudate nucleus by the internal capsule (Brain, 1985).

GLOSSOLALIA: speech in unknown or imaginary language, such as "speaking in tongues."

GLOSSOPHARYNGEAL NERVE (IX): serves tongue and pharynx; taste and gag reflex.

GLOVE AND STOCKING ANESTHESIA: see polyneuropathy.

GLYCOGEN: the chief carbohydrate storage material in animals; formed by and largely stored in the liver and to a lesser extent in muscles; depolymerized to glucose and liberated as needed.

GNOSIA: the faculty of perceiving and recognizing.

GOAL FORMULATION: refers to the complex process of determining what one needs or wants and conceptualizing some kind of future realization of that need or want; the capacity to formulate a goal or form an intention; involves motivation and awareness of oneself psychologically, physically, and of one's surroundings; impairment in the the capacity to formulate goals; apathety; unable to initiate activities; unable to carry out complex activities even though fully capable of doing so; unable to assume responsibilities requiring appreciation of long-term or abstract goals; unable to enter into new activities independently; poor grooming; disorientation to date, place, and time suggest an inability to be alert to or appreciate environmental cues; usually a result of frontal-lobe dysfunction.

GOAL FORMULATION TESTS: attention to external/situational cues: Problem of Fact Test (Stanford-Binet); Cookie Theft Picture test from the Boston Diagnostic Aphasia Examination; Planning Tests; maze learning tests.

GOAL IDEA: the idea to be reached in order to answer a question or solve a problem.

GOAT: Galveston Orientation and Amnesia Test.

GOLLIN FIGURES TEST: (Gollin, 1960) incomplete drawings to assess perceptual functions; sensitive to right parietal-lobe lesions.

GOLLIN INCOMPLETE FIGURES TEST: test of visual perception; sensitive to right parietal-cortex damage.

GONADOTROPIC HORMONE: secretion of anterior pituitary gland.

GONODS: a gamete-producing gland; an ovary or testis; normal gonadal function depends upon stimulation from gonadotropic hormones of the adenohypophysis (anterior pituitary gland).

GOODWIN PSYCHOSOCIAL ASSESSMENT BATTERY: (Goodwin, 1983b) a psychosocial predictive battery for post head-injured patients that uses the scaled scores from the WAIS-R Performance Scale subtests, Digit Span from the Verbal Scale subtest, and standardized scores from Trail Making Tests A and B at 6 months post-injury to predict psychosocial adjustment at 2 years post-injury.

GORHAM'S PROVERBS TEST: (Gorham, 1956) formalizes the task of proverb interpretation and scoring; written test; sensitive to bilateral and right frontal-lobe disease; sensitive to aging.

GRADENIGO'S SYNDROME: sixth nerve may be damaged by mastoiditis or middle ear infection which causes severe ear pain and a combination of 6th, 7th, 8th, and occasionally 5th nerve lesions.

GRANDIOSITY: an inflated appraisal of one's worth, power, knowledge, importance, or identity; when extreme, grandiosity may be of delusional proportions.

GRAND MAL EPILEPSY: *tonic spasm*: occurs first; characterized by muscle spasms which tend to be symmetrical on both sides of the body; head, mouth,and eyes may be turned to one side; upper limbs

G

adducted at shoulders and flexed at other joints; lower limbs extended with the feet inverted; breathing ceases during tonic phase, lasting from a few seconds to half a minute; *clonic*: tonic spasms become clonic with sharp, short, interrupted jerks; tongue may be bitten and mouth may foam; incontinence; unconscious state for variable time (minutes to half an hour) followed by sleepiness and confusion; headache after attack; may be ideopathic or a result of cerebral lesion in any lobe of the brain, most often in one frontal lobe or temporal lobe (Brain, 1985).

GRANULAR FRONTAL CORTEX: Brodmann's areas 9, 10, 45, 46, and 47; prefrontal lobe, or tertiary zones of the frontal unit; the integrated area of function (the superstructure) above all other parts of the cerebral cortex where the formation of intentions takes place (Luria, 1973a).

GRAPHEMES: basic units of writing in a given language which are combined to form written words.

GRAPHESTHESIA: inability to identify numbers or letters traced on the skin with a blunt object.

GRAPHOMOTOR APHASIA: the person cannot express himself in writing.

GRASHEY'S APHASIA: aphasia due to lessened duration of sensory impressions, causing disturbance of perception and association, without lack of function of the centers or conductivity of the tracts; seen in acute diseases and concussion of the brain.

GRAVE'S DISEASE: a disorder of the thyroid of unknown etiology, occuring most often in women, and characterized by exophthalmos, enlarged pulsating thyroid gland, marked acceleration of the pulse rate, a tendency to profuse sweats, nervous symptoms (including fine muscular tremors, restlessness, and irritability), psychic disturbances, emaciation, and increased metabolic rate.

GRAY COMMISSURE: a bundle of interneurons in the spinal cord, connecting opposite sides of the cord.

GRAY MATTER: mixture of capillary blood vessels and cell bodies of neurons; masses of cell bodies and dendrites in various parts of the CNS which appear gray because they are not myelinated.

GROOVED PEGBOARD TEST: (Kløve, 1963; Matthews & Kløve, 1964) a manual dexterity test taken from the Wisconsin Neuropsychological Test Battery (Harley et al., 1980) a complex version of the pegboard test; good test to study improvement in motor functions (Haaland et al., 1977; Meier, 1974).

GROPING FOR WORDS: see amnestic dysnomic aphasia, circumlocution.

GROWTH HORMONE: anterior pituitary; somatotropic hormone.

Gm.; gm.: gram.

gtt(s): drop(s).

GTT: glucose tolerance test.

GU: genitourinary.

GUSTATION: the sensation of taste.

GUSTATORY HALLUCINATIONS: hallucinations of taste; temporal-lobe disease/lesion; upper surface of temporal lobe in the depths of the Sylvian fissures.

GUSTATORY NEURAL PATHWAYS: three cranial nerves take part in the transmission process that carries impulses from taste receptors to the brain: facial nerve (VII), which innervates the anterior two-thirds of the tongue, the glossopharyngeal nerve (IX) which innervates the remaining one third; and the vagus nerve (X) which innervates the taste buds located in the pharynx; only a portion of the neural fibers in each is concerned exclusively with taste; the remaining nerve fibers are involved in tactile and temperature sensations in the head as well as in control of the muscles in the face and tongue; all three enter the brain at the medulla; some nerve fibers cross in the brainstem while others remain on the same side; all ascend to the thalamus and then continue to the somatosensory cortex (Brodmann's area 1).

GYN: gynecology.

GYRI TEMPORALES TRANSVERSI: transverse temporal gyrus: the transverse convolutions marking the posterior extremity of the superior temporal gyrus and lying mostly in the lateral sulcus; the more marked of these, the anterior transverse temporal gyrus (Heschl's convolution), represents the cortical center for hearing.

GYRUS: tortuous elevations (convolutions) of the surface of the cerebral hemisphere, caused by infolding of the cortex and separated by fissures or sulci.

GYRUS OF NEOCORTEX: ridge in the neocortex.

GYRUS PRECENTRALIS: precentral gyrus, primary motor cortex.

H

H-R-R PSEUDOISOCHROMATIC PLATES: (Hardy et al., 1955); screens for two rare forms of color blindness which would not be correctly identified by the Ishihara or Dvorine tests; also identifies two other common types of color blindness.

HALLERVORDEN-SPATZ SYNDROME: hereditary disorder characterized by marked reduction in the number of the myelin sheaths of the globus pallidus and substantia nigra with accumulations of iron pigment, progressive rigidity beginning in the legs, choreoathetoid movements, dysarthria, and progressive mental deteriora-

H

tion; transmitted as an autosomal recessive trait, usually begins in the first or second decade, with death occuring before age 30.

HALLUCINATIONS: dreamlike states in which familiar voices, music, scenes, etc. are experienced as being there (real), even when the patient knows that they could not be; perception for which there is no appropriate external stimulus, such as hearing voices that are not really there; see also auditory, gustatory, mood-congruent, mood-incongruent, olfactory, somatic, tactile, and visual hallucinations (Penfield, 1954).

HALLUCINATIONS (AUDITORY): an imaginary perception of sound, most commonly of voices, but sometimes of noises, music, etc.; *auditory*: Brodmann's area 22 of either hemisphere; lesion(s) of the temporal lobes where they involve the reticular activating and limbic systems; characteristic of psychosis.

HALLUCINATIONS (GUSTATORY): an imaginary perception of taste, unpleasant tastes being the most common.

HALLUCINATIONS (MOOD-CONGRUENT): imaginary perceptions considered real by the patient which are consistant with the mood.

HALLUCINATIONS (MOOD-INCONGRUENT): imaginary perceptions considered real by the patient which are inconsistant with the mood.

HALLUCINATIONS (OLFACTORY): imaginary perceptions of smell, most often unpleasant, which the patient considers real.

HALLUCINATIONS (SOMATIC): imaginary perceptions of a physical experience within the body which the patient considers real such as a feeling of electricity running through the body.

HALLUCINATIONS (TACTILE): an imaginary perception involving the sense of touch, often of things on or under the skin; formication is the sensation of something creeping or crawling on or under the skin; may be seen in alcohol withdrawal delirium, cocaine withdrawal, etc.

HALLUCINATIONS (VISUAL): imaginary perceptions involving sight which may be formed images, such as people, or unformed images, such as flashes of light; visual hallucinations should be distinguished from illusions which are misperceptions of real external stimuli; usually originate in the visual association areas, particularly the temporal lobes; may occur prior to a temporal-lobe epilepsy attack; frequently occur with toxic conditions; occasionally occur in schizophrenia.

HALLUCINOGEN: a substance that produces hallucinations.

HALLUCINOSIS OF LHERMITTE: not unpleasant, animated visual hallucinations with good insight; due to subthalamic and midbrain lesions.

HALSTEAD-REITAN TEST BATTERY - evaluation for malingering: malingerers may have poorer scores on the Speech Sounds Perception Test, the Finger Tapping Test, the tests for Finger Agnosia and Sensory Suppression, the Hand Dynamometer Test, and Digit Span from the WAIS-R; may do better than brain-damaged patients on the Category Test, the Tactual Performance Test, and Trail Making Test Part B.

HALSTEAD-REITAN NEUROPSYCHOLOGICAL TEST BATTERY: consists of 5 basic tests: 1. Category Test; 2. Tactual Performance test; 3. Rhythm Test; 4. Speech Sounds Perception Test; 5. Finger Oscillation test; often administered in conjunction with Trail Making tests, Aphasia Screening Test, the MMPI, WAIS-R, a sensory examination, and grip strength test; an Impairment Index is determined by tabulating the scores of specifically indicated tests that exceed the cutting scores.

HANDEDNESS: cerebral dominance for language and handedness are closely allied; cerebral dominance for language is significantly influenced by heredity; should be reported as strong or weak, left or right, or ambidexterous; see cerebral dominance for percentages in population.

HANDEDNESS TESTS: ask patient to show which hand would be used to hold a knife, throw a ball, stir coffee, or flip a coin; Halstead-Reitan cone.

Hct.: hematocrit.

HEADACHE: may be a result of a neurological disorder (migraine), tumor, infection, or psychological factors such as tension; may be caused by pressure, traction, displacement, or inflammation of the dura, large arteries of the brain, venous sinuses, branches of the fifth, ninth, and tenth cranial nerves, and the first to third cervical nerves.

HEADACHES ASSOCIATED WITH NEUROLOGICAL DISEASE: usually result from distortion of pain-sensitive structures as caused by tumor, head trauma, infection, vascular malformations, and severe hypertension; see also migraine.

HEADACHES-HYPERTENSION: most often located in the occipital region.

HEADACHES-TENSION: psychogenic or anxiety headaches characterized by sensations of tightness and persistent band-like pain in the forehead, temples, or occipital region; result from sustained contraction of the muscles of the scalp and neck caused by constant stress or tension, especially if poor posture is maintained for any period of time.

HEADACHES-TUMORS: pain located on the same side as the tumor.

HEAD TRAUMA: (MMPI interpretation) significantly elevated profiles suggestive of neurotic emotional disturbances involving depression, agitation, confusion, oversensitivity, poor concentration, and a loss of efficiency in carrying out everyday tasks (Casey & Fennell,

H

1981).

HEARING: see auditory, listening, aphasia, verbal perception, amusia, auditory inattention, eighth cranial nerve, vestibulocochlear nerve, or Gyri Temporales Transversi.

HEBB'S RECURRING DIGITS TEST: (Milner, 1970, 1971); a disguised learning test; sensitive to left temporal-lobe lesions and hippocampal dysfunction.

HEIDENHAIM'S SYNDROME: rapidly progressive disease characterized by cortical blindness, presenile dementia, dysarthria, ataxia, athetoid movements, and generalized rigidity.

HEMATOMA: massive accumulation of blood in tissue; local swelling or tumor filled with effused blood most often following a blow to the head; may be extradural, subdural, or intracerebral; may develop rapidly or slowly over several days.

HEMI-: a prefix signifying one half.

HEMIANESTHESIA: anesthesia affecting only one side of the body; also called unilateral anesthesia.

HEMIANOPIA: defective vision or blindness in one half of the visual field; see also absolute h., altitudinal h., bilateral h., binasal h., binocular h., bitemporal h., complete h., congruous h,, equilateral h., homonymous h., horizontal h., incomplete h., incongruous h., lateral h., lower h., macular sparing h., nasal h., quadrant h., quadrantic h., relative h., temporal h., true h., unilateral h., uniocular h., vertical h.

HEMIANOPSIA: hemianopia.

HEMIATAXIA: ataxia affecting one side of the body only; caused by subthalamic lesion of contralateral side; see also ballismus.

HEMIBALLISMUS: abrupt onset of wild flinging movements of the limbs on one side.

HEMICRANIA: partially absent brain.

HEMIHYPESTHESIA: abnormal decreased acuteness of sensation on one side of the body.

HEMIPLEGIA: paralysis or weakness of one side of the body; see alternate h., alternating oculomotor h. (Weber's syndrome), ascending h., facial h., faciobrachial h., faciolingual h., flaccid h., spastic h., Wernicke-Mann h.

HEMIPLEGIC GAIT: leg does not flex freely at knee and hip and is held stiffly; leg rotates outward and describes a semicircle (circumduction); foot drags, arm carried in a flexed position and does not swing.

HEMORRHAGE: the escape of blood from the vessels; bleeding.

HEMORRHAGE INTO TUMORS: rare; the only type of tumor that bleeds is a metastatic deposit from a malignant melanoma; symptoms are like sub-arachnoid hemorrhage.

HEMORRHAGIC CEREBRAL VASCULAR ACCIDENTS: see intracerebral hemorrhage, angioma, sub-arachnoid hemorrhage, hemorrhage into tumors.

HEPATOLENTICULAR DEGENERATION: Wilson's disease.

HEPATOSPLENOMEGALY: enlargement of the liver and spleen.

HERPES SIMPLEX ENCEPHALITIS: causes loss of much medial temporal and orbital brain tissue, usually including the hippocampal memory registration substrate, the amygdala with its centers for control of primitive drives, and that area of the frontal lobes involved in the kind of response inhibition necessary for goal-directed activity and appropriate social behavior; exceedingly dense memory defect with profound anterograde amnesia, usually considerable retrograde amnesia and severe social dilapidation (Hierons et al., 1978).

HESCHL'S GYRUS: see auditory system; Brodmann's area 41.

HETERONYMOUS HEMIANOPIA: hemianopia affecting the nasal or the temporal half of the field of vision of each eye.

HETEROPHORIA: failure of the visual axes to remain parallel after the visual fusional stimuli have been eliminated.

HETEROTOPIA: displaced islands of grey matter appearing in the ventricular walls or white matter; caused by aborted cell migration.

Hgb.: hemoglobin.

HICCUP SPEECH: see choreic and myoclonic dysarthrias.

HIDDEN FIGURES TEST: (Gottschaldt, 1928; Thurstone, 1944) tests the ability to hold a closure against distraction.

HIDDEN OBJECTS TEST: test of immediate memory and learning for spatial orientation and span of immediate memory; patient is asked to recall where and what objects have been hidden while patient observes (Strub & Black, 1977).

HIERARCHY OF BRAIN FUNCTION: 1. intact hindbrain and spinal cord (low decerebrate functioning); 2. midbrain, hindbrain, and spinal cord intact (high decerebrate functioning), voluntary and automatic behavior; 3. diencephalon (intact hindbrain, spinal cord, and midbrain), affect and motivation; 4. basal ganglia (intact hindbrain, spinal cord, midbrain, and diencephalon), self-maintenance, 5. cortex: sequencing, voluntary movement, and pattern perception.

HINDBRAIN: consists of sensory nuclei of the vestibular system overlying the fourth ventricle, motor nuclei of the cranial nerves beneath the ventricle, ascending sensory tracts from the spinal cord, descending fiber tracts to the spinal cord, and nuclei composing the reticular activating system; lower part of brainstem; includes medulla oblongata and cerebellum; also called the rhombencephalon.

HINDBRAIN FUNCTIONING: (low decerebrate animal with both the hindbrain and spinal cord intact); sensory input into the hindbrain comes predominantly from the head and is carried over cranial nerves IV and XII. Most of these nerves also have motor nuclei in the hindbrain whose efferent fibers control muscles in the head and neck; interneurons in the hindbrain have multiplied to form nuclei

H

as well as more complex coordinating centers such as the cerebellum; sensory input to the hindbrain is not limited to the cranial nerves since the spinal somatosensory system has access to hindbrain motor systems, just as the hindbrain has access to spinal motor systems.

HIPPOCAMPAL COMMISSURE: interconnects the hippocampal formations of the two hemispheres.

HIPPOCAMPAL LESIONS: both hippocampi are essential for normal memory, and the left and right hippocampi can function dissociated: the left is more important in the memory of verbal material, and the right is more important in the memory of visual and spatial material; *left hippocampal lesion*: impairment in recall of nonsense syllables and digit span (Corsi, 1972); *right hippocampal lesion*: impairment in tactile maze learning (Milner, 1965), visual maze learning facial recognition (Milner, 1968), spatial block span, and spatial postition (Corsi, 1972).

HIPPOCAMPAL MEMORY DYSFUNCTION: destruction of both hippocampi results in extremely dense, intractable amnesia as a result of failure to register new information.

HIPPOCAMPUS: (Brodmann's area 21) a nucleus of densely packed pyramidal cells in the medial temporal lobe of each cerebral hemisphere, lying in the floor of the inferior horn of the lateral ventricles; thought to be involved in the processing of short-term memory.

HISTOTOXIC ANOXIA: anoxia resulting from disturbance in the tissues that impairs utilization of oxygen; may be caused by cyanide poisoning.

HOARSENESS OF VOICE: see tenth cranial nerve; vagus nerve.

HOLMES-ADIE PUPIL: widely dilated, circular pupil that may react very slowly to very bright light; shows a more definite response to accommodation; both reactions are minimal and thought to be produced by slow inhibition of the sympathetic activity; usually unilateral; caused by degeneration of the nerve cells in the ciliary ganglion; often associated with loss of knee jerks; also called tonic pupil and Adie's syndrome.

HOLOPROSENCEPHALY: cortex forms a single undifferentiated hemisphere.

HOMEOSTASIS: the balanced state of the internal environment, which must remain relatively constant for optimal production of energy.

HOMOLATERAL: situated on, pertaining to, or affrecting the same side; ipsilateral.

HOMOLOGOUS: corresponding in structure, position, origin, etc.

HOMOLOGUE: any homologous organ or part; an organ similar in structure, position, and origin to another organ.

HOMONYMOUS FIELD CUT: loss of vision in the same part of the field of each eye.

HOMONYMOUS HEMIANOPIA: defective vision or blindness in the right or left halves of the visual fields of the two eyes; blindness of one entire visual field as a result of a lesion that completely severs the optic tract, the lateral geniculate body, or Brodmann's area 17; see also macular sparing homonymous hemianopia, anterior visual cortex lesion, lesion of opposite optic tract or internal capsule.

HOMOTOPIC: same points of the two hemispheres of the brain.

HOOPER VISUAL ORGANIZATION TEST: (Hooper, 1958) perceptual puzzle test requiring conceptual reorganization of disarranged pieces of objects; tests the same functions as the WAIS-R Object Assembly subtest.

HORIZONTAL HEMIANOPIA: altitudinal hemianopia; defective vision or blindness in a horizontal half of the visual field.

HORMONES: biochemical substances manufactured by endocrine glands; secreted directly into the circulatory system which carries them to various target organs; speed up or slow down chemical processes and may affect remote parts of the body; regulate metabolism and maintain homeostasis.

HORNER'S SYNDROME: damage to the sympathetic pathway produce abnormalities of the eyes as follows: reduced pupillodilator activity on the affected side; varying degrees of ptosis of the eyelid; may be loss of vasoconstriction causing a bloodshot eye; sweating over the forehead may be impaired; may be caused by massive damage to one hemisphere of the brain and producing Horner's syndrome on the same side as the lesion, brainstem lesions, vascular lesions, multiple sclerosis, pontine gliomas, brainstem encephalitis, cervical cord lesions, syringomyelia, cord gliomas, ependymonas primary, or metastatic malignancy of the lung apex, cervical rib, or avulsion of the lower brachial plexus; any lesions of the neck area: neoplastic infiltration, surgical procedures on the larynx or thyroid, malignant disease in the jugular foramen at the skull bases, or lesions of cranial nerves IX,X,XI, and XII.

hr.: hour.

H.S.; h.s.: hour of sleep; bedtime.

ht.: height.

HUMAN FIGURE DRAWING TESTS: relatively culture free and language independent; some measure of the intellectual functioning of patients whose ability to draw has remained essentially intact; Goodenough Draw-a-Person (D. B. Harris, 1963); A Lady Walking in the Rain (Taylor, 1959); House-Tree-Person; may be used to obtain rough estimates of the general ability of adults with verbal impairments.

HUMAN FIGURE DRAWINGS INTERPRETATIONS: drawings of left-hemisphere patients have fewer details, giving the drawings a

H

simplistic or poorly defined appearance; six characteristics of human figure drawings that are strongly associated with organicity: 1. lack of details; 2. parts loosely joined; 3. parts noticeably shifted; 4. shortened and thin arms and legs; 5. inappropriate size and shape of other body parts (except the head), and 6. petal-like or scribbled fingers; may be as childlike, simplistic, not closed, incomplete, crude, or unintegrated (Hécaen et al., 1951); asymmetry may appear either as a difference in the size of limbs and features of one side of the body relative to those on the other side, or in a tendency of the figure to lean to one side or the other; absence of a portion of the figure is more common with patients with somatosensory defects who may "forget" to draw the affected part although they perform well on visual field and visual attention tests (Cohn, 1953; Schulman et al., 1965); catastrophic reactions may manifest by brain-damaged patients.

HUMOR: right-hemisphere lesioned patients may have difficulty in appreciating the humor in cartoons probably as the result of not being able to integrate all the elements of the picture/story (Wapner et al., 1981); deficits in ability to comprehend humorous material: verbal humor — left-hemisphere lesion; non-verbal humor — right-hemisphere lesion (Gardner et al., 1975).

HUNGER: controlled by the hypothalamus through mediation of the forebrain bundle.

HUNTINGTON'S CHOREA/DISEASE: hereditary disease that involves degeneration of the basal ganglion structures, particularly the caudate nucleus and the putamen; usually involves atrophy of the frontal cortex and the corpus callosum (Berry, 1975; Lishman, 1978); symptoms include involuntary, spasmodic, often tortuous movements that ultimately become profoundly disabling; cognitive and personality disorders; irritability, anxiety, emotional lability, impaired social judgment, and impulsivity involving aggressive or sexual behavior common; apathy may be a result of an increasing inability to plan, initiate, or carry out complex activities (Caine et al., 1978); sometimes misdiagnosed in the early stages as schizophrenia; onset is usually in the 40th to 50th decade but may be as early as age 20 (Burch, 1979); death usually follows 10 to 15 years after diagnosis although some may live as long as 30 years (Walton, 1977).

HUNTINGTON'S DISEASE TEST INTERPRETATIONS: cognitive skills involving overlearned skills, such as reading and writing, word usage, and simple visual recognition, structured drawing (Gainotti et al., 1980) tend to be relatively well preserved; poor performance on tasks that require speed or mental tracking, that lack familiarity and structure (Aminoff et al., 1975; Fedio et al., 1979); WAIS/WAIS-R pattern shows highest scores on Information and Comprehension subtests; impairments on Arithmetic, Digit Span, Digit Symbol, and Picture Arrangement subtests (Josiassen, Curry, Roemer, De Bease,

H

& Mancall, 1982).

HYDROCEPHALUS: a condition characterized by abnormal accumulation of fluid in the cranial vault, accompanied by enlargement of the head, prominence of the forehead, atrophy of the brain, mental deterioration, and convulsions. It may be congenital or acquired and have a sudden onset or be slowly progressive; *communicating h.*: no obstruction in the ventricular system, and cerebrospinal fluid passes readily out of the brain into the spinal canal, but is not absorbed; h. *ex vacuo*: a compensatory replacement by cerebrospinal fluid of the volume of tissue lost in atrophy of the brain; *noncommunicating h.*: obstructive h. due to ventricular block; *otitis h.*: caused by spread of the inflammation of otitis media to the cranial cavity; *secondary h.*: resulting from meningitis.

HYPER-: a prefix meaning above, beyond, or excessive.

HYPERACTIVITY: afferent disorder; see hyperkinesia.

HYPERADRENOCORTICISM: a condition characterized by abnormally increased functional activity of the cortex of the adrenal gland; see also Cushing's syndrome.

HYPERCAPNIA: excess of carbon dioxide in the blood.

HYPERESTHESIA: underlying sensory deficit which elevates the perception threshold; once the stimulus is perceived it may have a severely painful or unpleasant quality (hyperpathia); see also paresthesia.

HYPERGLYCEMIA: a condition characterized by a high level of glucose in the blood; a symptom of diabetes mellitus.

HYPERGRAPHIA: excessive writing; often seen in temporal-lobe epileptics (Waxman & Geschwind, 1974).

HYPERINSULINISM: excessive secretion of insulin by the pancreas which may lead to hypoglycemia.

HYPERKINESIA: abnormal increased motor function or activity.

HYPERMETAMORPHOSIS: rapid drift of thought activity, leading to mental distraction and confusion, and forming a chief element in mania; excessive attentiveness to visual stimuli, as in the Klüver-Bucy syndrome; see also stimulus bound.

HYPERMETRIA: voluntary muscular movement that overshoots the intended goal.

HYPERNATREMIA: excessive amount of sodium in the blood associated with fluid intake, usually dehydration; symptoms include cerebral edema leading to severe brain dysfunction of increasing somnolence, stupor, and coma leading to decerebrate rigidity; seizures may manifest.

HYPEROPIA: far sightedness.

HYPEROSMIA: abnormally increased sensitivity to odors.

HYPERPATHIA: severely painful or unpleasant quality to sensate stimulation; see also thalamic pain and hyperesthesia, paresthesia.

H

HYPERPHAGIA: ingestion of a greater than optimal quantity of food; over-eating; a condition characterized by constant hunger; a symptom of diabetes mellitus.

HYPERPOLARIZATION: inhibitory condition in neural transmission.

HYPERPOLARIZATION OF AXON: increased resting potential in neural transmission.

HYPERPROSEXIA: a condition in which the mind is occupied by one idea to the exclusion of others.

HYPERPYREXIA: a highly elevated body temperature.

HYPERSECRETION: above normal level of secretion.

HYPERSEXUALITY: see temporal-lobe epilepsy; amydala; Klüver-Bucy syndrome; temporal lobe, bilateral excision; frontal-lobe syndrome.

HYPERSOMNIA: prolonged states of sleep; can be aroused, but if left alone, immediately falls asleep; see also encephalitis lethargica, trypanosomiasis, severe myxedema, Kleine-Levin syndrome, Pickwickian syndrome, narcolepsy, cataplexy.

HYPERTENSION and COGNITIVE IMPAIRMENTS: deficits in visual memory and complex concept formation tasks (Goldman et al., 1974, 1975).

HYPERTENSION: high blood pressure.

HYPERTENSIVE CEREBRAL HEMORRHAGE: see subcortical stroke.

HYPESTHESIA: diminution of all sensation.

HYPERTHYROIDISM: excessive functional activity of the thyroid gland characterized by increased basal metabolism, goiter, and disturbances in the autonomic nervous system; sometimes called Grave's disease.

HYPERTONIA: a condition of excessive muscle tone; increased resistance of muscle to passive stretching.

HYPERTRICHOSIS: excessive growth of hair.

HYPERVENTILATION SYNDROME: an emotional disorder in which rapid deep breathing caused by emotional tension, anxiety, or acute fear produces giddiness and clouding of consciousness, and sometimes apprehension, confusion, numbness of the hands and face, muscular cramps of the hands and feet, and a sense of air hunger.

HYPNAGOGIC HALLUCINATIONS: vivid hallucinations when falling asleep lasting 1-2 minutes.

HYPNOPOMPIC HALLUCINATIONS: hallucinations persisting after sleep; applied to visions or dreams that persist prior to complete awakening.

HYPNOSIS: an artificially induced passive state in which there is increased amenability and responsiveness to suggestions and commands, provided that these do not conflict seriously with the subject's own conscious or unconscious wishes.

HYPO-: a prefix meaning beneath,, under, or deficient.

HYPOCHONDRIASIS: an unrealistic interpretation of physical signs or sensations as abnormal leading to a fear or belief of having a disease.

HYPOGLOSSAL NERVE (XII): controls the tongue muscles; see also 12th cranial nerve.

HYPOGLYCEMIA: an abnormally diminished content of glucose in the blood, which may lead to tremulousness, cold sweat, piloerection, hypothermia, and headache, accompanied by confusion, hallucinations, bizarre behavior, and ultimately convulsions and coma; if severe the patient may survive in a state clinically similar to coma vigil; may be caused by hyperinsulinism.

HYPOINSULINISM: results in hyperglycemia (diabetes mellitus).

HYPOKALEMA: loss of intracellular potassium; impairs neuromuscular function; causes muscle weakness and fatigability; may be total flaccid paralysis; may be confusion, impaired consciousness, and delirium which may lead to coma; may be caused by adrenocortical adenoma, ingestion of cortisone, ingestion of diuretic medications, vomiting or diarrhea.

HYPOKINETIC ANOXIA: see stagnant anoxia.

HYPOMAGNESIA: depletion of magnesium in the blood; sometimes observed in small infants fed a diet limited to milk; may be associated with protein-calorie malnutrition, malabsorption syndrome, alcoholism, cirrhosis of the liver, and diabetic acidosis; causes an increase in neuromuscular activity; symptoms may include confusion, irritability, state of agitation, muscle twitching, hallucinations, and coma; seizures sometimes occur.

HYPOMANIA: a mild form of manic excitement.

HYPOMETRIA: voluntary muscular movement that undershoots the intended goal.

HYPONATREMIA: depletion of sodium in the blood associated with fluid intake; symptoms may include fatigue, nausea, vomiting, and abdominal cramps; may progress to confusion, delirium, epileptic seizures, and coma; brain-damage may occur and be fatal in some patients.

HYPOPHYSIS: the pituitary gland; an epithelial body of dual origin located at the base of the brain in the sella turcica.

HYPOPLASIA: incomplete development of an organ so that it fails to reach adult size.

HYPOSECRETION: reduced level of secretion, usually below normal.

HYPOTENSION: low blood pressure.

HYPOTHALAMUS: located next to the third ventricle; not included in the limbic system functionally, although much of the expression of activity in the limbic system occurs via connections with the hypo-

H

thalamus; composed of 22 small nuclei and the fiber systems that pass through it and the pituitary gland; a principal component of the diencephalon; has right and left lobes; rostral to the midbrain tegmentum; connected by numerous fiber systems to the thalamus, basal ganglia, and limbic system; the main afferent connections of the hypothalamus are derived from the fornix, are distributed to all the hypothalamic nuclei, and terminate in the mammillary body; efferent connections include ascending projections into the limbic system, the cortex, and thalamus; descending projections go to the tegmentum, reticular formation, and the cranial nerve nuclei; olfactory information reaches the hypothalamus via the medial forebrain bundle which also receives information from other areas of the limbic system and forms the main longitudinal tract between the various hypothalamic nuclei as it lies along the lateral border of the area; cortical activity reaches the hypothalamus directly and also via the thalamus; from below, the hypothalamus receives visceral and gustatory sensation via both the dorsal and longitudinal fasciculus and the reticular formation; much of the visceral sensation relayed to the cortex via the mammillo-thalamic tract and thalamus; controls fluid balance and thirst mechanism, body temperature regulation, sweating mechanisms, appetite, satiety, feeding reflexes, peristalsis, sex, and the various secretions associate with eating and digestion; regulates endocrine activity via the pituitary glands, consummatory motor reflexes, modulation of muscle tension, and the autonomic nervous system: the posterior portion controls the SNS; the anterior portion regulates the PNS; controls the activity of the adrenal medulla; participates in the mediation of general arousal and sleep (working with the ARAS and nonspecific thalamic nuclei); mediates both defensive and aggressive behavior, pleasure, fear-anger and punishment effects as well as positive reinforcement effects; the anterior nuclei including the supraoptic and paraventricular nuclei are particularly concerned with fluid balance via the antidiuretic hormone secretion and control of the thirst mechanism; the central nuclei are concerned with body temperature regulation by control over skin blood vessels and sweating mechanisms; the posterior hypothalamus contains the dorsal nuclei, the posterior hypothalamic nucleus, and the supramammillary and mammillary nuclei.

HYPOTHALAMIC LESIONS: damage to the anterior and central nuclei areas may cause diabetes insipidus, complete adipsia, hyperpyrexia, pulmonary edema or acute gastric erosions; the anterior and central nuclei are particularly likely to be damaged by pituitary tumors, craniopharyngiomas, head injuries, and intracranial surgery in this region; lesions to the posterior hypothalamus are unusual and may be associated with total loss of appetite leading to gross emaciation or gross overeating with obesity and altered personality often characterized by extremely bad temper and aggression; lesions in the lateral area are characterized by somnolence, disturbances of body temperature control, and occasionally altered appetite; the lateral hypothalamic area has inter-connecting pathways running through it so that the clinical signs may indicate damage to either the nuclei or the tracts.

HYPOTHERMIA: abnormally low temperature of the body; may be a result of dysfunction of the CNS or of the endocrine system.

HYPOTHYROIDISM: deficiency of thyroid activity; *adults*: most common in women and characterized by decrease in basal metabolic rate, tiredness, and lethargy, sensitivity to cold, and menstrual disturbances; if untreated, may progress to myxedema; *infants*: cretinism; *juveniles*: less severe mental developmental retardation and mild symptoms of the adult form.

HYPOTONIA: diminished tone of the skeletal muscles; diminished resistance of muscles to passive stretching.

HYPOTONIC: slack limb(s).

HYPOVENTILATION SYNDROME: obesity-hypoventilation syndrome; heterogeneous group of disorders with differing clinical manifestations: hypersomnolence/obesity caused by nighttime sleep apnea with hypoxemia and hypercapnia causing arousal with return of normal respiration, leading to chronic sleep deprivation and daytime somnolence; occasionally life-threatening; part of the Pickwickian syndrome.

HYPOXEMIA: deficient oxygenation of the blood; hypoxia.

HYSTERICAL GAIT (HEMIPLEGIC): see hysterical gait, monoplegic.

HYSTERICAL GAIT (MONOPLEGIC): patient does not lift foot off the floor while walking; drags foot or slides it along like a skate; circumduction absent; Babinski sign absent; legs are rigid with pseudocontractures or flaccid; the patient may look like he/she is walking on stilts; may use crutches or remain in bed.

I

IATROGENIC: any adverse condition in a patient occurring as the result of treatment by a physician or surgeon.

ICP: intracranial pressure or intermittent catheterization program.

ICSH: interstitial-cell-stimulating hormone, secreted by the anterior pituitary gland in males.

ICTAL/ICTUS: a seizure, stroke, blow, or sudden attack.

IDEATIONAL APRAXIA: loss of ability to make proper use of an

I

object, due to lack of perception of its proper nature and purpose; called also sensory apraxia.

IDEA OF REFERENCE: an idea, held less firmly than a delusion, that events, objects, or other people in the person's immediate environment have a particular and unusual meaning specifically for him or her.

IDENTITY: the sense of self, providing a unity of personality over time; disturbances in identity or sense of self are seen in schizophrenia, borderline personality disorder, and identity disorder.

IDEOKINETIC/IDEOMOTOR APRAXIA: an interruption between the ideation center and the center for the limb; simple movements can be performed but not complicated ones; called also limb-kinetic a. and transcortical a.

IDEOMOTOR APRAXIA: unable to use objects appropriately and at will; commonly associated with lesions near or overlapping speech centers and often appears concomitantly with communication disabilities; see also ideokinetic a.

IDIOPATHIC: unknown etiology.

IDIOPATHIC NORMAL PRESSURE HYDROCEPHALUS: hydrocephalus in which the cause is not apparent; onset often insidious; course progressive.

ILLINOIS TEST OF PSYCHOLINGUISTIC ABILITIES (ITPA): delineates areas of deficit in communication-related functions; some subtests of the ITPA may be used with adult brain-injured patients: Visual Closure, Visual Sequential Memory, Visual Reception, or Auditory Reception.

ILLNESS - DENIAL OF: see anosodiaphoria, asomatognosia.

ILLUSIONS: a misperception of a real external stimulus; perceptual distortions (Penfield, 1954); four kinds: 1. auditory (sounds seem louder, fainter, more distant, or nearer; superior-temporal gyrus dysfunction (Brodmann's area 22) of either hemisphere; 2. visual illusions (objects are nearer, farther, larger, or smaller); right temporal-lobe dysfunction; 3. illusions of recognition in which the present experience seems either familiar (déjà vu) or strange, unreal, and dreamlike: right temporal-lobe dysfunction; and 4. emotional illusions such as feelings of fear, loneliness, or sorrow: either temporal-lobe dysfunction.

I.M.: intramuscular.

IMMATURE BEHAVIOR: lesion of the dorsolateral frontal lobe.

IMMEDIATE MEMORY: working memory; 30 seconds to several minutes duration; first stage of short-term memory storage; fixation of the information selected for retention by the registration process.

Imp.: impression.

IMPERSISTENCE: inability to maintain an action such as holding one's tongue out and saying "ahhh" for several seconds or standing on one foot.

IMPOTENCE: lack of power, chiefly of copulative power in the male; *atonic*: due to paralysis of the motor nerves without evidence of lesion of the central nervous system; *paretic*: due to lesion in the central nervous system, particularly in the spinal cord; *psychic*: dependent on mental complex; symptomatic: due to some other disorder, such as injury to nerves in the perineal region, by virtue of which the sensory portion of the erection reflex arc is interrupted.

IMPRESSION APHASIA: see Wernicke's aphasia.

IMPRESSIVE SPEECH: Luria's term for receptive speech.

IMPULSE CONTROL-LACK OF: may be caused by a lesion to the posterior-orbital parts of the frontal lobes, medial forebrain tracts, or lateral hypothalamus.

INABILITY TO SHRUG: spinal accessory nerve (XI).

INAPPROPRIATE AFFECT: expression of emotions that are inconsistent with the cognitive expression, e. g., laughing while talking about something sad.

INARTICULATE: not having joints; disjointed; not uttered like articulate speech.

INATTENTION: may be caused by a parietal-lobe lesion; see extinction, cortical inattention, unilateral inattention, suppression, polymodal neglect, unilateral neglect.

INCOHERENCE: speech that is not understandable due to a lack of logical or meaningful connection between words, phrases, or sentences; disrupted organization of thought with fragmentation, repetition, and perseveration.

INCOMPETENT: a legal term referring to persons who cannot be considered responsible for their actions.

INCOMPLETE HEMIANOPIA: hemianopia affecting less than an entire half of the visual field.

INCONGRUOUS HEMIANOPIA: hemianopia in which the defects in the field of vision in the two eyes differ in one or more respects, as in extent or intensity.

INCONTINENCE: inability to control excretory functions, as defecation (fecal) or urination (urinary).

INDIFFERENCE: orbital frontal-lobe dysfunction/damage.

INDOLEAMINE: serotonin is the most important indoleamine; biomine neurotransmitters produced by the Raphè nucleus.

INDUCTION TEST (level XIV): (Stanford-Binet subtest) a serial reasoning task.

INERTIA: remaining at rest or in the same straight line unless acted upon by some external force; indisposition to motion, exertion, or change; deficit in active properties; sluggish; slow to move or act.

INFARCT: an area of dead or dying tissue (necrosis) resulting from an obstruction of the blood vessels normally supplying the area or part.

I

INFECTION: invasion of the body by disease-producing (pathogenic) microorganisms and the reaction of the tissues to their presence and to the toxins generated by them; infections of the nervous system usually spread from infection elsewhere in the body — especially the the ears, nose, and throat; they also may be introduced directly into the brain as a result of head trauma, skull fractures, or surgery; infections of the nervous system are particularly serious because they cause neurons and glia to die, resulting in lesions; may interfere with blood supply to neurons, producing thrombosis, hemorrhage of capillaries, or infarcts; may cause a disturbance of glucose or oxygen metabolism that may kill brain cells; may alter the neural cell membranes, thus altering the electrical properties; may interfere with the basic enzymatic processes of the cell, producing any number of abnormal conditions; the byproducts of the body's defense system (pus) may impair neuronal functioning by significantly altering the extracellular fluids surrounding a neuron and thereby altering the neuronal function or occupy space causing pressure on the brain; often causes edema which compresses the brain.

INFERIOR CEREBELLUM LESIONS: see cerebellum/cerebellar.

INFERIOR COLLICULI: mediates whole body movements/reflexes to auditory stimuli; one of two structures of the lower portion of the tectum; see also auditory system.

INFERIOR FRONTAL OCCIPITAL FACICULUS: a collection of association fibers in the inferior part of the extreme capsule near the uncinate fasciculus, connecting various inferior gyri of the temporal and frontal lobes.

INFERIOR LONGITUDINAL FASCICULUS: a bundle of association fibers interconnecting the cortex of the occipital and temporal lobes, extending through the occipital and temporal lobes of the cerebrum, and consists chiefly of geniculocalcarine projection fibers.

INFLEXIBLE BEHAVIOR: (perseveration); bilateral prefrontal lesions.

INFORMATION SUBTEST (WAIS-R): Information and Vocabulary subtests are the best WAIS-R battery measures of general ability (learning capacity, mental alertness, speed, and efficiency); Information tests verbal skills, breadth of knowledge, and particularly in older populations, remote memory; reflects formal education and a motivation for academic achievement (Saunders, 1960a); in brain-injured populations, the Information subtest tends to appear among the least affected WAIS-R battery subtests (O'Brian &Lezak, 1981; Sklar, 1963); can often serve as the best estimate of original ability; markedly low Information subtest score suggests left hemisphere involvement, particularly if verbal tests generally tend to be relatively depressed and the patient's history provides no other good predictor of the hemispheric side of a suspected brain lesion (Reitan,

1955; Smith 1966; Spreen & Benton, 1965); may give spuriously high ability estimates for overachievers.

INFORMATION SUBTEST in dementia: may be a relatively normal score; the test explores overlearned material which often survives a dementing process for a long time past the patient's ability to care for self.

INGENUITY TEST: Stanford-Binet subtest, levels I and II); a complex reasoning test involving arithmetic operations and concepts; may expose subtle difficulties in formulating problems or in conceptual tracking.

INHIBITION: a checking or preventing of the expression of impulses or desires; thought to be controlled by the prefrontal area.

INNERVATED: connected with the nervous system.

INSIGHT: the level of self-understanding, appreciation of condition, and logic of expectations state of being fully aware of the nature and degree of one's deficits; an individual's understanding of the origin and mechanisms of his attitudes and behavior.

INSOMNIA: want of sleep; impairment in duration, depth, or restorative properties of sleep; see also initial, middle, and terminal insomnia.

INSOMNIA-PRIMARY: life-long loss of restful sleep in the absence of neurosis, depression or other psychiatric or medical diseases with effects of partial sleep deprivation; patients with primary insomnia become sleep pedants or sleep hypochondriacs; fewer hours of sleep than normal, less REMS, more stage II (NREM), body movements, more rapid pulse, peripheral vasocontriction, higher body temperature, and heightened physiologic arousal.

INSOMNIA (INITIAL): difficulty in falling asleep.

INSOMNIA (MIDDLE): awakening followed by difficulty in returning to sleep but eventually doing so.

INSOMNIA (TERMINAL): awakening at least two hours before one's usual waking time and being unable to return to sleep; also called early morning awakening; a frequent symptom of severe depression.

INSULA: a triangular area of the cerebral cortex which forms the floor of the lateral cerebral fossa; covered over and hidden from view by the juxtaposition of the opercula, which forms the lateral sulcus; also called the island of Reil; a lesion may cause agrammatism.

INSULIN: hormone secreted by islet cells of the pancreas; enables body cells to metabolize blood sugar; hypoinsulinism results in hyperglycemia (diabetes mellitus); hyperinsulinism leads to hypoglycemia.

INTEGRATIVE FUNCTIONS OF CORTEX: granular frontal cortex.

INTENTIONS: granular frontal cortex.

INTENTION TREMOR: a tremor which arises or which is intensified when a voluntary, coordinated movement is attempted.

INTER-ICTAL: during a seizure.

I

INTERFERENCE-VISUAL TEST: see Visual Interference Test.

INTERNAL CAPSULE: a fanlike mass of white fibers that separates the lentiform nucleus laterally from the head of the caudate nucleus, the dorsal thalamus, and the tail of the caudate nucleus medially; consists of an anterior limb, a genu, a posterior limb and retrolentiform and sublentiform parts; carries both afferent and efferent fibers of the cerebral cortex.

INTERNAL CAPSULE LESION: corticospinal motor neuron paralysis; face, arm, leg equally involved.

INTERNAL CAROTID ARTERY: originates from the common carotid artery in the neck and branches to the caroticotympanic rami, ophthalmic, posterior communicating, anterior choroid, anterior cerebral, and middle cerebral arteries; serves the middle ear, brain, pituitary gland, orbit, and choroid plexus.

INTERNAL CAROTID ARTERY OCCLUSION: may be completely occluded without causing symptoms; usually causes recurrent transitory disturbances due to localized cerebral ischemia such as aphasia, mental confusion, or contralateral hemiparesis or parathesia causing "stuttering hemiplegia" for a year or two; may also cause transitory amblyopia of the eye on the same side, focal or generalized epilepsy; often followed by a sudden stroke due to extensive infarction of the affected hemisphere; symptoms may include transitory crossed homonymous hemianopia, hemiplegia, and loss of spatial and discriminative sensibility on the opposite side of the body; left-sided, may cause aphasia, both receptive and expressive (Brain, 1985).

INTERNAL CAROTID ARTERIAL INFARCTION: often in a patient with cerebral arteriosclerosis; thrombosis of the internal carotid artery is usually followed by an infarct in the distribution of the middle cerebral artery; because of collateral circulation there may be no symptoms, and in others, major symptoms; lesions most often occur in the internal carotid artery at the origin of the vessel at the common carotid artery in the neck; symptoms include stupor or coma, flaccid hemiplegia with decreased deep tendon reflexes on the affected side, dysphasia, homonymous visual field defects, facial weakness, hemihypesthesia, and a unilateral extensor plantar response; may produce death from respiratory arrest as a result of swelling and intracranial pressure (Reitan & Wolfson, 1985).

INTERNEURON: located between sensory neurons entering the spinal cord and the motor neurons leaving the spinal cord; hindbrain interneurons are multiplied to form nuclei as well as more complex coordinating centers such as the cerebellum.

INTEROCEPTIVE STIMULI: stimuli originating in the viscera, as distinguished from exteroceptive stimuli which originate outside the body.

INTERTEST SCATTER: variability between scores of a set of tests.

INTERNUCLEAR OPHTHALMOPLEGIA: see disconjugate eye movements.

INTEROCEPTOR: any one of the sensory nerve terminals which are located in and transmit impulses from the viscera.

INTRACEPHALIC: within the brain.

INTRACEREBELLAR: within the cerebellum.

INTRACEREBRAL: within the cerebrum.

INTRACEREBRAL HEMORRHAGE: usually a rupture of one of the more peripheral lenticulo-striate arteries in the region of the external capsule which may extend into the sylvian fissure or into the lateral ventricle; symptoms included sudden fulminating headache with rapidly deepening loss of consciousness and tentorial herniation; the ipsilateral pupil and then both pupils dilate and become fixed to light; death usually follows within 15 minutes to a few hours; see also subcortical stroke.

INTRACISTERNAL: within a cistern, especially the cisterna cerebellomedularis.

INTRACRANIAL HEMORRHAGE - brainstem: there are several ways the brainstem can be affected: hemorrhage into the pons causes death within hours; the cerebral peduncle may be involved and produces a midbrain lesion; if the 4th ventrical is involved, acute brainstem dysfunction may follow with cardiac and respiratory arrest; hemorrhage into the cerebellum distorts the brainstem and death usually follows unless there is a surgical evacuation; subarachnoid bleeding may cause similar symptoms as the cerebellum hemorrhage such as occipital headache, vomiting, ataxia, impaired consciousness, gaze palsies, bilateral pyramidal signs and periodic respiration followed by death.

INTRADURAL HEMATOMA: a hemhorrage within or beneath the dura.

INTRAFUSAL FIBERS: fibers that, along with extrafusal fibers, make up skeletal muscles; the reciprocal action of the two kinds of fibers produces muscle tension, which is regulated by the stretch reflex.

INTRUSIONS: inappropriate recurrence of a response or type of response from a preceding test item, test, or procedure; may be due to an anticholinergic reaction; may be seen in Alzheimer's patients (Fuld et al., 1982) or frontal-lobe dysfunction; may also be referred to as perseverative responses.

INVOLUNTARY MOVEMENTS: (akathisia) consist of continual changes in posture for no apparent reason; distortion of posture; seen in Parkinson's disease and extrapyramidal reaction to neuroleptic drugs; a condition of motor restlessness ranging from a feeling of inner disquiet to inability to sit or lie quietly or to sleep, along with tremors of the extremities.

INVOLUNTARY NERVOUS SYSTEM: autonomic nervous system.

ION: e; electrically charged particles.

IPSILATERAL: same side.

I.Q.: intelligence quotient.

IRRITABILITY: may be attributable to subcortical stroke or brain damage.

ISCHEMIA: deficiency of blood in a part due to functional constriction or actual obstruction of a blood vessel.

ISCHEMIC SCORE: (Hatchinsky et al., 1975; Harrison et al., 1979) a thirteen-item scored check list which may be answered from behavioral observations, patient and family information, and clinical data; the higher the score, the more likely a multi-infarct dementia is present rather than a primary degenerative dementia.

ISHIHARA TEST: (Ishihara, 1954); color perception test, particularly for color blindness.

ISLET CELLS OF PANCREAS: secrete insulin.

ISOLATION SYNDROME: see transcortical aphasia.

ISOMORPHIC REACTIONS: equal or similar movements (similar to perseveration) (Luria, 1973b).

ISTHMUS: a narrow connection between two larger bodies or parts.

ISTHMUS OF CINGULATE GYRUS: the constricted portion of the cingulate gyrus, connecting with the parahippocampal gyrus in the region of the splenium corpus callosum.

ITPA: Illinois Test of Psycholinguistic Abilities.

IV: intravenous; interventricular.

IVP: intravenous pyelogram.

J

JACKSONIAN MARCH: see focal seizures, Jacksonian motor seizures.

JACKSONIAN MOTOR SEIZURE: rolandic area foci; usually rolandic cortex (Brodmann's area 4); sometimes premotor cortex (Brodmann's area 6); begins with a tonic contraction or a clonic rhythmic twitching of extremity or face on one side, spreads (marches) up limb; may occur in bursts, or paroxysms; see also focal epileptic seizures.

JACKSON'S STRIP: precentral gyrus, primary motor cortex.

JACKSON'S SYNROME: paralysis of the tenth, eleventh, and twelfth cranial nerves, with paralysis of the soft palate, larynx, and one-half of the tongue; associated with paralysis of the sternomastoid and trapezius muscles.

JAKOB-CREUTZFELT ISEASE: dementia coupled with parkinsonism and motor neuron disease; see Creutzfeldt-Jakob syndrome.

JAMAIS VU: objects appear far away or unreal (symptom of psychomotor epilepsy).

JARGON APHASIA: a form of expressive aphasia with utterances of meaningless phrases; form of aphasia with so many paraphasic errors that the discourse is unintelligible or difficult to follow; see also Wernicke's aphasia.

JERKY MOVEMENTS: see cerebellar diseases.

JOM: juvenile-onset diabetes mellitis.

JOKOB DISEASE: see Creutzfeldt-Jakob syndrome.

JUGMENT TESTS: WAIS-R Comprehension subtest items; proverbs.

JUGMENT OF LINE ORIENTATION TEST: (Benton et al., 1975, 1978, 1983) a spatial orientation test; examines the ability to estimate accuracy of angular orientation line pairs to numbered radii forming a semicircle; sensitive to posterior right-hemisphere brain-damage.

JUGULAR FORAMEN: 9th, 10th, and 11th cranial nerves enter the internal part of the foramen lying on the medial side of the sigmoid sinus. The foreman angles forwards and laterally under the petrous bone which is excavated by the slight ballooning of the sigmoid sinus as it bends downwards to become the jugular bulb. The three cranial nerves emerge in front of the jugular bulb lying between it and the carotid artery which enters the carotid canal just anteriorly; the 12th (hypoglossal) nerve exits through the anterior condylar canal and comes into close relationship with the three other nerves outside the skull; the cervical sympathetic nerve which ascends into the area on the carotid artery does not exit from the skull via the foramen.

JUGULAR FORAMEN SYNROMES: Vernet's Syndrome; Collet-Sicard Syndrome; Villaret's Syndrome.

K

K: potassium.

KASANIN-HANFMANN CONCEPT FORMATION TEST: (Hanfmann, 1953) test of abstract problem solving.

KATZ ADJUSTMENT SCALE: (Katz & Lyerly, 1963); consists of five subscales which assess different behavioral aspects of the patient's life as given by the relatives; scored on a 4-point rating scale.

Kg.: kilogram.

KIMURA BOX TEST: test of apraxia.

KINDLING: a technique devised by Goddard (1980) to study epilepsy;

K

certain portions of the limbic system are given from one to two seconds of electrical stimulation each day; initially, no observable effect, but will begin to produce epileptic attacks. After the shocks are continued for a long period of time, the seizures may begin to occur spontaneously.

KINESOGENIC: chorea initiated by a sudden voluntary movement.

KINESTHETIC: muscle movement sense.

KINETIC MELODY: smooth execution of series of sequential motor movements (Luria, 1973b).

KLANG/KLANGING: see clang associations.

KLEINE-LEVIN SYNDROME: periodic hypersomnolence lasting for periods of 2-3 weeks and hyperphagia; attacks 2-3 times a year; onset usually in adolescence with striking male predominance; sometimes associated with psychosis.

KLINEFELTER'S SYNDROME: a condition characterized by the presence of small testes, with fibrosis and hyalinization of seminiferous tubules, impairment of function and clumping of Leydig cells, and by increase in urinary gonadotropins; associated with an abnormality of the sex chromosomes in which there is an extra X chromosome (XXY instead of XY); impaired WAIS-R Verbal IQ; Performance Scale unaffected; delayed speech development; delayed emotional development; and school maladjustment.

KLÜVER-BUCY SYNDROME: 1. loss of fear; 2. indiscriminate dietary behavior (hyperbulimia) including ingestion of plastics, feces, etc.; 3. greatly increased autoerotic, homosexual, and heterosexual activity, with inappropriate object choice; unable to compete appropriately in social situations; 4. hypermetamorphosis, or a tendency to attend to and react to every visual stimulus; 5. tendency to examine all objects by mouth; shows compulsive oral behavior; and 6. visual agnosia; inability to identify friends and relatives; some of these features may reflect memory loss, continued eating and sexual activity being due to incomplete recollection of previous indulgences; caused by medial temporal-lobe damage resulting from bilateral anterior temporal lobectomy or a neurological disease such as meningoencephalitis; apparently requires that the amygdala and inferior temporal cortex be removed bilaterally.

KNOX CUBE IMITATION TEST: a test from the Arthur Point Scale of Performance battery (Arthur, 1947); may be both verbal and nonverbal contributions; ease of administration and simplicity of the required responses recommend this task for memory testing of patients with speech and motor disabilities and low stamina (Inglis, 1957); test examines the sequential, time-dependent functions of the left hemisphere (Horan et al., 1980).

KOHS BLOCKS: sensitive to postcentral lesions (Benton, 1969a; Luria, 1973a) and to degenerative disorders (Botez & Barbeau, 1975; Botez,

Botez, Levielle et al., 1979); may be useful to demonstrate mild visuoconstructive deficits in very bright patients.

KORSAKOFF'S PSYCHOSIS: chronic alcoholics may retain the ability for some new learning, but have difficulty with retrieval; usually a permanent sequela to an attack of Wernicke's encephalopathy; particular tendency to upset temporal relationships; gross memory defects (Butters & Cermak, 1974; Butters et al., 1977; Kapur & Butters, 1977; Ryan & Butters, 1980a; Talland, 1968); confabulation (Howieson, 1980a); affective blandness and passivity; defective ability to consolidate, retrieve, and utilize newly registered data (Albert et al., 1979; Buschke & Fuld, 1974; Butters & Cermak, 1975, 1976, 1980; Talland 1968); may be able to perform Digit Span, Subtracting Serial Sevens, and other tasks involving immediate memory and attention, although not likely to resume interrupted activities and show little, if any, learning curve on repetitive tasks (Talland, 1965a); tend to be oblivious to chronology in their recall of remote events so that they report impossible sequences unquestioningly and without guile (Lezak et al., 1983; Lhermitte & Signoret, 1972): slowed perceptual processing, premature responding, diminished ability to profit from mistakes, and diminished ability to perceive and use cues (Oscar-Berman, 1980); behavioral defects specifically and consistently associated with Korsakoff's syndrome are disorientation for time and place, apathy characterized by a virtually total loss of initiative, disinterest, and a striking lack of curiosity about the past, present, or future; emotional blandness with a capacity for momentary irritability, anger, or pleasure that quickly dissipates when the stimulating condition is removed or the discussion topic changed; the memory defects of the Korsakoff's syndrome render the severely impaired patient dependent and call attention to the central organizing function of retention and recall for emotional and intellectual behavior (Lezak, 1983); may show slow improvement in memory, orientation, and general responsiveness when given large doses of thiamine early in the course of the disease (Berglund et al., 1979), but many reach a plateau without regaining enough capacity to maintain social independence; on the Wechsler Memory Scale the MQ may be 20-30 points below IQ (Butters & Cermack, 1980).

KORSAKOFF-WERNICKE DISEASE: (Talland, 1968) six major symptoms in otherwise normal appearing functioning — normal IQ, alert and attentive, appears motivated, and generally lacks other neurological signs of cerebral deficit; usually normal EEG: 1. anterograde amnesia; unable to form new memories; especially poor at learning paired-associate lists; 2. retrograde amnesia: loss of old memories; 3. confabulation — made up stories about past events rather than admit memory loss which are often based on past

L

experiences and are therefore often plausible; 4. meager content in conversation; 5. lack of insight into memory defect; and 6. apathy; indifference and incapacity to persevere in ongoing activities; loses interest in things quickly and appears indifferent to change; symptoms may appear suddenly within the space of a few days; cause: thiamine deficiency resulting from prolonged intake of large quantities of alcohol; progressive syndrome which can be arrested with massive doses of thiamine, but cannot be reversed; prognosis poor; thiamine deficiency damage is thought to result in damage to the dorsomedial thalamus which produces memory loss; may perform well on digit repetition tasks but performs poorly on random letter tasks or cancellation tasks.

KURU: a chronic, progressive, uniformly fatal nervous system disorder caused by a virus and transmissible to subhuman primates; found exclusively among the Fore and neighboring people of New Guinea; chief symptoms are truncal and limb ataxia, a shivering-like tremor, and dysarthria; strabismus and extrapyramidal symptoms may also be found; pathologically, the brain shows the changes of spongioform enchephalopathies: neuronal loss, astrogliosis, and status spongiosus; amyloid plaques present in about two thirds of the cases; neuropsychological manifestations typical to viral encephalitis (Reitan & Wolfson, 1985).

KYPHOSCOLIOSIS: backward and lateral curvature of the spinal column.

L

L: lumbar; left; liter.

lab.: laboratory.

LABIALS: speech sounds formed during articulation (m, b, p).

LABILE/LABILITY: emotional instability; a tendency to show alternating states of gaiety and somberness or anger; see also emotional lability.

LACK OF DRIVE/ INITIATIVE/ WILL POWER: abulia.

LACK OF INSIGHT: impaired or abolished state of being fully aware of the nature and degree of one's own deficits.

LACK OF SPONTANEITY: frontal lobe dysfunction/damage.

LACONIC: brief or terse in speech or expression; using few words.

LACONIC SPEECH: pauses between utterances; inability to sustain a monologue and narrative.

LACTOGENIC HORMONE (PROLACTIN): mediates milk production and brings corpus luteum into a fully functional state; secreted by the anterior pituitary gland.

LAMARKISM: a theory that acquired characteristics can be transmitted genetically to progeny; now discounted.

LANGUAGE - SUBCORTICAL COMPONENTS: (Penfield & Roberts theory, 1959) the left posterior thalamus, especially the pulvinar, functions to coordinate the activity of the cortical speech zones; Ojemann (1975) and Cooper and associates (1973) theory: left pulvinar, ventrolateral thalamus and the lateral posterior-lateral central complex have a unique role in language not shared by other subcortical structures.

LANGUAGE COMPREHENSION DEFICIT: may be a result of lesion(s) in any of the language zones of the left hemisphere (parietal, temporal, or frontal lobes).

LANGUAGE COMPREHENSION DISORDERS: Brodmann's area 22; left temporal lobe.

LANGUAGE DISORDERS: Brodmann's areas 39 and 40, left; aphasia refers to a disorder of language apparent in speech, writing (agraphia), or reading (alexia) produced by injury to brain areas specialized for these functions; disturbances of language due to severe intellectual impairment, loss of sensory input, paralysis; incoordination of the musculature of the mouth (anarthria) or hand are not considered to be aphasic disturbances; see also auditory comprehension, visual comprehension, articulation, word finding, paraphasia, grammar and syntax disorders, repetition, verbal fluency, writing, and the various types of aphasia.

LANGUAGE MODEL (WERNICKE-GESCHWIND MODEL): involves Broca's area, Wernicke's area, arcuate fasciculus, precentral and postcentral face area, angular gyrus, and auditory and visual cortex; *language pathways*: spoken word is heard in Brodmann's areas 41 and 42, comprehended in Wernicke's area (Brodmann's area 22), and results in hearing and comprehending the word (cognition) which is transmitted to Broca's area followed by transmission to the face area and to the cranial nerves resulting in speech; the written word is received in Brodmann's area 17 (visual) and is transmitted to Brodmann's areas 18 and 19 (visual association areas) followed by transmission to Brodmann's area 39 (angular gyrus) and to Wernicke's area (Brodmann's area 22) resulting in reading.

LATERAL: away from the midline or median plane; opposite of medial.

LATERAL CEREBELLAR LESION: see cerebellar lesions.

LATERAL CORTICOSPINAL MOTOR TRACT: connects with motor neurons in the dorsolateral portion of the ventral zone of the spinal cord and with interneurons in the dorsolateral portion of the intermediate zone of the spinal cord.

LATERAL EYE MOVEMENTS: abducens nerve (VI).

L

LATERAL FISSURES OF THE NEOCORTEX: begins in a cleft on the anterior-inferior surface of the cortex and differentiates the temporal lobe from the other parts of the cortex.

LATERAL GENICULATE NUCLEUS: an area in the thalamus where the optic nerve synapses with a set of neural fibers that project to the visual area in the occipital lobe of the cortex.

LATERAL HEMIANOPIA: vertical hemianopia; defective vision or blindness in a lateral half of the visual field.

LATERAL HYPOTHALAMUS: an area in the hypothalamus believed to play a role in the control of eating, drinking, and nonaffective attack behavior.

LATERAL LEMNISCUS: a tract that transmits auditory information from the superior olive to the inferior colliculus.

LATERAL MOTOR SYSTEM: controls movements of the fingers, hands, and arms.

LATERAL MEDULLARY LESION: see brainstem lesions, lateral medullary syndrome.

LATERAL MEDULLARY SYNDROME: caused by an infarction of a wedge-shaped area of the lateral aspect of the medulla and the inferior surface of the cerebellum; may be due to thrombosis of the posterior inferior cerebellar artery or of one vertebral artery; onset characterized by severe vertigo and sometimes vomiting; dysphagia; occasionally pain or parethesia, e.g., a sensation of hot water running over the face; some cerebellar deficiency with nystagmus, hypotonia, and incoordination on the side of the lesion; ipsilateral paralysis of the soft palate, pharynx, and vocal cord; Horner's syndrome (miosis and ptosis) present on the affected side; dissociate sensory loss; analgesia and thermo-anesthesia on the face on the same side as the lesion and on the trunk and limbs on the opposite side; persistent neuralgic pain in the face, on the same side, and sometimes of the limbs and trunk on the opposite side (Brain, 1985).

LATERAL SPINOTHALAMIC TRACT: a bundle of nerve fibers ascending the lateral part of the spinal cord and ending in the thalamus; thought to convey temperature and pain information.

LATERALITY: recent studies have shown that laterality of function can be affected by environmental factors as well as genetically determined factors such as gender and handedness; the cerebral organization of some left-handers and females appears to have less functional asymmetry than males; laterality is relative and not absolute, because both hemispheres play a role in nearly every behavior; although the left hemisphere is especially important for the production of language in most people, the right hemisphere also has some language capabilities (Kolb & Whishaw, 1980); the right hemisphere is most often found to process music and forms.

LAZY-EYE: see amblyopia ex anopsia.

L

LBBB: left bundle branch block.

L-DOPA: drug used to treat Parkinson's Disease.

LE: lower extremities.

LEARNING A CODE TEST: (Lhermitte & Signoret, 1972, 1976) Korsakoff patients are unable to perform on this test.

LEARNING A LOGICAL ORDER TEST: (Lhermitte & Signoret, 1972, 1976) Korsakoff patients are unable to perform on this test.

LEARNING A PLACE IN SPACE TEST: (Lhermitte & Signoret, 1972, 1976); Korsakoff patients perform poorly; bilateral hippocampal lesioned patients are unable to perform.

LEARNING LOGICAL AND SEQUENTIAL ORDER TESTS: (Lhermitte & Signoret, 1972, 1976) Learning a place in space test, learning a code test, learning a logical order test.

LEARNING SLOWNESS - RESPONSE SETS: may be caused by aging, a dementing process, frontal-lobe disease, Korsakoff's syndrome, or head injury; the first four items of the Block Design subtest (WAIS-R) are easy for persons with average or better constructional ability; typical response patterns for persons with impaired constructional ability may be: first two items failed, or passed only on the second trial while the succeeding two or three or more items are passsed, each more rapidly than the last (Newcombe, 1969; Smith, 1966); split-brain patient: often unable to perform on Block Design because he/she can use only one hemisphere and each hemisphere contributes to the adequate realization of the design; neither hemisphere alone is competent in this task (Geschwind, 1979); left parietal lesioned patients: tend to show confusion, simplification, and concrete handling of the design, although orderly; typically work from left to right, and their construction usually preserves the square shape of the design; their greatest difficulty is often in placing the last block (which will typically be on their right) (McFie, 1975); right-sided lesioned patients: may begin at the right of the design and work left; visuospatial deficits show up in disorientation, design distortions, and misperceptions; some patients with severe visuospatial deficits lose sight of the squared or self-contained format of the design altogether; left visuospatial inattention may compound design-copying problems and result in two- or three-block solutions to the four-block designs in which the whole left half or one left quadrant of the design has been omitted; both right and left hemisphere damaged patients make many more errors on the side of the lesion; errors at the top of the constructions may indicate temporal lobe components; errors at the bottom of the construction have parietal lobe components (Kaplan, 1986).

LEARNING TEST BATTERY: (Meyer & Falconer, 1960) test for retention of newly learned material.

LEFT PARIETAL-LOBE SENSITIVE TESTS: WAIS-R Block De-

L

sign.

LEFT SIDED NEGLECT: usually caused by a lesion in the right inferior parietal lobe; may also be due to lesions to the frontal lobe and cingulate cortex as well as to subcortical structures including the superior colliculus and lateral hypothalamus (and others).

LEFT TEMPORAL-LOBE SENSITIVE TESTS: Verbal-memory tests such as Associate Learning test and the Logical Memory test from the Wechsler Memory Scale, Similarities (WAIS-R), Rey-Osterrieth Complex Figures or Taylor's Complex Figure, Hebb's Recurring Digits (Milner, 1970), Constant Trigrams (Milner, 1970. 1972), Wicken's Release from PI Test (Craik & Birdwistle, 1971; Wickens, 1970).

LEITER INTERNATIONAL PERFORMANCE SCALE: devised especially for testing verbally handicapped and foreign language-speaking children; sometimes useful for adult brain-damaged patients; provides some differentiation of performance levels for some functions such as serial reasoning and two-dimensional construction; the examiner must rely on own content analysis when interpreting a patient's performance; includes nonverbal analogues of Block Design, Block Counting, and Similarities, test of perceptual recognition, size and number estimation, and comprehension of sequences and progressions.

LENTICULAR APHASIA: see commissural aphasia.

LESION: any pathological or traumatic discontinuity of tissue or loss of functions of a part, especially when involving a small, well-defined area.

LETTER SPAN: (Botwinick & Storandt, 1974; Newcombe, 1969); although similar in concept to digit span tests, brain-damaged patients produce lower average scores than on digit span — forward; sensitive to left-hemisphere damage (temporal or temporoparietal lobes).

LEUCOPENIA: see leukopenia.

LEUCOTOMY: see leukotomy.

LEUKODYSTROPHIES: a number of rare familial diseases which occur most commonly in infancy and childhood as well as conditions resulting in abnormal metabolism and formation of myelin; characterized by a degree of destruction of axons, relative preservation of nerve cells, and absence of inflammation; most common: metachromatic leukodystrophy (MLD) caused by an inherited autosomal recessive trait characterized by a genetically determine enzymatic defect; *symptoms*: gradual intellectual deterioration, episodes of moodiness and withdrawal, possible delusions and hallucinations; outbursts of rage; frequently given a psychiatric diagnosis incorrectly (Reitan & Wolfson, 1985).

LEUKOPENIA: reduction of the number of leukocytes in the blood, the count being around 5000.

LEUKOTOMY: cutting of the white matter in the oval center of the frointal lobe of the brain; prefrontal lobotomy.

LH: lutenizing hormone.

LICHTHEIM'S APHASIA: spontaneous speech is lost but the ability to repeat words is retained.

LIFE SATISFACTION INDEX: (Neugarten et al., 1961) a low score suggests depression; primarily designed for older people.

LIMBIC LOBE: limbic system.

LIMBIC SYSTEM: formally called the rhinencephalon; group of paleo-cortical structures, nuclei, and connecting fibers which ring the di-encephalon; amygdala, hippocampus and hippocampus gyrus, for-nix, the uncus, cingulate gyrus, part of the insula, the septal area, the isthmus, Broca's olfactory area, and the orbital surface of the frontal pole; the hippocampal gyrus overlays the hippocampus at the posterior end of the temporal lobe immediately behind the bulge overlying the amygdala; the main fiber tract from the hippocampal area is the fimbria which is joined by other fibers from adjacent areas to form a dense bundle called the fornix which sweeps posteriorly and then up and over anteriorly to distribute to all areas of the hypothalamus, but particularly to the mammillary body and parts of the thalamus; some fimbria fibers decussate directly to the opposite hippocampus and there are also important cross connections be-tween the amygdala on each side through the anterior commissure; involved in some cognitive functions, but primarily is concerned with motivational and emotional activities; has been called the "emo-tional brain;" controls the experience of emotion.

LIMBIC SYSTEM LESIONS: damage in the region of the amygdala is associated with rage reactions, hyperphagia, and increased sexual activity; lesions in the region of the uncus are associated with olfactory and gustatory hallucinations; temporal-lobe seizures may spread to the limbic system structures; the cingulate gyrus lies above the corpus callosum; connecting pathways traverse the isth-mus posteriorly and extend forward to Broca's olfactory area; psy-chosurgery (leucotomy, lobotomy, cingulotomy) performed on these pathways and the connections from the cingulate gyrus to the thalamus produces emotional blunting of phobic anxiety states and chronic pain syndromes.

LINE BISECTION TEST: (Diller et al., 1974; Kinsbourne, 1974; Schenkenberg et al., 1980); sensitive to right-hemisphere lesions; errors most often made by patients with visual field defects who tend to under estimate the size of the line; primarily a test for visual unilateral inattention/ neglect opposite to the defective field; right-hemisphere damaged patients neglect about a third of the lines.

LINE ILLUSION TEST: see Muller-Lyer line illusion test.

L

LINE TRACING TASK: (Talland, 1965a) timed test of scanning; examines fine motor regulation; tracking behavior problems tend to show up in difficulties with angles, overshooting lines at corners, perseveration of an ongoing response, and inability to decrease size when indicated (Lezak, 1983).

LINGULA: a general term for a small tongue-like structure.

LINGUALS: formed during articulation (l, t).

LINGUO OR PHARYNGEAL APRAXIA: often accompanies Broca's aphasia; manifested in faulty efforts to smack the lips and to make other purposeful or facial movements.

LIPID STORAGE DISEASES: cerebromacular degeneration caused by accumulation of lipid in the ganglion cells of the retina of the eye; result of inherited autosomal recessive trait causing enzyme deficiency which represents a metabolic abnormality; includes Tay-Sachs disease, Niemann-Pick disease (Reitan & Wolfson, 1985).

LISSENCEPHALY: brain fails to form sulci and gyri and corresponds to a 12-week old embryo.

LITERAL PARAPHASIA: faulty pronunciation.

LITTLE'S DISEASE: congenital spastic stiffness of the limbs; a form of cerebral spastic paralysis dating from birth and may be associated with various disorders, including birth trauma, fetal anoxia, or illness of the mother during pregnancy; characterized by muscular weakness, walking difficulties, and usually, by convulsions, bilateral athetosis, and mental deficiency; also called spastic diplegia.

LLE: lower left extremity.

LLQ: lower left quadrant.

LMP: last menstrual period.

LOA: loosening of associations.

LOC: level of care.

LOCKED-IN SYNDROME: paralysis of all muscles except eye movements; inability to communicate with others except by eye movements; see medullary vascular lesions.

LOCOMOTOR ATAXIA: see late syphilis, tabes dorsalis.

LOGICAL MEMORY SUBTEST: (WMS) tests immediate recall of verbal ideas with two paragraphs; sensitive to learning deficits involving complex or novel information (Kaszniak et al., 1979; Kear-Colwell, 1973; Wilson et al., 1982) .

LOGORRHEA: protracted uncontrollable talking.

LONG-TERM MEMORY: located primarily in the medial temporal lobe; the storage of information in a code that is resistant to retrograde interference.

LONG-TERM MEMORY DEFICIT: lesion in Brodmann's area 21, hippocampus (and possibly the amygdala).

LONG-TERM MEMORY vs SHORT-TERM MEMORY: (Kolb & Whishaw theory 1980) may be parallel processes in which material is stored separately in both; the parietal lobe appears to be involved in short-term memory and the temporal lobe in long-term memory.

LONGITUDINAL EVALUATION OF HEAD-TRAUMA VICTIMS: (Eson et al., 1978); a series of measures taken from the Boyd Developmental Progress Scale and the Vineland Social Maturity Scale that are used to document the return of adaptive behaviors following severe head-injury.

LOOSE ASSOCIATIONS: see flight of ideas, formal thought disorder; derailment.

LORDOSIS: anterior concavity in the curvature of the lumbar spine as viewed from the side; the term is used to refer to abnormally increased curvature (hollow back, saddle back, swayback).

LOW BLOOD PRESSURE: hypotension.

LOWER HEMIANOPIA: defective vision in the lower half of each eye.

LOWER NEURON LESION (7th nerve): causes paralysis of whole face; see seventh nerve lesion.

LUE: left upper extremity.

LUMBAR PUNCTURE: see cerebrospinal fluid studies.

LUPUS ERYTHEMATOSUS, SYSTEMIC: a generalized connective tissue disorder, affecting mainly middle-aged women, ranging from mild to fulminating, and characterized by skin eruptions, arthralgia, leukopenia, visceral lesions, fever, and other constitutional symptoms.

LUQ: left upper quadrant.

LURIA/CHRISTENSEN'S BLOCK COUNTING: taken from Yerkes and available in Christensen's Luria test; test of spatial reasoning; no norms available.

LURIA'S FUNCTIONAL UNITS: the cortex is divided into two function units: 1. the posterior portion of the neocortex (parietal, temporal, and occipital lobes) is the sensory unit which receives sensory impressions, processes them, and stores them as information; 2. the anterior cortex (frontal lobe; motor unit); formulates intentions, organizes them into programs of action, and executes the programs. In both cortical units there is a hierarchical structure with three cortical zones arranged functionally one above the other.

LURIA'S MATH REASONING PROBLEMS: (Christensen, 1979) involve little math skills; use intermediate operations that are not specified; requires inhibition of the impulsive direct method; require comparisons between elements of the problem that require reasoning ability to solve.

LURIA-TYPE COMPUTATIONAL QUESTIONS: (Christensen, 1979) inability to respond correctly to the simplest and automatic levels such as addition, division, and multiplication suggests an impairment in symbol formulation characteristic of aphasic disorders or a severe breakdown in conceptual functions; more complex math

M

operations, such as carrying, test the immediate memory span, attention, and mental tracking functions.

LURIA-TYPE TESTS: (for planning and perseverative behavior); copying and maintaining alternating letters or repetitive sequential patterns of hand movements with separate trials for each hand; may be caused by trauma, fetal anoxia, or illness of the mother during pregnancy; characterized by muscular weakness, walking difficulties, and usually, by convulsions, bilateral athetosis, and mental deficiency; also called spastic diplegia.

LUTEINIZING HORMONE (LH): secreted by the anterior pituitary gland; completes follicular maturation and rupture (ovulation); brings about development of the corpus luteum; increases estrogen release in females; LH is called interstitial-cell-stimulating hormone (ICSH) in males; mediates the synthesis and release of androgens in males.

M

M. A.: mental age.

MACQUARRIE TEST FOR MECHANICAL ABILITY: paper and pencil test; examines visuomotor speed and accuracy, visuospatial estimation, and visual tracking; individual subtest items may be compared; when visuospatial functions are impaired but motor activity remains intact and under good control; large differences in performance levels will appear in low tracing and location scores and higher scores on the motor speed and accuracy tasks.

MACQUARRIE TEST FOR MECHANICAL ABILITY BLOCK COUNTING SUBTEST: see block counting subtest of the Macquarrie test for Mechanical Ability.

MACROGYRIA: gyri are broader and less numerous than normal.

MACULA COMMUNIS: a thickened area on the wall of the otic vesicle which divides into the macula sacculi (saccule) and macula utriculi (utricle); vestibular receptors in the middle ear involved in upright posture and orientation.

MACULA CORTEX LESION: caused by damage to the tip of the occipital pole; homonymous macular defects are always exactly congruous.

MACULA OF THE RETINA: group of retina cells responsible for central vision.

MACULAR REGION OF THE VISUAL SYSTEM: occipital lobe.

MACULAR SPARING: sparing of the central visual field when one occipital lobe is destroyed; the macular region of the visual system

M

receives a double vascular supply, from both the middle and posterior vertebral arteries, making it more resilient to large hemispheric lesions and/or the foveal region of the retina projects to both hemispheres so that even if one occipital lobe is destroyed, the other receives projections from the fovea; macular sparing helps to differentiate lesions of the tract or thalamus from cortical lesions, since macular sparing occurs only after lesions (usually large) of the visual cortex.

MACULAR SPARING HEMIANOPIA: lesion of the occipital cortex.

MAGICAL THINKING: the individual believes that his or her thoughts, words or actions will cause or prevent a specific outcome in a way that defies normal laws of cause and effect.

MAIN RADIATION LESION: causes a complete homonymous hemianopia.

MALARIA: caused by protozoa, Plasmodium genus, which are transmitted by the bites of infected mosquitoes. Cerebral malaria occurs when the plasmodia infect the capillaries of the brain, producing local hemorrhages and subsequent degeneration of neurons.

MALIGNANT: tumors having the properties of anaplasia, invasion, and metastasis; tumors that tend to become progressively worse and to result in death.

MALINGERING: conscious and unconscious motivations may contribute to symptoms which resemble neurological disorders, but may not actually be based in fact (pseudosymptoms); secondary gain may exacerbate symptoms; identifying malingering may not always be clear-cut, but should be suspected if there are inconsistencies in the history or examination; indications of malingering may show up in some of the following test results: Bender-Gestalt, Benton Visual Retention Test, Halstead-Reitan, MMPI, Porch Index of Communicative Ability;, and Rorschach. Specific tests to unearth malingering: Memory of 15 items (Lezak, 1983, pp. 618; Rey, 1964), Dot Counting (Rey, 1941), Wechsler Memory Scale Associate Learning (Gronwall, quoted in Lezak, 1983), Word Recognition (Rey, 1941), and Symptom Validity Test (Pankratz, 1979; Pankratz at al., 1975).

MALIGNANT NEUROLEPTIC SYNDROME: a life-threatening reaction to neuroleptics characterized by diaphoresis, hyperpyrexia, confusion, tremors, delirium, and autonomic symptoms such as tachycardia.

MANDIBULARIS NERVE: mandibular nerve; general sensory; one of three divisions of the trigeminal nerve, passing through the foramen ovale to the infratemporal fossa. Origin: trigeminal ganglion; extensive distribution to muscles of mastication, skin of face, mucous membrane of mouth, and teeth.

MANIC-DEPRESSIVE ILLNESS: an affective disorder in which there is a mood disturbance involving either elation or depression; more

M

commonly referred to as Bipolar Disorder; frequently the manic phase involves psychosis involving flight of ideas, grandiosity, pressured speech, neologisms, paranoid ideation, delusions, religiosity, agitation, auditory hallucinations, loss of sleep and appetite, poor concentration, speeded ideation, etc.; the depressed stage may include loss of appetite, loss of sleep or hypersomnia, auditory hallucinations, suicidal ideation, paranoia, and delusions; not all these symptoms may be present, but sometimes, other psychotic symptoms will be included.

MANNERISM: a rapidly performed, semi-automatic grimace or gesture.

MANUAL DEXTERITY: see motor performance, alternating hand movement defects, Finger Tapping Test, Purdue Pegboard Test, Grooved Pegboard Test, motor tests for ataxia.

MARCHE À PETITS PAS: uncertainty of balance and short-stepped gait; lesion(s) of extrapyramidal structures; see also Parkinson's Disease, Wilson's Disease, extrapyramidal, basal ganglia, cerebellum.

MARCUS-GUNN PUPIL: abnormal pupillary response; when stimulated the reaction is slower, less complete, and so brief that the pupil may dilate again (pupillary escape phenomena).

MARIE'S DISEASE: see acromegaly, Marie-Tooth Disease.

MARIJUANA USE: personality changes in heavy users: affective blunting, mental and physical sluggishness, apathy, restlessness, some mental confusion, and defective recent memory (Evans, 1975; Kolansky & Moore, 1972; Lishman, 1978); also spelled mariahuana, mariguana, marihuana.

MASOCHISM: pleasure derived from suffering physical or mental pain.

MASS ACTION HYPOTHESIS (CORTICAL FUNCTION): the entire brain participates in every behavior, and therefore the removal of any cortical tissue produces, with respect to any task, a deficit that is proportional to the amount of tissue removed (Lashley 1939).

MATTIS ORGANIC MENTAL SYNDROME SCREENING EXAM: (Mattis, 1976) an extensive structured examination with a scoring system which evaluates dementia; can be administered in 15 to 20 minutes; it evaluates 10 areas of cognitive functioning: state of consciousness, insight, affect, estimate of premorbid intellectual abilities, general information, verbal abstraction, attention, memory, language, and construction.

MAXILLARIS NERVE: maxillary nerve; general sensory; one of the three terminal divisions of the trigeminal nerve, passing through the foramen rotundum; extensive distribution to skin of face and scalp, mucous membrane of maxillary sinus and nasal cavity, and teeth.

MAZE LEARNING DEFICITS: (Milner, 1965; 1969); inability to learn pathways in a maze may be due to bilateral hippocampal lesions as well as frontal-lobe lesions; frontal-lobe lesioned patients may show rule-breaking behavior.

mcg.: microgram.

MC GILL PICTURE ANOMALY TEST: right temporal-lobe lesioned patients are usually unable to identify anomalies or oddities in the complex pictures.

MEANINGFUL PICTURES TEST: (Battersby et al., 1956); visual neglect/ inattention test.

MEASLES: see subacute sclerosing panenchephalitis.

MECHANICAL REASONING TEST: bicycle drawing test; MacQuarrie Test of Mechanical Ability.

MEDIAL: pertaining to the middle; closer to the median plane or the midline of a body or structure; the middle layer of structures.

MEDIAL CEREBELLAR LESION: disruption of ability to stand upright and walk.

MEDIAL GENICULATE NUCLEI: a nucleus within the medial geniculate body, composed of central and dorsal parts which receive ascending auditory fibers and project to the auditory cortex.

MEDIAL LONGITUDINAL FASCICULUS: controls lateral eye gaze.

MEDIAL LONGITUDINAL FISSURE: the deep fissure that extends inferiorly to the corpus callosum; separates the brain into right and left hemispheres; also called longitudinal fissure.

MEDIAL TEMPORAL-LOBE: controls long-term memory; Brodmann's area 21; particularly the hippocampus and the amydala.

MEDULLARY INFARCTS: motor deficits, disturbances of respiratory and vasomotor control centers, disruption of other aspects of vital functions, changes or deficits in pain and temperature sensitivity, vertigo, vomiting, and varying degrees of paralysis of the palate, pharynx, and vocal cords (Reitan & Wolfson, 1985).

MEDULLA: a general term for the inmost part of an organ or structure.

MEDULLA LESION: may cause Wallenburg's syndrome; crossed paralysis; see also brainstem lesions.

MEDULLA OBLONGATA: the truncated cone of nerve tissue continuous above with the pons and below with the spinal cord; lies anterior to the cerebellum; upper part of its posterior surface forms the floor of the lower part of the fourth ventrical; contains ascending and descending tracts, and important collections of nerve cells that deal with vital functions, such as respiration, circulation, special senses, primitive visceral reflexes such as heart rate, and blood pressure; significant injury to the medulla oblongata usually results in death.

MEDULLOBLASTOMA: midline tumor of cerebellum; causes severe equilibrium disturbance; see also under tumor.

MEDULLOBLASTOMA OF CEREBELLAR VERMIS: causes cerebellar gait.

M

MELANIN: the dark amorphous pigment of the skin, hair, and various tumors, the choroid coat of the eye, and the substantia nigra of the brain.

MELANOMA: a tumor made up of melanin-pigmented cells. the term used alone refers to a malignant melanoma.

MELATONIN: inhibits production of gonadatropic hormone releasing factors; prevents premature sexual maturation; hyposecretion leads to the development of completely adult-like secondary sexual characteristics in children; hypersecretion leads to failure to develop sexually.

MEMORY: the retention of learned experiences; two types: 1. primary or short-term; 2. secondary or long-term; see further discussion on specific types.

MEMORY DISTURBANCE/DISEASE: usually follows bilateral damage to the medial temporal lobe and its connections to the mammillary body and upper brainstem; see also Korsakoff's psychosis, ECT, dementia, anoxia, hypoglycemia, limbic encephalitis, bilateral posterior cerebral artery occlusion, head injuries, atrophy.

MEMORY - AUDITORY: Brodmann's area 22.

MEMORY - IMMEDIATE RECALL: steps: 1. initial registration; 2. short-term holding; 3. verbal repetition; all steps are carried out by the language cortex surrounding the Sylvian fissure.

MEMORY - LONG-TERM: (Broadbent, 1958) the knowledge of a former state of mind after it has already once dropped from consciousness.

MEMORY - PRIMARY: (James, 1890, p. 648) endures for a very brief period of time; (Broadbent, 1958); short-term memory.

MEMORY - RECENT: presumes intact registration, retention, and short-term storage; limbic structures are required to insure long-term storage and retrieval of memories from the cortex; structures required: hippocami, amygdala, mamillary bodies, dorsal medial nuclei of thalami, and any essential subcortical links.

MEMORY - RECENT, IMPAIRMENT: if limbic structures are damaged in isolation there may be: 1. severe anterograde amnesia, 2. moderate/ severe retrograde amnesia, 3. confabulation, 4. intact short-term memory; defects may be found following a bilateral temporal lobectomy, herpes simplex encephalitis, bilateral hippocampal infarction, Korsakoff's disease, bilateral destruction of the mamillary bodies and the dorsal medial nucleus of the thalamus; Alzheimer's dementia will cause defects in new learning; in head trauma: if the temporal lobes are concussed against the bony middle fossa, there is disruption of the hippocampal function which disturbs memory storage and retrieval. may also be caused by a dorsolateral frontal-lobe lesion (Milner, 1974).

MEMORY - REMOTE: stored in the appropriate cortex; does not require the limbic system for retrieval from storage; lost only by destruction of the cortex by any one of the degenerative diseases (Alzheimer's, Pick's, senility).

MEMORY - SECONDARY: the knowledge of a former state of mind after it has already once dropped from consciousness (Broadbent, 1958); long-term memory.

MEMORY - SHORT-TERM: (Broadbent, 1958) endures for a short period of time; the language system must be intact; aphasia can cause disruption, particularly in conduction aphasia; primary deficit is the inability to repeat.

MEMORY TESTS: Wechsler Memory Scale (WMS), Revised Wechsler Memory Scale, Learning Test Battery, Memory Test Battery, Randt Memory Test, Remote Memory, Recall of Public Events, Facial Recognition Test, Old-Young Test, Television Titles.

MEMORY EXAMINATION: (Lezak, 1983) testing should include span of immediate retention, learning capacity, retention of newly learned material, and efficiency of retrieval of both recently learned and long-stored information (remote memory); tests may include a WAIS-R battery, a mental status examination which includes items involving remote personal memory, verbal retention task, personal orientation, a test of configural recall and retention, and a test of learning ability that gives a learning curve; pronounced deficits on the general review of memory should be explored in detail with systematic comparisons between functions, modalities, and the length, type, and complexity of the content.

MEMORY FOR DESIGNS TESTS: (Graham & Kendall, 1960); Stanford-Binet subtests and WMS; sensitive to right-hemisphere damage.

MEMORY FOR STORY AND PARAGRAPH TESTS: Stanford-Binet subtests, Logical Memory subtest from the Wechsler Memory Scale, Babcock Story Recall Test, The Cowboy Story.

MEMORY IMPAIRMENT: bilateral removal of the medial temporal lobes, including the hippocampus and amygdala results in anterograde amnesia; Brodmann's area 21 (Milner, 1972); "memory problems" may mean any number of specific disabilities involving registration, attention, tracking, immediate memory span, learning or retrieval in one or more modalities (Gronwall & Wrightson, 1981), or a condition in which the patient has stored and can retrieve required memories, but seems unable to do so without response-directed questioning or cuing (Schachter & Crovitz, 1977). What patients and families call "memory problems" may result from diffuse damage and reticular formation dysfunction, damage to the memory system, frontal-lobe lesions, or any combination of these (Lezak, 1983); those activities that have a large attentional component, such as immediate memory span, tend to improve quickly and reach a

M

plateau within the first six months to a year after injury (Gronwall & Vigoroux et al., 1971); activities such as new learning that involve the memory system tend to improve over a longer period of time (O'Brien & Lezak, 1981; Vigoroux et al., 1971); deficits having to do with retrieval rather than registration and learning may either improve as specific verbal or visuospatial functions return, making stored information and response patterns available again; if the deficits have resulted from extensive frontal-lobe or subcortical damage, only minimal improvement can be expected soon after return of consciousness (Lezak, 1978b).

MEMORY OF FORMS: a tactile memory test; Seguin-Goddard formboard test (Teuber & Weinstein, 1954).

MEMORY PROCESS: steps: registration; retention/storage; retrieval; basic types: immediate; recent or short-term; remote or long-term.

MEMORY TESTS: sensitive to right temporal-lobe lesions: McGill picture anomalies, Rey complex figures test, Bender-Gestalt, Wechsler Memory Scale (drawing subtest); sensitive to left temporal-lobe lesions: Wechsler Memory Scale (paired associate & logical stories), Rey auditory learning test.

MEMORY THEORY (Hebb, 1949): short-term memory is an active process of limited duration, whereas long-term memory involves an actual structural change in the nervous system; neurons in the brain are interconnected with many other neurons, and, in turn, each neuron receives input from many synapses upon its dendrites and cell body. The resulting neuronal loops contain neurons whose output signal may be either excitatory or inhibitory. Many of the loops probably run from the cortex to the thalamus or other subcortical structures, such as the hippocampus, and back to the cortex (Lorente de No, in Hebb, 1949). Hebb's theory postulates that each psychologically important event, sensation, percept, memory, thought, emotion, etc., is conceived to be the flow of activity in a given neuronal loop. Synapses in a particular path become functionally connected to form a cell assembly. If two neurons are excited together, they become linked functionally. Cell assembly is a system that is initially organized by a particular sensory event, but is capable of continuing its activity after the stimulation has ceased. To produce functional changes in synaptic transmission, the cell assembly must be repeatedly activated. After the initial sensory input the assembly reverberates; repeated reverberation produces the structural changes. Thus, short-term memory is reverberation of the closed loops of the cell assembly; long-term memory is more structural, a lasting change in synaptic connections. For the structural changes to occur there must be a period in which the cell assembly is left relatively undisturbed for 15 minutes to an hour. This process of structural change was called consolidation by Hebb

(1949); the hippocampus was assumed to be especially important to the process of consolidation. Any cell assembly could be excited by others (the basis for thought or ideation). The essence of an "idea" is that it occurs in the absence of the original environmental event that it corresponds to.

MENINGES: the three membranes that envelop the brain and spinal cord: the dura mater, pia mater, and arachnoid.

MENINGIOMA: growths attached to the meninges and grow entirely outside the brain; well encapsulated; most benign of all brain tumors; often multiple; disturb brain function by producing pressure on the brain; often produce seizures; usually lie over the hemispheres, but some may occur between the hemispheres; may erode the overlying bone; if removed completely, they do not usually recur.

MENINGITIS: infection of the cerebrospinal fluid with inflammation of the pia mater and arachnoid tissue, the subarachnoid space, and superficial tissues of the brain; highest incidence in children under five (70%) and people over seventy (20%); symptoms may include fever and headache, followed by drowsiness, confusion, loss of consciousness, nuchal rigidity, sometimes seizures, motor deficits, cranial nerve palsies, irritability, stupor, coma, and death; Reitan & Wolfson (1985) have found residual neuropsychological deficits in neurologically "recovered" patients; types include acute bacterial m., pneumococcal m., meningococcal m., tuberculous m.

MENTAL DISORDER: (DSM III-R) a clinically significant behavioral or psychologic syndrome or pattern that occurs in an individual and that typically is associated with either a painful symptom (distress) or impairment in one or more important areas of functioning; when the disturbance is limited to a conflict between the individual and society, this may represent social deviance, but is not necessarily a mental disorder.

MESENCEPHALON: primitive division of the brain; midbrain; includes the tectum, tegmentum, & cerebral aqueduct.

MESIAL: nearer the median line.

MESIAL FRONTAL-LOBE: the middle portion of the frontal-lobe.

MESION: the plane that divides the body into right and left symmetrical halves.

METABOLITE: any substance produced by metabolism or by a metabolic process.

METAMORPHOPSIA: disturbance of vision in which objects are seen as distorted in shape.

METASTASIS: the transfer of disease from one organ or part to another organ or part not directly connected; may be due to the transfer of pathogenic microoganisms or to transfer of cells, as in malignant tumors.

METASTATIC: refers to metastasis.

M

METENCEPHALON: includes the cerebellum, pons, fourth ventrical; part of the hindbrain; anterior portion of the rhombencephalon.

mg.: milligram.

MICHIGAN NEUROPSYCHOLOGICAL TEST BATTERY: (Smith, 1980) a well-balanced battery of tests, some unpublished, which takes about 3 hours to administer; no norms; not standardized.

MICROENCEPHALY: development of the brain is rudimentary and the person has low-grade intelligence.

MICROGLIA: small, non-neural, interstitial cells of mesoderm origin that form part of the supporting structure of the CNS; various forms; may have slender branched processes; migratory and act as phagocytes to waste products of nerve tissue.

MICROGRAPHIC: small and cramped handwriting of patients with Parkinsonian tremor; sometimes seen in temporal-lobe epilepsy.

MICROPOLYGYRIA: gyri are more numerous, smaller, and more poorly developed than normal.

MICROPSIA: visual images (hallucinations) that seem too small.

MICTURITION: urination; cortical center: medial surface of the frontal lobes.

MIDBRAIN: consists of two main subdivisions: 1. the tectum which lies above the aqueduct and forms the dorsal aspect; and 2. the tegmentum which lies below the aqueduct rostral to the pons; the basis pedunculi are on the ventral aspect; in the middle part of the tegmentum, sensory fibers ascend in its dorsal and lateral areas; motor fibers descend in the ventral portions; the central part contains nuclei and fiber systems that are of crucial importance in the mediation of both positive (pleasure) and negative (fear and anger) emotions; the tegmentum is important in determining levels of consciousness (wakefulness, arousal, and attention).

MIDBRAIN LEVEL: contains auditory and optic levels which allow animals to receive simple sensory input that originates at some distance; these sensory systems are linked with voluntary motor systems that allow the animal to respond to distant stimuli by moving toward or away from them; contains programs that allow animals to chain together a number of movements to form complex behaviors of the automatic type.

MIDBRAIN OCCLUSIONS: rare; characterized by palsy of the third cranial nerve and contralateral hemiparesis. Thrombosis of the superior cerebellar artery involves the junction of the midbrain and pons and frequently produces homolateral cerebellar signs; nystagmus and facial paresis; pain and temperature sensation on the opposite side of the body may also be impaired (Reitan & Wolfson, 1985).

MIDBRAIN VASCULAR LESIONS: dorsolateral infarction: Horner's syndrome on the same side and total loss of sensation on the opposite side of the body; severe cerebellar deficit on the same side if the superior cerebellar peduncle is damaged; paramedian infarction: incomplete 3rd nerve palsy; damage to the red nucleus interrupts the dentato-rubro-thalamic tract from the opposite cerebellar hemisphere causing severe cerebellar signs in the limbs opposite the 3rd nerve palsy (Benedikt's syndrome); basal infarction: the 3rd nerve fascicle will be destroyed causing a complete 3rd nerve palsy; damage to the cerebral peduncle will result in hemiplegia of the opposite limbs including the face (Weber's syndrome).

MIDDLE CEREBRAL ARTERY: one of two major divisions of the internal carotid artery; the other division is the anterior cerebral artery; irrigates the anterior and middle portions of the cortex as well as the subcortical structures of this same area; joins with the anterior cerebral artery to form the anterior communicating artery.

MIDDLE CEREBRAL ARTERY OCCLUSIONS: occlusion of the main trunk: causes massive infarction of the bulk of the hemisphere; coma frequent; occlusion of the dominant hemisphere: a global dysphasia; occlusion of the non-dominant hemisphere: severe dyspraxia and possibly denial of the existance of the left side; precentral and central branch occlusions cause a flaccid monoplegia of the arm and face; both pyramidal and extrapyramidal mechanisms may be destroyed producing a flaccid type of weakness of the face and arm, with little or no potential for recovery; hemianaesthesia and complete hemianopia usually present; occlusion of the perforating artery (Capsular C.V.A): occlusion of one of the lenticulostriate vessels is both frequent and has the most favorable outcome; may cause pseudobulbar palsy which may go unnoticed until the corticobulbar fibers on the other side are damaged and the cranial nerve nuclei are deprived of all control; speech, chewing and swallowing become impossible; significant recovery is unusual; often seen in diabetic or hypertensive patients; occlusion of the main motor pathways of the capsule: the only evidence of cortico-bulbar fiber damage is a mild upper motor neuron facial weakness; both limbs on contralateral side become flaccid but may recover; rarely any sensory deficit or field defect; no dysphasia; there may be dysarthria; occlusion of the terminal branch of the dominent hemisphere: the precentral artery supplies the motor areas for the face and arm and Broca's speech area; occlusion causes flaccid paralysis of the face and arm, total dysarthria, and inability to write; central artery occlusion: causes weakness of the face, arm, and mild dysphasic difficulties.

MIGRAINE: a headache characterized by aching throbbing pain, frequently unilateral, and often coincident with pulse beat; often preceded by a visual disturbance (aura) that occurs within a restricted region of the visual field; may be zone of flashing, whirling, or shimmering light that slowly increases in size, lasting 15 to 30

M

minutes; the aura is presumed to occur because vasoconstriction of one or more cerebral arteries has produced ischemia of the occipital cortex; the headache begins when the vasoconstriction reverses, thus ending the visual disturbance, and vasodilation occurs; the pain is localized in one side of the head and can be accompanied by nausea and vomiting; may last for hours to days; occurrence generally drops with aging and usually ceases in middle age; triggered by environmental factors: anxiety, the termination of anxiety, fatigue, bright light, and sometimes allergies.

MIGRAINE HEADACHE-TREATMENT: usually treated with ergotamine compounds and caffeine; biofeedback training has been used successfully to ward off an attack; treatment usually involves a totally dark room and avoidance of circumstances that are known to precipitate the attacks.

MILL HILL VOCABULARY SCALE: sensitive to dominant hemisphere disease (Brooks & Aughton, 1979a,b).

MILLARD-GUBLER SYNDROME: pontine vascular lesion involving the sixth and seventh cranial nerves as well as the fibers of the corticospinal tract; a crossed paralysis; facial palsy combined with a contralateral weakness or paralysis of the arm and leg, and paralysis of the outward movement of the eye.

min.: minimum; minute.

MINIMAL BRAIN DYSFUNCTION: a behavioral syndrome diagnosed in up to 5 to 10% of school-age children characterized by hyperactivity, distractability, and short attention span, as well as certain perceptual-cognitive signs; may be due to a deficiency in catecholaminergic function; levels of homovanillic acid in the cerebrospinal fluid have been found to be significantly lower (Shaywitz, Cohen, & Bowers, 1977); often associated with with perinatal hypoxia; symptoms tend to lessen with age, but persist into adult life (Wood, Reimherr, Wender, & Johnson, 1976); may be ameliorated by continual use of pharmacological stimulants, especially catecholaminergic agonists such as amphetamine, methylphenidate, and caffeine (Bradley, 1950; Millichap, 1973, in Goldstein, 1984).

MINI-MENTAL STATE: (Folstein et al., 1975); a brief and simple test of cognitive functions which has been standardized; useful to track changes in intellectual functioning in progressive dementias and psychiatric patients.

MINIMAL REFLEX ACTIVITY: slight flexion or extension of the foot; some toe twitches; extension of the large toe; anal and bladder reflexes for waste secretion may be present.

MINKUS COMPLETION TEST: tests syntactical construction, word usage, and reading comprehension (Terman & Merrill, 1973).

MINNESOTA MULTIPHASIC PERSONALITY INVENTORY: (Dahlstrom et al., 1975; Hathaway & McKinley, 1951; Welsh &

Dahlstrom, 1956;); untimed 566-item true-false paper and pencil questionnaire; general pattern tendencies include: nonpsychiatric patients with CNS disease tend to have an elevated "neurotic triad" (Hs, D, and Hy) (Dikmen & Reitan, 1974) and higher than average Sc scores and Pt scores (Mack, 1979); elevation of scales 2, 8, and 1 characterize profiles of traumatically injured patients (Casey & Fennell, 1981); head injured often have elevated 2 and 8 scales (Heaton et al., 1978); generally, brain-damaged patients have elevated profiles, reflecting the frequent incidence of emotional disturbance in these patients (Filskov & Leli, 1981); the Sc scale may be one of the highest scores in the profiles of epileptic patients (Doehring, 1962; Kløve 1974); multiple sclerosis patients may have high neurotic triad scores (Dahlstrom & Welsh, 1960); malingerers may produce severely disturbed-appearing profiles; brain-damaged patients often have T-scores above 70 on scales 2, 7, and 8; malingerers may exceed T-scores of 70 on scales F, 1, 3, 6, 7, 8, and 10 (Heaton et al., 1978).

MINNESOTA PAPER FORM BOARD TEST: (Likert & Quasha, 1970); test of perceptual organizing behavior; calls on perceptual scanning and recognition as well as the ability to perceive fragmented percepts as wholes.

MINNESOTA PERCEPT-DIAGNOSTIC TEST: (Fuller, 1969; Fuller & Laird, 1963) tests for the presence of a tendency toward rotation in drawings; may be useful in discriminating brain-damaged patients.

MINNESOTA TEST FOR DIFFERENTIAL DIAGNOSIS OF APHASIA: — revised edition (Schuell, 1972); focuses on different aspects of each of five areas, defined by factor analysis in which aphasic patients commonly have problems: auditory disturbances, visual and reading disturbances, speech and language disturbances, visuomotor and writing disturbances, and disturbances of numerical relationships and arithmetic processes; takes from one to three hours to administer; can be used for planning therapy (Osgood & Miron, 1963; Zubrick & Smith, 1979); not standardized.

MINOR HEMISPHERE: the nondominant hemisphere; usually the right hemisphere in right handed persons.

MIOSIS: extreme constriction of the pupils caused by pontine lesions.

ml.: milliliter.

mg.: milligram.

mm.: millimeter.

MMPI: Minnesota Multiphasic Personality Inventory (MMPI); although differential diagnosis of brain dysfunction with the MMPI has been disappointing (Goldstein, 1984), it can provide information regarding level of adjustment (Russell, 1977).

MNEMIC PROCESSES: memory processes.

M

mo.: month.

MOBILE SPASM: see athetosis.

mod.: moderate.

MODIFIED CARD SORTING TEST: (Nelson, 1976) multiple stimulus cards are removed to simplify the Wisconsin Card Sorting Test; test of concept formation and cognitive flexibility.

MODIFIED WORD LEARNING TEST: (Walton & Black, 1957) rewards speed of learning; high degree of accuracy in identifying organic conditions.

MONGOLISM: see Down's syndrome.

MONOCULAR BLINDNESS: loss of sight in one eye as a result of destruction of the retina or optic nerve of that eye.

MONOPLEGIC: paralysis of one side; see also hemiplegic.

MOOD: emotional tone; prevailing emotional state without reference to the stimuli; a pervasive and sustained emotion that may color the person's perception of the environment; examples include: sadness, happiness, anger, apathy, anxiety, depression, elation; see also dysphoric, elevated, euphoric, euthymic, expansive, and irritable mood.

MOOD (DYSPHORIC): unpleasant mood such as depression, anxiety, or irritability.

MOOD (ELEVATED): a mood more cheerful than normal; it does not imply pathology.

MOOD (EUPHORIC): an exaggerated feeling of well-being; implies a pathological mood.

MOOD (EUTHYMIC): mood in the normal range, which implies the absence of depressed or elevated mood.

MOOD (EXPANSIVE): lack of restraint in expressing one's feelings, frequently with an overvaluation of one's significance or importance; may also be in combination with elevated or euphoric mood.

MOOD (IRRITABLE): internalized feeling of tension associated with being easily annoyed or provoked to anger.

MOOD-CONGRUENT: a state of emotion which is appropriate to the situation or environmental stimuli.

MOOD-INCONGRUENT: a state of emotion which is not appropriate to the situation or environmental stimuli; inappropriate affect.

MOONEY'S CLOSURE TEST: (Mooney & Ferguson, 1951; Mooney, 1957); sensitive to right-hemisphere lesions, particularly right-temporoparietal areas; test of visual perception.

MORPHINE: the principal and most active alkaloid of opium; narcotic analgesic; constricts pupil.

MOTIVATION: see tegmentum; drive.

MOTOR APHASIA: Broca's a., ataxic a., frontocortical a, verbal a; expressive a.

MOTOR APRAXIA: loss of ability to make proper use of objects although its proper nature is recognized; also called cortical or innervation a.

MOTOR COMMAND AREA (PRIMARY): Brodmann's area 4.

MOTOR CORTEX UNIT (LURIA): frontal lobes; primary zone: motor strip; Brodmann's area 4; final cortical motor command area; secondary zone: premotor area; Brodmann's area 6; motor programs are prepared in the secondary zone for execution by the primary zone; tertiary zone: prefrontal or granular frontal cortex; Brodmann's areas 9, 10, 45, 46, 47; formation of intentions; Luria describes the tertiary zone of the frontal unit as the most highly integrated area of function (the super-structure above all other parts of the cerebral cortex).

MOTOR DISCONNECTION SYNDROME: the motor system is largely crossed; commissurotomy of the corpus callosum produces several kinds of motor difficulties: any task involving either a verbal command for the left hand to follow or verbal material for the left hand to write, a form of apraxia and agraphia ensues because the left hand does not receive instructions from the left hemisphere; apraxia and agraphia would not ensue from right-sided stimuli because the right side has access to the speech hemisphere; if the right hand (left-hemisphere control) were asked to copy a geometric design, it might be impaired because it is disconnected from the right hemisphere; each hand and arm function independently in the commissured patient so that if the two arms must be used in cooperation to perform a task there would be severe deficits in coordination (Zaidel & Sperry, 1977).

MOTOR EPILEPSY: (simple motor epilepsy) a convulsion originating in the precentral motor cortex; begins with clonic movements of a small part of the opposite side of the body, usually the thumb and index finger, the angle of the mouth, or the great toe; movement becomes more violent, spreads on the same side, with loss of consciousness; followed by transitory weakness of muscles involved lasting from a few hours to two days; weakness known as Todd's paralysis (Brain, 1985).

MOTOR FIBER PATH: bundles of motor fibers which make up the internal capsule originate in the primary motor cortex, descend through the basal ganglia, sweep down the ventral aspect of the brainstem, and upon reaching the spinal cord, synapse with spinomotor neurons; make voluntary movement possible.

MOTOR FUNCTION TESTS - FRONTAL-LOBE LESIONS: lesions of the pre- and postcentral gyri reduce strength and finger-tapping speed on the contralateral side to the lesion; motor sequencing can be assessed with the facial sequence test.

MOTOR FUNCTION TESTS: hand dynamometer, finger tapping speed, and movement sequencing.

M

MOTOR HOMUNCULUS: a character drawing of anatomical stuctures over a drawing of precentral gyrus (primary motor cortex).

MOTOR IMPERSISTENCE: the inability to sustain certain discrete voluntary motor acts on command; tends to occur with right hemisphere or bilateral cortical damage (Joynt et al., 1962; Joynt & Goldstein, 1975).

MOTOR IMPERSISTENCE TESTS: keeping eyes closed or keeping tongue extended; fixating gaze in lateral visual fields, keeping mouth open, fixating on examiner's nose (during confrontation testing of visual fields), sustaining "ah" sound, and maintaining grip.

MOTOR PERFORMANCE: observation of motoric symptoms may implicate cerebellar, frontal lesion(s), or sensory deficits of a parietal nature; motor dysfunctions of interest to neuropsychologists are those movements that are responses to a command or imitation of movements, coordinated movements (at command), cognitively maintained or changed movements, timed or regulated movements, sequential movements, and integration of speech, thought, and movements.

MOTOR REGULATION TESTS: see self-regulative tests or fine motor regulation tests.

MOTOR RESTLESSNESS: see akathisia.

MOTOR STRIP: precentral gyrus; Brodmann's areas 4 & 6.

MOTOR STRIP (AREA): includes that part of the precentral convolution which contains Betz cells (Brodmann's area 4); extends anteriorly into Brodmann's area 6, the secondary motor area of the superior frontal convolution, and posteriorally into the anterior parietal lobe, where it overlaps the sensory areas.

MOTOR SYSTEMS: see cortical motor systems, subcortical motor systems, ventromedial system, pyramidal tract, motor cortex, ventromedial tract.

MOTOR SYSTEM LESIONS (LEVEL 1): Brodmann's area 4; lesions in this level produce severe, chronic deficits in fine motor controls and also reduce speed and strength of limb movements.

MOTOR SYSTEM LESIONS (LEVEL 2): Brodmann's areas 4, 6, & 8 of frontal cortex and areas 5 & 7, parietal; cortical lesions in this level of control do not abolish limb or axial movements since subcortical structures can still operate to produce basic limb and axial movements; alter more complex aspects of limb and axial movements, producing more subtle deficits; lesions in Brodmann's areas 5 & 7 contribute to apraxias; lesions in Brodmann's areas 6 & 8 appear to impair the smooth transition of separate axial, limb, and hand movements into a fluid series of movements.

MOTOR SYSTEM LESIONS (LEVEL 3): prefrontal cortex; produce alterations in basic aspects of personality and social behavior;

interfere with planning and execution of complex behavioral programs. People with prefrontal lesions are seldom able to hold jobs and have difficulty looking after many daily activities. They are typically late for appointments and are often unable to maintain close relationship even with their immediate families.

MOTOR SYSTEM - CORTICAL: 3 levels of function: 1. Brodmann's area 4; axons largely synapse directly on spinal motor neurons or cranial nerve motor nuclei; specialized for controlling fine hand, finger, and facial movements; 2. Brodmann's areas 4, 6, & 8 of the frontal cortex and 5 & 7 of the parietal cortex; contribute to two descending systems: one controlling limb movements, the other, body movements; all neurons of the limb-controlling system synapse in the red nucleus, although they may synapse earlier — primarily in the basal ganglia; lesions in area 5 & 7 contribute to apraxias; 3. prefrontal cortex; receive input from the tertiary zones of the parietal and temporal cortex; send efferents to cortical neurons in both the first and second levels as well as to the basal ganglia and brainstem nuclei of the motor system; controls/monitors the overall motor programs and adds flexibility to motor output by modifying behavior with respect to specific internal and external factors; provides the highest control of affective behavior and is able to effect control of basic emotional behavior by virtue of its intimate connections with the limbic system; the three levels of cortical motor control are hierarchical with respect to final motor output, the first level being closest to it and the third level being most removed. Whereas the first level synapses directly upon spinal motor neurons, the second level and, to a greater extent, the third level have multiple synapses en route to the spinal motor neurons; lesions in the first level are easily specified; at the other two levels, the effects of cortical lesions become progressively more difficult to define because there are subcortical levels of control before the final motor output in the spinal cord and cranial nerve nuclei.

MOTOR TRACTS: see lateral motor system, lateral corticospinal tract, rubrospinal motor tract, ventromedial motor system, ventromedial corticospinal tract, tectospinal tract, medial reticulospinal tract, vestibulospinal tract, lateral reticulospinal tract, medial longitudinal tract.

MOURNING REACTION: naturally follows the experience of personal loss of a capacity whether it is due to brain injury, a lesion in the nervous system, or amputation of a body part (Lezak, 1983).

MOVEMENT PROGRAMMING IMPAIRMENT: dorsolateral frontal-lobe lesion (Kolb & Milner, 1980; Luria, 1973a).

MQ: Mental Quotient; most usually associated with the total score of the Wechsler Memory Scale.

MULLER-LYER LINE ILLUSION TEST: left-sided lesions tend to be

M

associated with an accentuation of illusion (Barton, 1969; Houlard et al., 1976); more errors are made with advancing age.

MULTI-INFARCT DEMENTIA: progressive stepwise degenerative course as a result of multiple strokes (small strokes) that eventually lead to diffuse softening and degeneration of cerebral tissue (Torack, 1978; Walton, 1977); often due to arteriosclerosis; may resemble Alzheimer's disease but usually has an acute onset and progresses in a stepwise manner; symptoms may fluctuate from hour to hour, or day to night with nocturnal confusion; cognitive deficits usually precede personality deterioration; usually included motor dysfunction such as gait disturbances and rigidity; hypertension is frequently a precipitating factor (Ladurner et al., 1982); also called arteriosclerotic dementia; arteriosclerotic psychosis.

MULTILINGUAL APHASIA EXAMINATION: (Benton & Hamsher, 1978) provides for a systematic, graded examination of receptive, expressive, and immediate memory components of speech and language functions; subtests may be used separately to examine specific impairments.

MULTIPLE SCLEROSIS: early signs may include a sixth nerve palsy, diplopia; demyelinizing disease; cause unknown; progressive degenerative nervous system disease caused by patchy deterioration of the myelin sheath around nerve fibers which disrupt the normal transmission of nerve impulses; thought to be a breakdown in the patient's autoimmune system (Matthews, 1978); characterized by irregularly recurring acute episodes, each one taking an additional toll; weakness or loss of control of a limb; dysarthria with characteristic spasmodically paced speech (scanning speech); eye muscle imbalance causing double vision; blindness, usually transient in one eye; loss of sphincter control; patchy painless sensory changes such as numbness (Walton, 1977); wide variation in rate and extent of mental and physical decline; depression may be common, but many also show euphoric moods which may mask or fluctuate with an underlying depression (Surridge, 1969); depression and preoccupation with their physical disabilities tend to characterize mild cases when cognitive functioning is intact (Peyser et al., 1980); those with mild physical impairments may deny that they have worries or problems; with severe cognitive dysfunction, the patient may display unbounded optimism with a thoroughly unrealistic assessment of his disability, his situation, and the future; emotional lability, irritability, and distractibility are common as the disease progresses; fatigue usually present from the onset.

MULTIPLE SCLEROSIS TEST INTERPRETION: impairment of conceptual reasoning (Beatty & Gange, 1977; Lishman, 1978; Staples & Lincoln, 1979), short-term recall and new learning (Beatty & Gange, 1977; Rao et al., 1982; Vowels, 1979); WAIS-R and Halstead

Battery show depressed scores primarily on timed motor subtests, tests of cognitive function that have important motor components, and sensory discrimination tests (Goldstein & Shelly, 1974; Ivnick, 1978; Kaplan & Tsaros, 1979); many patients with only mild neurological signs may show no cognitive impairment at all (Vowels, 1979); optic nerve damage (afferent pathway lesion) results in an abnormal pupillary response called the Marcus Gunn pupil in which there is a pupillary escape phenomena.

MULTIPLE SCLEROSIS AND THE BRAINSTEM: internuclear ophthalmoplegia, isolated 6th nerve palsies, bilateral vestibular pathway damage with rotatory nystagmus on lateral gaze and vertical nystagmus on upward gaze, combination of bilateral cerebellar and pyramidal signs.

MUSCLE MOVEMENT SENSE: kinesthetic sense.

MUSCLE RESISTANCE: see rigidity, cogwheel phenomenon.

MUSCLE TENSION REGULATION: muscles automatically tense and relax according to particular stimuli; in every skeletal muscle there are two types of contracting fibers, extrafusal and intrafusal which lie side by side; they are attached and work in synchrony, shadowing each other's movement; muscle tension is initiated when added weight causes extrafusal fibers to stretch and in the process causes intrafusal fibers to lengthen; stretching of the intrafusal fibers, in turn, causes the receptors in the nuclear bag to stretch and produces neural impulses that travel to the spinal cord and then back to the extrafusal fibers whose contraction produces muscle tension.

MUSCULAR DYSTROPHY: a group of genetically determined painless degenerative myopathies characterized by weakness and atrophy of muscle without involvement of the nervous system.

MUSCULAR RIGIDITY: consists of increased muscle tone simultaneously in both extensor and flexor muscles; particularly evident when limbs are moved passively at a joint; move in a series of interrupted jerks (cogwheel phenomenon) rather than as a smooth motion; the rigidity may be sufficiently severe to make all movements difficult; seen in Parkinson's disease and extrapyramidal reaction to neuroleptic drugs.

MUSICAL HEARING DEFECT (timbre & tonal memory): right secondary auditory cortex.

MUTILATED PICTURES TEST: (Stanford-Binet) may be used to assess the capacity for visual organization with severely impaired brain-lesioned patients.

MUTISM: a condition of being without speech.

MYASTHENIA GRAVIS: severe muscle weakness and paralysis perhaps as a result of a deficiency of acetylcholine in the neuromuscular junctions preventing fibers from depolarizing or perhaps an excess

N

of acetylcholine esterase; early signs may be diplopia and ptosis of the eyelid.

MYOCARDIAL ANOXIA: a failure of coronary blood flow to keep up with myocardial needs.

MYCOTIC INFECTIONS: fungal infection that may invade the brain whose resistance has been reduced by various diseases such as tuberculosis or malignant tumors.

MYDRIASIS: abnormal dilatation of pupils resulting from midbrain lesions and is a frequent finding in cases of deep coma.

MYELENCHEPHALON: spinal brain; part of the hindbrain or rhombencephalon; includes medulla oblongata and fourth ventricle.

MYELODYSPLASIA: defective development of any part of the spinal cord (especially the lower segments).

MYOCLONIC DYSARTHRIA: see choreic dysarthria.

MYOCLONIC SPASMS: massive seizures that consists of a sudden flexion or extension of the body and often begin with a cry.

MYOCLONUS: involuntary and arrhythmic movement which is much faster than chorea often triggered by sensory stimuli such as flickering light, series of loud sounds, or startle response.

MYOPIA: near sightedness.

MYOTONIA: increased muscular irritability and contractility with decreased power of relaxation; tonic spasm of muscles.

MYXEDEMA: a condition characterized by a dry, waxy type of swelling with abnormal deposits of mucin in the skin and other tissues, associated with hypothyroidism; edema is of nonpitting type; facial changes are strikingly distinctive, with swollen lips and thickened nose; see also thyroid disease.

N

N/A; NA: not applicable.

NALOXONE HYDROCHLORIDE: see Narcan.

NAMING: able to identify objects by name; a characteristic looked for when assessing aphasia; difficulty in finding the names of objects is characteristic of anomic aphasia (amnesic aphasia); circumlocution may be substituted for correct name of object; deficits in naming may result from 1. inability to identify distinguishing characteristics of an object, 2. inability to develop the auditory form of the word, 3. inability to select the appropriate word from those expressing ideas closely associate with it; may be a result of a lesion in the angular gyrus (not a proven theory)(Kolb & Whishaw, 1980).

NAMING OBJECTS FROM MEMORY: (Stanford-Binet subtest)

suitable for severely impaired brain-damaged patients.

NARCAN: trade name of naloxone hydrochloride; a synthetic congener of oxymorphone; used as a narcotic antagonist.

NARCISSISM: self-love; normal at an early stage of psychosexual development, but when dominant in adulthood is pathological.

NARCOLEPSY: uncontrollable sleepiness, occurs many times a day for about 15 minutes at a time; person easily awakened; may have blurring of vision, diplopia, and ptosis; cataplexy (70%); sleep paralysis (50%); hypnagogic hallucinations (25%).

NASAL HEMIANOPIA: hemianopia in the medial vertical half of the visual field of vision (the half nearest the nose) loss of vision of nasal field as a result of a lesion of the lateral chiasm.

NASOGUTTURAL SOUNDS: nk and ng; formed during articulation.

NC: no code.

NE: norepinephrine.

NECKER CUBE ILLUSION TEST: test of perceptual fluctuation/ reversals; most often scored by the "rate of apparent change" (L. Cohen, 1959); brain-injured patients show fewer reversals; right-hemisphere lesioned patients reported fewer reversals than left-hemisphere lesioned patients; bilateral frontal-lobe injured patients see more reversals but reversal rate is slow (Teuber, 1964; Yacorzynski, 1965); no right-left lesion differential with frontal-lobe lesions.

NECROSIS: death of tissue, usually as individual cells, groups of cells, or in small localized areas.

neg.: negative.

NEGLECT OF BODY AND BODILY CONDITION: see asomatognosia.

NEOCEREBELLUM: outermost lateral portion of the cerebellum; projections from the lateral nuclei of the cerebellum go to the ventral thalamus and from there to the precentral motor cortex; has access to the corticospinal tract that controls more distal movements of the arms and fingers as well as proximal movements of the body.

NEOCEREBELLUM LESIONS: produce weakness and a tendency to fatigue, difficulty in localizing or pointing to body parts correctly, and a variety of deficits in the control of the extremities such as overshooting the mark when pointing, flailing at the joints, staggering, and an inability to carry out repeated rhythmical movements.

NEOCORTEX: comprises most of the forebrain by volume; consists of four to six layers of cells (grey matter) beneath which their axons form pathways (white matter); comprises 80% of the human brain; area of up to 2500 sq. cm.; thickness of 1.5 to 3.0 mm.; the wrinkled surface of the neocortex consists of clefts (fissures or sulci) and ridges (gyri); consists of two nearly symmetrical hemispheres, the left and the right, separated by the medial longitudinal fissure; each hemi-

N

the right, separated by the medial longitudinal fissure; each hemisphere is subdivided into four lobes: frontal, parietal, temporal, and occipital.

NEOLOGISMS: fragmented words, made up words; new words invented by the patient, distortions of words, or standard words to which the subject has given new meaning.

NEONATORUM ANOXIA: anoxia of the newborn.

NEOPALLIUM: that part of the pallium (cerebral cortex) showing stratification and organization characteristic of the most highly evolved type of cerebral tissue.

NEOPLASM: see Tumor (neoplasms).

NERVE CLASSIFICATION: 3 types: sensory, motor, mixed; sensory and motor are only in the 12 cranial nerves, all other nerves are mixed.

NERVES - MIXED: (motor & sensory): Trigeminal (chewing & face sensitivity); Glossopharyngeal (tongue & pharynx); Vegas (heart & blood vessels); Facial (facial movement & taste).

NERVES - MOTOR: Hypoglossal (tongue movement); Spinal Accessory (neck & visceral movement); Oculomotor (eye movements); Trochlear (eye movements); Abducens (eye movements).

NERVES - SENSORY: Olfactory (smell); Optic (vision); Auditory (hearing & balance sense).

NERVE PALSY: see brainstem lesions.

NERVOUS SYSTEM: (2 major divisions): 1. central nervous system (CNS) which serves the brain and the spinal cord; 2. the peripheral nervous system (PNS) which serves the body (somatic) and the autonomic nervous system (ANS) which serves the visceral parts of the body which in turn breaks down into the sympathetic nervous system (SNS) and the parasympathetic nervous system (PNS).

NEURASTHENIC SYNDROME: see posttraumatic syndrome.

NEUROCYTOMA: see tumor.

NEUROHYPOPHYSIS: posterior lobe of the pituitary gland.

NEUROMA: a tumor or new growth largely made up of nerve cells and nerve fibers.

NEURON: basic unit of the nervous system; 3 types: 1. sensory (PNS) which carry impulses from receptors towards the CNS, afferently; 2. motor (PNS) which carry impulses from the CNS to effectors, efferently; 3. interneurons in the CNS.

NEURONAL ACTIVITY: the spread of a nervously significant change of state within a neuron; unmyelinated fiber conducts impulses via a progression of ionic movements between neighboring areas; myelinated fibers conduct impulses by ionic movement, skipping from one node of Ranvier to the next.

NEURONAL AXON: the part of the cell body that sends information.

NEURONAL CELL BODY (SOMA): metabolic activities.

N

NEURONAL COMPONENTS: cell body (soma), axon, and dendrites.

NEURONAL DENDRITES: the part of the cell body that receives information.

NEUROPSYCHOLOGICAL BATTERY FOR EPILEPSY: (Dodrill, 1978a,b,c) a modified version of the Halstead-Reitan test battery which also includes tests of memory, motor control, concentration, and mental flexibility.

NEUROPSYCHOLOGICAL EVALUATION TESTS: (not a complete list; tests most often reviewed, only) WAIS-R; Halstead-Reitan battery; Luria's Neuropsychological Investigation; McGill picture anomalies, Mooney faces, Rey complex figures, Wechsler Memory Scale, delayed recall of stories, paired associates and drawings, right-left differentiation, Semmes body-placing test, object naming, Token test, Corsi recurring blocks, Hebb recurring blocks, Wisconsin card-sorting test, Chicago word-fluency test, Dynamometer, Kimura box test, Bender-Gestalt. Most well-established institutions have developed batteries which may included some or all of the tests mentioned above. For example, see the Montreal Neurological Institute battery (Kolb & Whishaw, 1980), the Boston Diagnostic Aphasia Exam or the Michigan batteries.

NEUROPSYCHOLOGICAL TEST BATTERY: (Miceli et al., 1977; 1981) consists of six tests: Word Fluency (Benton, 1968); Phrase Construction (see Lezak, 1983 p. 341); Rey's 15 Word Memory Test; Modified Raven's Coloured Progressive Matrices; Immediate Visual Memory; Copying Drawings. Sensitive to right-left, anterior-posterior localization (Miceli et al., 1981).

NEUROPSYCHOLOGY: a specialty within the field of psychology that focuses primarily on neurobehavioral functioning.

NEUROSENSORY CENTER COMPREHENSIVE EXAM FOR APHASIA: (Spreen & Benton, 1969) sensitive to moderately and severely aphasic patients (Greenberg, 1979); insufficient standardization; not useful for examining mild impairments (Lezak, 1983).

NEUROTIC DISORDER: a mental disorder characterized by a psychic symptom or group of symptoms that is distressing to the individual and is recognized by him or her as unacceptable and alien (ego-dystonic); not caused by organic factors; reality testing is grossly intact; behavior does not actively violate gross social norms; relatively enduring or recurrent without treatment and is not limited to transitory reaction to stressors;

NEUROSYPHILIS: occurs in 6%-7% of persons with untreated primary or secondary syphilis; categories include: chronic basal meningitis, meningovascular syphilis, general paresis, tabes dorsalis, gumma of the brain (Reitan & Wolfson, 1985).

NEUROTIC PROCESS: a specific process involving the following sequences: 1. unconscious conflicts between opposing desires or

N

between desires and prohibitions, which cause 2. unconscious perception of anticipated danger or dysphoria (dejection), which leads to 3. use of defense mechanisms that result in 4. either physical symptoms, personality disturbance, or both.

NEUROTRANSMITTER DEGRADATION: the free neurotransmitter within the synapse may be degraded to control internal neurotransmitter concentrations.

NEUROTRANSMITTER INACTIVATION OR REUPTAKE: in some synapses the neurotransmitter is inactivated in the area of the synaptic space; in others it is taken back up into the synapse; in some both mechanisms may be active.

NEUROTRANSMITTER RECEPTOR INTERACTION: the released neurotransmitter crosses the synaptic space and binds to specialized receptors on the post-synaptic membrane where it initiates depolarization or hyperpolarization of the post-synaptic membrane.

NEUROTRANSMITTER RELEASE: released only by telodendria, not the dendrites.

NEUROTRANSMITTER STORAGE: stored in the synapse in one or more of several ways, at least one of which is in vesicles available for release into the subsynaptic space.

NEUROTRANSMITTER SYNTHESIS: precursor chemicals obtained from food or manufactured in the cell are transported down the axon into the synapse where they are synthesized into the neurotransmitter.

NEUROTROPIC VIRUS: a virus that has a special affinity for cells of the central nervous system as in poliomyelitis and rabies.

NEW ADULT READING TEST: test of premorbid intellectual verbal abilities (Nelson & O'Connell, 1978).

N.F.B.S.: non-fasting blood sugar.

nil.: nothing.

NINTH CRANIAL NERVE: (Glosso-Pharyngeal) primarily sensory except for motor supply to the stylo-pharyngeus muscle; *origin*: several rootlets from the lateral side of upper part of the medulla oblongata, between the olive and the inferior cerebellar peduncle; *branches*: typanic nerve, pharyngeal, stylopharyngeal, tonsillar, and lingual rami, ramus to the carotid sinus, and ramus communicating with the auricular ramus of the vagus nerve; supplies the tongue, pharynx, and parotid gland.

NINTH CRANIAL NERVE LESION: may cause severe pain in the throat when fluid or food is swallowed.

NMR: nuclear magnetic resonance scanning.

NOC: nocturnal; at night.

NOMINAL APHASIA: marked by the defective use of name of objects; see also anomia, dysnomia, anomic a., amnestic dysnomia.

NONCOMMUNICATING HYDROCEPHALUS: hydrocephalus due

to ventricular block; also called obstructive h.

NONDOMINANT (RIGHT) FRONTAL LOBE - LESIONS: causes impaired learning of spatial patterns.

NONFLUENT APHASIA: lesion in Broca's area; little speech is produced, and is uttered slowly, with great effort and poor articulation; see also Broca's a.

NONPARALYTIC MOTOR DYSFUNCTION: apraxia; parietal lobe.

NONSENSE SYLLABLES TESTS: (Newcombe, 1969; Talland, 1965a) sensitive to left-hemisphere lesions.

NONVERBAL AUDITORY PERCEPTION: recognition, discrimination, and comprehension of nonsymbolic sound patterns, such as music, tapping patterns, and the meaningful noises of sirens, dog barks, and thunderclaps are subject to impairment much as is the perception of language sounds (Frederiks, 1969). Defects of nonverbal auditory perception tend to be associate with lesions of the right-temporal lobe (Gordon, 1974; Milner, 1962, 1971).

NONVERBAL AUDITORY PERCEPTION TESTS: Seashore Rhythm Test, Luria-Nebraska battery, Seashore Test of Musical Talent.

NONVERBAL MEMORY: Rey Complex Figure test.

NOREPINEPHRINE: (NE) Hormone secreted by the adrenal medulla along with epinephrine, mimics SNS activity; triggers ACTH release, and stimulates liver to convert glycogen to glucose; chemical neurotransmitter.

NORMAL PRESSURE HYDROCEPHALUS: (NPH) pressure build up in the lateral ventricles, gradually enlarging them (Adams, 1980); reversable by a shunt operation; results from obstruction of the flow of cerebral spinal fluid, usually by scarring from old trauma or infection, or from hemorrhage or tumor (Pincus & Tucker, 1978; Wells, 1978); main area of damage is in the midbrain reticular formation (Torack, 1978); if not treated, leads to confusion, disorientation, incontinence, and increasing mental debilitation, gait disturbance, and memory impairment; may resemble Alzheimer's disease but the order of appearance of symptoms may distinguish between them; incontinence and a clumsy, wide-base gait commonly an early symptom (Benson, 1975). Mental changes involve disorientation, confusion, decreased attention span, and both mental and motor slowing, with good preservation of cognitive functions, judgment, and self-awareness; depression is not uncommon; may be distinguished from Alzheimer's disease by the sequence of symptoms: Alzheimer's course — early memory impairment with incontinence and loss of ability to walk in terminal stage where NPH the sequence is reversed; *testing*: in early stages, lowered scores on the Wechsler Intelligence Scales will be on Arithmetic, Digit Span, and the timed tests, reflecting slowing, impaired attention and mental tracking; patient performs no better with two hands than one on tests such as

N

block construction and pegboard tests (Botez et al., 1975) also called communicating hydrocephalus because there is "communication" between the expanded ventricles and the lumbar sac with normal intraventricular pressure.

NORMOCEPHALIC: normal brain size.

NPH: normal pressure hydrocephalus.

NREM: non-rapid eye movement; usually said of sleep stage.

NUCHA: nape, scruff, or back of neck.

NUCLEAR MAGNETIC RESONANCE (NMR) SCANNING: a method of scanning the brain in which there is no limitation of X-ray exposure and differentiates between grey and white matter better than the CT-scan; no apparent hazard to the patient; successive projection of an axis and repeated through 180 degrees for each slice; fat and bone marrow appear white; tissue or fluids appear black; cortical bone appears black (Brain, 1985).

NUCLEUS: large number of cell bodies grouped together.

NUCLEUS AMBIGUOUS: the nucleus of origin of motor fibers of the vagus, glossopharyngeal, and accessory nerves that supply the striated muscles of the larynx and pharynx; consists of an intermittent cell column in the middle of the lateral funiculus of the medulla oblongata, between the caudal end of the medulla and the level of exit of the glossopharyngeal nerve.

NUMBER SPAN: (Barbizet & Cany, 1968) tests the span of new verbal learning.

NUMBNESS OF FACE: may be a lesion of the Trigeminal nerve (V).

NUMBNESS OF HANDS AND FINGERS: (following a few hours sleep) see acroparesthesia.

NYCTALOPIA: poor twilight or night vision associated with vitamin A deficiency or pigmentary degenerations of the retina.

NYSTAGMUS: involuntary, rhythmic, rapid movement of the eyeball which may be horizontal, vertical, rotatory, or mixed; weakness in maintaining the conjugate deviation of the eyes or an imbalance in the postural control of the eye movements; the laterally deviated eyes drift slowly back to the central postion (pathological component), and flick quickly back to regain position (said to be the direction of the nystagmus (e.g., defined in the direction of the fast movement); the quick recovery flick is thought to be generated in the pons; the absence of opticokinetic nystagmus (pathological condition) may be a result of a lesion in the pursuit gaze pathway or the opposite parieto-occipito-temporal cortex; other causes of nystagmus: alcohol, head-injury, all sedative drugs, especially barbiturates, glutethimide, and anticonvulsants, and especially diphenylhydantoin (Epantutin), primdone (Mysoline), and carbomazepine (Tegretol).

NYSTAGMUS (HORIZONTAL, COURSE): pathognomic of disease

in cerebellopontine angle.

NYSTAGMUS (VERTICAL): pathognomic of disease in the tegmentum of the brainstem and possibly of cerebellar connections.

O

100-HUE AND DICHOTOMOUS TEST FOR COLOR VISION: (Farnsworth, 1943); can be used to identify color agnosias and to screen for the purely sensory disorder.

obj.: objective.

OBJECT AGNOSIA - visual: unable to identify objects even though primary senses are intact; see astereognosis or visual object agnosia.

OBJECT AND PICTURE MEMORY SPAN: verbal mediation of object and picture stimuli may confound the results if used strictly as a visual retention test.

OBJECT ASSEMBLY SUBTEST: (WAIS-R) two dimensional space constructional task; test of speed of visual organization and motor response as well as capacity for visual organization; the speed component renders it relatively vulnerable to brain damage generally; lowest association with general intellectual ability of all the Performance Scale subtests and is second only to Digit Span in weakness on this factor; relatively pure measure of visuospatial organization ability; requires little abstract thinking; ability to form visual concepts quickly and translate them into rapid hand responses is essential for an average or better score; sensitive to posterior lesions, particularly right-hemisphere lesions (Black & Strub, 1976; Long & Brown, 1979) correlates with Block Design; patterns of variations of Block Design and Object Assembly scores relative to one another and to other tests allow the examiner to infer the different functions that contribute to success on these tasks.

OBJECT CLASSIFICATION TEST: (Payne & Hewlett, 1960) modification of the Color Form Sorting Test; test of conceptual functioning.

OBJECT RECOGNITION BY TOUCH: stereognosis.

OBJECT SORTING TEST: (Goldstein & Scheerer, 1941, 1953; Weigl, 1941); test of conceptual functioning; sensitive to frontal-lobe lesions.

OBSESSIONS: recurrent, persistant ideas, unwanted thoughts, images, or impulses which invade consciousness; characteristic of obsessive compulsive disorder and may also be seen in schizophrenia.

OBSTINATE PROGRESSION: see Parkinson's disease.

OBSTRUCTIVE HYDROCEPHALUS: see noncommunicating hydrocephalus.

O

OCCIPITAL LOBE: terminus of the geniculocalcarine pathways which are essential for visual sensation and perception; lies astride the calcarine fissure at the rear of the head; macular vision cells are located at the extreme tip; peripheral field cells lie anteriorally; lower field cells in upper half; upper field cells in lower half; separated from the parietal cortex medially by the parieto-occipital sulcus. On the lateral surface of the brain there are no definite boundaries between the occipital, parietal, and temporal lobes. The areas are sometimes referred to as the parietal-occipital area and the temporal-occipital area. Only the lateral gyrus is obvious in the occipital cortex.

OCCIPITAL LOBE ASSOCIATION AREA LESION(S): cause visual agnosias.

OCCIPITAL LOBE (BILATERAL-LESIONS): cause cortical blindness; a state of blindness without change in optic fundi or pupillary reflexes; visual illusions, hallucinations, and metamorphopsias may also occur.

OCCIPITAL LOBE (DOMINANT-HEMISPHERE LESIONS): (Brodmann's areas 18 & 19); loss of visual recognition with retention of some degree of visual acuity (visual agnosia); unable to recognize objects visually, but able to do so by tactile or other extravisual sense; alexia (word blindness); can see letters and words but cannot recognize their meaning; involvement of the subcortical white matter may cause visual object agnosia; may interfere with reading and writing, and cause acalculia.

OCCIPITAL LOBE (NONDDOMINANT - HEMISPHERE LESIONS): agnosia for recognition of faces (prosopagnosia); agnosia for a complex of objects of elements which are perceived individually, but not as a whole (simultanagnosia); color agnosia; and Balint's syndrome (inability to look at and grasp an object, and inattention).

OCCIPITAL-LOBE PATHOLOGY: seizures with flashing light aura, visual field defects, alexia, visual agnosia, homonymous visual field defects, dyslexia.

OCCIPITAL-LOBE SEIZURES: sensation of lights, darkness, color, seeing stars, moving lights in the eye contralateral to the side of lesion.

OCCIPITAL-LOBE (UNILATERAL-LESIONS): result in homonymous defects in the contralateral visual fields — usually a loss of vision in part or all of the homonymous fields; perceived forms and contours may change (metamorphopsia) and/or an illusory displacement of images from one side of the visual field to the other (visual allesthesia) or abnormal persistence of visual image after the object has been removed (palinopsia).

OCULAR: pertaining to or affecting the eye.

OCULAR APRAXIA; head turns and the eyes go in the opposite direction.

O

OCULAR DISTURBANCES: see cerebellar disease, ocular dysmetria, nystagmus, ocular apraxia, oculargyric crisis, hemianopia, occipital-lobe lesions, dyslexia, alexia, Horner's syndrome, object agnosia.

OCULAR DYSMETRIA: overshooting of the eyes on attempted fixation, followed by several cycles of oscillations of diminishing amplitude until precise fixation is attained; occurs in diseases of the cerebellum or its pathways.

OCULOGYRAL CRISIS: fixed deviation of the eyes in an upwards direction; lateral deviation or downward deviation occurs less frequently; over-activity of the basal ganglia; may be a feature of post-encephalitic Parkinsonism; compulsive thoughts or actions and confusional state may coexist; other causes include phenothiazine hypersensitivity, post head-injury states, and neurospyphilis.

OCULOMOTOR (alternating) HEMIPLEGIA: see Weber's syndrome.

OCULOMOTOR NERVE (cranial nerve III): motor and parasympathetic; several groups of nerve cells ventral to the aqueduct of Sylvius at the level of the superior colliculi; fibers go to the ipsilateral eye except those innervating the superior rectus muscle; originates in the brainstem, emerging medial to cerebral peduncles and running forward in the cavernous sinus; enters orbit through the superior orbital fissure; branches supply the levator palpebrae superioris, all extrinsic eye muscles except the lateral rectus and superior oblique; controls eye movement, reaction to light, lateral eye movements, and eyelid movement.

OEDEMA: see edema.

OLFACTORY CEREBRAL SYSTEM: uncrossed neuronal paths; input from each nostril goes to the ipsilateral side of the brain; the two olfactory centers are connected by the anterior commissure; if the anterior commissure is severed, olfactory input to the right nostril cannot gain access to the left-hemisphere speech zone and anosmia results.

OLFACTORY HALLUCINATIONS: lesion of the inferior and medial parts of temporal lobe, around the hippocampal convolution or uncus (uncinate seizure).

OLFACTORY NERVE (cranial nerve I): the nerves of smell consisting of about 20 bundles which arise in the olfactory epithelium and pass through the cribriform plate of the ethmoid bone to the olfactory bulb.

OLIGODENDROGLIA: the non-neural cells of ectodermal origin forming part of the adventitial structure (the neuroglia) of the CNS; vinelike prolongations form an incomplete investment for the myelin sheaths in the white matter, and with microglia they

O

form the perineuronal satellites in the gray matter; insulate and speed transmission of central nervous system neurons.

OMEGA SIGN: a particular type of wrinkling of the forehead observed in severely depressed patients; the wrinkling is located between the eyebrows and takes the form of the Greek letter, omega.

ONCOLOGY: the sum of knowledge concerning tumors; the study of tumors.

ONTOGENY: the development of the individual organism.

ONTOLOGY: the study of the nature of being in reality.

OPERANT MOVEMENTS: also called voluntary, instrumental, appetitive, or purpositive movements.

OPHTHALMICUS NERVE: sensory; one of the three terminal divisions of the trigeminal nerve serving the eyeball and conjunctiva, lacrimal gland and sac, nasal mucosa and frontal sinus, external nose, upper eyelid, forehead, and scalp.

OPHTHALMOPLEGIA: paralysis of the eye muscles.

OPIATE DRUGS: most effective pain-relieving agents available; may mimic the postsynaptic stimulation from endogenous, natural opiate-like substances in the brain called endorphins; morphine, codeine, heroin.

OPPOSITE ANALOGIES TEST: Stanford-Binet subtest, age levels from IV to SA III; test of conceptual functioning.

OPPOSITE SIDE: contralateral.

OPSOCLONUS: sustained, irregular, conjugate "dancing" movements of the eyes in a horizontal, rotary, and vertical direction or a fast-frequency flutter; may be associated with cerebellar disease, a viral infection, or occult neuroblastoma; also called nystagmus.

OPTIC APHASIA: inability to name objects seen due to a interruption of the connection between the speech and visual centers.

OPTIC ATAXIA: characterized by inaccurate reaching for objects and localizing stimuli in space such as past-pointing; problem of perceptual-motor coordination in the mechanism of localization or visually guided movements; Balint (1909) noted this difficulty as part of a syndrome that included paralysis of gaze with an inability to shift the eyes and inattention to objects and events in other parts of the visual field; lesion of Brodmann's area 7 (Ratcliff, 1972); finger localization and finger naming are impaired (Damasio & Benton, 1979).

OPTIC CHIASMA: the part of the hypothalamus formed by the decussation, or crossing, of the fibers of the optic nerve from the medial half of each retina.

OPTIC CHIASMAL FUNCTION: to bring information from the halves of each retina that look to the right and the halves that look to the left together in the same optic tract.

OPTIC DISC: see blind spot.

OPTIC - GNOSTIC DEFECTS: visual simultaneous perception is limited to one or two points or objects at a time; usually due to a lesion of the occipital secondary or association areas.

OPTIC NERVE (cranial nerve II): see occulomotor cranial nerve; vision.

OPTIC PATHWAYS: the macula of the retina is situated to the side of the optic nerve head; macular fibers crowd into the temporal half of the disc to get into the appropriate position in the optic nerve and complete the shift to the center of the optic nerve as it joins the chiasm; the optic nerve splits such that the lateral fibers go straight back into the optic tract on the same side and the medial fibers decussate to the other side; information derived exclusively from the left or right side of vision arrives in the optic tract and is conveyed in the inner and outer halves of the tract; information from the same point on each retina must be relayed to immediately adjacent parts of the visual cortex; process starts with the rotation of the fibers in the optic tract through 90 degrees which brings the fibers from the lower and upper fields together in the medial and lateral halves of the tract respectively; posterior tract fibers fan out towards the six layers of the geniculate body; the macula fibers occupy a central wedge of the geniculate body with the lower fields represented medially and upper fields laterally; fibers sweep out into the hemisphere as two diverging fans (optic radiation) which later join to reach the occipital (calcarine) cortex which lies astride the calcarine fissure; cells subserving the peripheral fields lie anteriorly, and those subserving macular vision are concentrated at the extreme tip; upper fields are represented in the lower half and the lower fields in the upper half of the cortex.

OPTIC PEDUNCLE LESION: causes a complete homonymous hemianopia.

OPTIC RADIATION: fanning of optic nerve fibers through each hemisphere, coursing through the temporal and parietal lobes to rejoin in the occipital lobes; each passes through a geniculate body.

OPTICAL ILLUSION TESTS: Rubin Vase; Double Necker Cube; Muller-Lyer Line.

ORAL APRAXIA: see buccofacial apraxia.

ORBITAL AREA (FRONTAL LOBES) LESION(S): cause impaired social behavior, altered sexual behavior, reduced spontaneity; may show abnormal sexual behavior such as public masterbation by reducing inhibitions, although the actual frequency of normal sexual behavior may not be affected; also see affective

O

behavior control.

ORBITAL FRONTAL CORTEX: see frontal lobes.

ORIENTATION: the awareness of self in relation to one's surroundings; requires intact attention, perception, and memory abilities; sensitive to brain dysfunction (Schulman et al., 1965); usually impaired for time and place with generalized cortical dsyfunction such as senile dementia, acute OBS, limbic system involvement, or RAS; good orientation does not necessarily indicate lack of cerebral dysfunction.

ORIENTATION DEFICITS: frontal- lobe lesioned patients are impaired at an egocentric task and not an allocentric task (personal vs extrapersonal); parietal-lobe lesioned patients are impaired at an allocentric task and not egocentric task (Semmes et al., 1963) (environmental vs personal); left frontal-lobe and left parietal-lobe lesioned patients are more severely affected than right-hemisphere lesioned patients. Teuber (1964) hypothesises that deficits in personal orientation result from an absence of corollary discharge.

ORIENTATION SUBTEST: (WMS) test of time and place.

ORIENTATION TESTS: *place*: type of place the patient is currently, name of the place, location of the place, distance from home, direction from home or direction to another city or State; *time*: date and time of day, appreciation of temporal continuity; *person*: name and birthdate of the patient; Temporal Orientation Test; Temporal Disorientation Questionnaire; Time Estimation Test; Discrimination of Recency task; Spatial orientation; Perceptual Functions: Judgment of Line Orientation; Body Orientation; Personal Orientation Test; Body Center Test; Right-Left Orientation; Standardized Road-Map; Test of Direction Sense; Distance Estimation tasks; mental transformations in space; (mental rotations, inversions,etc.); Mental Reorientation task; Spatial Orientation Memory Test; Spatial Dyscalculias; Topographical Orientation; Geographic Orientation Tests.

ORGAN OF CORTI: the spiral organ lying against the basilar membrane in the chochlear duct that contains the special sensory receptors for hearing; served by the 8th cranial nerve.

ORGANIC BRAIN SYNDROME: (OBS) declining interest in daily living and environment, various physical complaints with no basis in physical exam; frequently presents, initially, as emotional and behavioral change; the most common emotional change is depression, later, disorientation and memory impairments.

ORGANIC DRIVENESS: hyperactivity and distractability; lesions in the reticular substance of the pons and medulla oblongata.

ORTHOGANAL: a line or plane which is not linear.

ORTHOSTATIC HYPOTENSION: faintness associated with changes in body position from recumbent to standing; also called postural hypotension.

OSCILLIPSIA: illusory movement of the environment in which objects seem to move back and forth, to jerk, or to wiggle.

OVEREATING: see bulimia, hyerphagia, Kleine-Levin syndrome, Pickwickian syndrome.

OVERLAPPING FIGURES TEST: (Christensen, 1979; Ghent, 1956; Luria, 1966) assesses inability to perceive more than one object at a time or shift gaze; inability may accompany a left-posterior lesion; slowing or inertia of gaze, perseverated responses, or confused responses that are more likely to be associated with an anterior lesion; may reflect left visuospatial inattention.

OVERSHOOTING GOAL: see hypermetria, dysmetria, cerebellar disease or lesions, past-pointing, ataxia.

OVERVALUED IDEA: an unreasonable and sustained belief or idea that is maintained with less than delusional intensity; differs from an obsessional thought in that the person holding the overvalued idea does not recognize its absurdity and thus does not struggle against it.

OXYTOCIN: stimulates smooth muscle; mediates uterine contractions (labor); mediates milk ejection reflex of lactating females; secreted by posterior pituitary gland.

P

p̄: after; following.

PACED AUDITORY SERIAL ADDITION TEST (PASAT): (Gronwall & Sampson, 1974; Gronwall & Wrightson, 1974); a multiple/double simultaneous tracking task; highly sensitive to brain-damage and postconcussion disorders; very sensitive to deficits in information processing ability (Gronwall & Wrightson, 1981), mental response slowing, and tracking deficits.

PACHYMENINX: dura mater.

PAIN DENIAL: see asymbolia for pain.

PALEOCEREBELLUM: the dominant cerebellar structure; projections from the paleocerebellum nuclei go to the red nucleus, and possibly to other brainstem nuclei; involved in the control of limb movements through the lateral spinal system, and body movements through the ventromedial system.

PALEOCEREBELLUM LESION: increase in rigidity of the limbs

P

which disrupts digital movement more than proximal movement.

PALIKINESIA: pathologic repetition of movements.

PALILALIA: a condition characterized by the repetition of a phrase or word with increasing rapidity.

PALINGRAPHIA: pathologic repetition of letters, words, or parts of words in writing.

PALINOPSIA: abnormal persistence of visual image after the object has been removed.

PALINPHRASIA: pathologic repetition of, in speaking, of words or phrases.

PALSY: paralysis.

PANIC ATTACK: sudden onset of intense apprehension, fear, and terror; often associated with feelings of impending doom; symptoms include shortness of breath, palpitations, chest pain, choking, and fear of going crazy or losing control.

PANTROPIC VIRUS: attacks other body tissue in addition to the central nervous system as in mumps and herpes simplex.

PAPER CUTTING TESTS: (Paterson & Zangwill, 1944) sensitive to parieto-occipital lesions.

PAPER CUTTING subtests: Stanford-Binet subtest levels IX, XIII, & AA; sensitive to visuospatial perception; sensitive to right-hemisphere lesions.

PAPER FOLDING TEST: Triangle subtest from the Stanford-Binet which is sensitive to spatial factor, speed of closure, and verbal reasoning (Beard, 1965).

PAPER FORM BOARD TEST (MINNESOTA): (Likert & Quasha, 1970); test of perceptual organizing behavior; calls on perceptual scanning and recognition, and the ability to perceive fragmented percepts as wholes.

PAPILLEDEMA: venous congestion and edema with elevation of disk margins; swelling of the optic papilla due to raised intracranial pressure, malignant hypertension, cerebral edema, raised C.S.F., protein, metabolic disorders, or other circulation disorders; may take up to 6 weeks to resolve swelling in the central retina as viewed with an ophthalmoscope; may indicate the presence of brain tumors or increased pressure in the brain; visual acuity little affected until late.

PARASITIC INFECTIONS OF CNS: include toxoplasmosis, cerebral amebiasis, cerebral malaria, cysticercosis, trypanosomiasis, and a number of diseases caused by invasion of the larval stages of trematodes and nematodes such as echinococcosis, schistosomiasis, paragonimiasis, trichinosis, and agiostrongyliasis; see also rickettsial diseases (see Reitan & Wolfson, 1985 for more detail).

PARAGRAMMATISM: impairment of speech, with confusion in the use of and order of words and grammatical forms.

PARAGRAPHIA: the writing of an incorrect word.

P

PARAGRAPH RECALL TEST: provides a measure of the amount of information that is retained when more is presented than most people can remember on one hearing; comparison of a patient'a memory span on a paragraph test with that on sentences shows the extent to which an overload of data compromises functioning; the difference between immediate and delayed recall of a paragraph is is an indirect measure of episodic memory (Wood et al., 1982); more sensitive to the memory defects of amnesic patients than are immediate recall scores, test of old learning, or digit learning; verbatim scoring has been found to differentiate hemisphere side of lesion in immediate recall trials and be more sensitive to lesion lateralization on delayed recall trials (Mills & Burkhart, 1980).

PARAGRAPH RECALL TESTS: Stanford-Binet subtests, Logical Memory subtest from the Wechsler Memory Scale, Babcock Story Recall Test, The Cowboy Story.

PARALALIA: any disturbance of the faculty of speech, especially the production of a vocal sound different from the one desired, or the substitution in speech of one letter for another.

PARALALIA LITERALIS: impairment of the power to utter the sounds of certain letters; see also stuttering, literal dysphasia.

PARALEXIC ERRORS: word or syllable substitution when reading; see also paraphasia, neologisms.

PARALOGISM: the use of meaningless or illogical language by the psychotic.

PARALYSIS: loss or impairment of motor function in a part due to lesion of the neural or muscular mechanism; 5 types: 1. affection of lower motor neurons; 2. disorder of upper motor (corticospinal and cortico-brainstem) neurons; 3. abnormalities of coordination (ataxia) due to lesions in the cerebellum; 4. abnormalities of movement and posture due to disease of the extrapyramidal motor system; and 5. apraxic or nonparalytic disturbances of purposive movement due to involvement of the cerebrum; *voluntary muscles*: loss of contraction due to interruption of one of the motor pathways from the cerebrum to the muscle fiber; further distinguished as traumatic, syphilitic, toxic, etc., according to the nerve, part, or muscle specially affected; see also hemiplegia, palsy, paraplegia, and paresis.

PARALYSIS AGITANS: a form of parkinsonism of unknown etiology usually occurring in late life, although a juvenile form has been described; slowly progressive disease characterized by masklike facies, characteristic tremor of resting muscles, slowing of voluntary movements, festinating gait, peculiar posture, and weakness of the muscles; lesion in the substantia nigra and/or corpus striatum; see Parkinson's disease/syndrome.

PARAMEDIAN ZONES OF MIDBRAIN: tegmentum; instrumental in controlling vertical gaze.

P

PARANEOPLASTIC DISEASES: see cerebellar lesions.

PARANOID IDEATION: ideations of less than delusional proportions, involving suspiciousness or the belief that one is being harrassed, persecuted, or unfairly treated.

PARAPHASIA: the production of unintended syllables, words, or phrases during the effort to speak (Goodglass & Kaplan, 1972); paraphasia differs from difficulties in articulation in that sounds are correctly articulated, but they are the wrong sounds, and either distort the intended word or produce a completely unintended word; disturbances in understanding language through auditory and visual speech forms; substantive elements of speech missing or substituted by errors in which the desired response is only approximated; see also neologisms.

PARAPHASIAS: see literal paraphasia, verbal paraphasia; anomic a., conduction a.; amnestic - dysnomic a.; neologisms; Wernicke's a.; posterior sylvian lesion.

PARAPHASIC SPEECH: see conduction aphasia, paraphasias.

PARAPLEGIA: paralysis of both lower extremities.

PARAPLEGIC GAIT: each leg is advanced slowly and stiffly with restricted motion at the knee and hip; legs are extended or slightly bent at knees and may be strongly adducted at hips, tending to cross (scissors gait).

PARASITE: an organism that lives upon or within another living organism at the host's expense; most common kinds of parasitic disease caused by parasitic infestation; amebiasis and malaria.

PARASITIC INFESTATIONS: see amebiasis and malaria.

PARASYMPATHETIC NERVOUS SYSTEM: division of the autonomic nervous system made up of the ocular, bulbar, and sacral divisions; (PNS); part of the ANS; predominates during physiological state of rest and relaxation; mediates specific visceral reflexes resulting from stimulation such as tearing when a foreign body is in an eye, salivation when food is in the mouth, penile erection as a result of palpitation, etc.; controlled by the anterior hypothalamus.

PARASYMPATHETIC PATHWAY (EYE): travels from the eye (retina) to the optic chiasm where the optic nerve splits and travels in the right and left optic tracts to the right and left lateral geniculate bodies; 10% of the fibers reaching the geniculate bodies subserve the light reflex and are relayed in the periaqueductal grey to both Edinger-Westphal nuclei; light falling on either eye excites both nuclei and causes constriction of both pupils (consensual light reflex); the Edinger-Westphal nuclei are also stimulated by the adjacent third nerve nuclear mass which controls the medial rectus muscles; when both medial rectus muscles are activated in an attempt to converge the eyes, the Edinger-Westphal nuclei become active and constrict the pupils, this being the suggested basis of the accommodation reflex; the parasympathetic fibers are carried in the third nerve to the orbit and lie in a superficial and dorsal position; the final relay of the pathway is in the ciliary ganglion in the posterior orbit, which gives origin to eight to ten short ciliary nerves, which subdivide into sixteen to twenty branches that pass around the eye to reach the constrictor muscle of the pupil; lesions in the retina, optic nerve, chiasm, and minor nerve damage to the optic nerve cause afferent pathway lesions causing a Marcus Gunn pupil; other diseases affecting the parasympathetic control of the pupil include multiple sclerosis, Parinaud syndrome, Argyll-Robertson pupil, and Holmes-Adie pupil.

PARASYMPATHOLITIC REACTION: see anticholinergic reaction.

PARATHORMONE: a hormone that increases blood calcium and reduces blood phosphate; prevents loss of each; hyposecretion or hypersecretion produces very severe disturbances of nervous and muscular function; produced by the parathyroid gland.

PARATHYROID GLAND: produces parathormone hormone.

PARENCHYMA: the essential elements of an organ; a general term to designate the functional elements of an organ, as distinguished from its framework.

PARESIS: partial paralysis (weakness).

PARESTHESIA: painful sensation which becomes excruciating when limb is touched (thalamic pain); unpleasant abnormal sensations after loss of normal sensations due to nerve damage; see hyperesthesia, hyperpathia.

PARETIC DYSARTHRIA: due to neural or bulbar (medullary) weakness or paralysis of the articulatory muscles (lower motor neuron paralysis); shriveled tongue lies inert on the floor of the mouth, and the lips are relaxed and tremulous; drooling because of dysphagia; difficulties with vibratives (r); seen in myasthenia gravis, diphtheria, poliomyelitis, and progressive bulbar palsy.

PARIETAL LOBES: sensory cortex; demarcated anteriorly by the central fissure, ventrally by the Sylvian fissure, dorsally by the cingulate gyrus, and posteriorly by the parietal-occipital sulcus; five major gyri: superior and inferior, the postcentral (behind the central sulcus), and the supermarginal and angular (on either side of the lateral fissure; principal regions of the parietal lobe include the postcentral gyrus (Brodmann's areas 1, 2, & 3), the superior parietal lobule (Brodmann's areas 5 & 7), the inferior parietal lobule (Brodmann's areas 40 & 43), and the angular gyrus (Brodmann's area 39); the postcentral convolution is the terminus of somatic sensory pathways from the opposite half of the body; perception of position in space and relationship of the various parts of the body to one another; speech function is in the supramarginal and angular gyri and in the adjacent temporal lobe.

P

PARIETAL-LOBE AFFERENT FIBERS: the principal afferents to the parietal lobe project from the lateral and posterior thalamus, hypothalamus, and primary and secondary sensory areas.

PARIETAL-LOBE - ANTERIOR ZONE: Brodmann's areas 1, 2, 3, & 43, and portions of 5 & 7; primary and secondary somatosensory cortex.

PARIETAL-LOBE EFFERENT FIBERS: the major projections go to the frontal and temporal association cortex, as well as to subcortical structures including the lateral and posterior thalamus and the posterior region of the striatum, midbrain, and spinal cord; no direct sensory projections go to the frontal lobe but sensory input to the frontal lobe is made through the corticocortical projections; the descending projections to the striatum and spinal cord, in particular, probably function as a guidance control system in the control of movements in space.

PARIETAL-LOBE FUNCTIONAL AREAS: anterior zone (Brodmann's areas 1, 2, 3, & 43 and portions of Brodmann's areas 5 & 7); the primary and secondary somatosensory cortex and the posterior zone (portions of Brodmann's areas 5 & 7 and areas 39 & 40) which is the association cortex of the parietal lobe.

PARIETAL-LOBE (DEEP LESION): impairment of all forms of sensation contralaterally as well as a contralateral homonymous hemianopia, often incongruous and greater in the inferior quadrants; lesions in the angular gyrus of the dominant hemisphere result in an inability to read.

PARIETAL-LOBE (DOMINANT SIDE, LARGE LESION): Gerstmann's syndrome; inability to write (agraphia), inability to calculate (acalculia), failure to distinguish right from left, and loss of recognition of various fingers and toes; true agnosia; also present: fluent aphasia and dysnomia (word-finding problems); lesion encompasses the angular gyrus.

PARIETAL-LOBE, LEFT SIDE, MOTOR FUNCTIONS: control function; provides a system for accurate internal representation of moving body parts and important for controlling changes in their spatial positions (Kimura, 1979); apraxia results from a disturbance in this function of controlling accurate positioning of limb and oral musculature; identification of the current position of the limb is a prerequisite for moving the limb to another position otherwise changes of position are awkward and frequently in error.

PARIETAL-LOBE LESIONS: cause mainly a defect in sensory discrimination with variable impairment of primary sensation (e.g., perception of painful, tactile, thermal, and vibratory stimuli is more or less normal, whereas distinction between single and double stimuli, sense of position, distinction point threshold, and localization of sensory stimuli are impaired or lost), and extinction (if both sides of the body are touched simultaneously, only the stimulus on the normal side is perceived; sometimes called cortical sensory defect); nondominent hemisphere: geographical confusion, sensory inattention, attention hemianopia, construction apraxia, sensory seizures, aphasia, dressing apraxia; global reduction of all forms of somatic sensation on the opposite side of body; inattentiveness to sensory stimuli on one side of body, astereognosis, autotopagnosia, asymbolia for pain.

PARIETAL-LOBE LESIONS AND MEMORY: (Warrington & Weiskrantz theory, 1973) left parietal lobe may have an important role in the storage of short-term memory.

PARIETAL-LOBE (NONDOMINANT SIDE, LARGE LESION): unawareness of hemiplegia and hemianesthesia (anosognosia); lack of recognition of left arm and leg, neglect of the left side of the body (as in dressing) and of external space on the left side (contralateral neglect), and constructional apraxia (an inability to perform the movements of constructing simple figures) due to a disturbance in the motor control of drawing or constructional abilities because of inadequate sensory-spatial representation; deprives the frontal motor system of sufficient information to carry out the appropriate movements; drawings are distorted, blocks are assembled in bizarre designs; maps lack spatial organization, etc. (Kolb & Whishaw, 1980); personality or behavior disturbances involving spatial orientation; overdevelopment of speech, to verbosity, which bears the character of empty reasoning masking the true defect of disorientation in space (Luria 1973); impaired freehand drawing, copying, or cutting out paper figures, addition of extra strokes to drawings; drawings lack accurate spatial relationships; topographical disability (unable to draw maps of well-known regions from memory); can recognize objects shown in familiar views, but impaired at recognizing objects shown in unfamiliar views; left-sided anosognosias and anosodiaphorias (indifference to the existence of disease).

PARIETAL-LOBE LESIONS (TERTIARY ZONES): severe disturbances in the integration and analysis of sensory information; impairment of cross-modal matching or the impairment of cognition; disturbance of gross movements of the arms (in space); severe bilateral apraxia when limb movements are required; mild apraxia when facial movements are required.

PARIETAL-LOBE (POSTERIOR ZONE): portions of Brodmann's areas 5 & 7, and areas 39 & 40; association cortex of the parietal lobes.

PARIETAL-LOBE, RIGHT SIDE, MOTOR FUNCTIONS: motor control of drawing or constructional abilities.

PARIETAL-LOBE TEST BATTERIES: Borod et al., 1980; Goodglass & Kaplan, 1972.

P

PARIETAL-OCCIPITAL APHASIA: combined alexia and apraxia with dysgraphia.

PARIETO-OCCIPITAL SULCUS: minor sulcus of the cerebral cortex, located in the posterior, superior portion of the brain which arbitrarily divides the parietal lobe from the occipital lobe; an overlap zone for visual and spatial functions.

PARIETAL RADIATION LESION: causes an inferior quadrantic homonymous hemianopia.

PARIETAL-TEMPORAL ASSOCIATION AREAS, LEFT: processes symbolic-analytic information, such as is found in language and arithmetic, in which the incoming sensory stimulation stands for, or abstractly symbolizes, something else; auditory, visual, and somatic input of a real object is intergrated and represented by an abstract stimulus that itself has auditory, visual, and somatic properties; this ability for cross-modal matching the various attributes of a real stimulus into an abstract, symbolic representation is the necessary foundation for the evolution of language (Geschwind, 1979; Luria & Hutton, 1977). They hypothesized that the function is performed by the angular and supramarginal gyri (approximately Brodmann's areas 39 & 40); short-term memory for verbal material.

PARIETAL-TEMPORAL ASSOCIATION AREAS, RIGHT: specialized for processing analysis of visual, auditory, and somatic input as to type and source (e.g. spatial characteristics) of sensory inputs; complex cognitive processes involving the integration of all sensory modalities for any given stimulus and evolving a picture in the mind of the stimulus as it is located in the environment; this ability is thought to develop in children at about age 10 (Piaget, 1971); short-term memory for spatial location of particular sensory inputs.

PARIETAL-TEMPORAL LOBE LESION, LEFT: disturbance of abstract symbolic integration; behaviors such as talking, reading, writing, etc., are disturbed; agraphia; dyslexia; dysphasia; apraxia; inability to combine blocks to form a design; dyscalculia; poor short-term memory; inability to distinquish right from left; hemianopia; finger agnosia; Gerstmann's syndrome.

PARIETAL-TEMPORAL-OCCIPITAL ASSOCIATION AREAS: posterior association cortex; located in front of visual association areas and behind the primary sensory strip; runs from the longitudinal fissure laterally to the areas adjacent to and just above the temporal lobe; functionally they comprehend cortical mediation for all behavior involving vision, touch, body awareness, verbal comprehension, spatial localization and for abstract and complex intellectual function of math reasoning and the formulation of logical propositions; cognition, thought, reasoning; also called the tertiary zone.

PARINAUD SYNDROME (EYE): pupils are dilated and fixed to light;

often coupled with loss of upward gaze; due to lesions compressing or infiltrating the tectum in the area of the superior collicular bodies causing interference with the decussating light reflex fibers in the periaqueductal area.

PARKINSON'S DISEASE/SYNDROME: progressive neuronal degeneration of basal ganglionic structures, particularly the substantia nigra; content of the striatum is depleted, presumably due to a loss of neurons in the substantia nigra and degeneration of the nigrostriatal tract to which they give rise and to the loss of the neurotransmitter substance, dopamine, which is produced by cells of the substantia nigra nucleus; possible disturbance of the ventromedial system at the level of the basal ganglia; symptoms include resting (static) tremor, muscular rigidity (cogwheel phenomenon), micrographia (also called amyostatic syndrome), akinesia , involuntary movements (akathisia); disorders of posture; disorders of righting; absence of arm swinging, bradykinesia, masked fascies (poverty of facial expression), dysarthric speech, general loss of grace, agility, poor fine motor coordination, marche à petits pas, difficulty in starting to walk and, once started, difficulty in stopping (festinating gait); etiologies may include encephalitis, multi-infarct dementia, toxic reactions, or familial tendencies (Kessler, 1978); mental changes occur in only about 1/3 of all patients (Wells, 1982); also called paralysis agitans; see Reitan & Wolfson (1985) for a detailed discussion of this syndrome.

PARKINSON'S DISEASE - COGNITIVE CHANGES: changes normally found in patients with frontal-lobe or basal-ganglia lesions; deficits on tests of extrapersonal orientation, personal orientation, the Wisconsin card-sorting test, and memory tests; verbal IQ usually normal; impairment of cognitive functioning may include slowed scanning on visual recognition tasks (Wilson et al., 1979); diminished conceptual flexibility (M. L. Albert, 1978; Bowen, 1976); slowing on motor response tasks that may reflect both bradykinesia and central defect of motor programming (Bowen, 1976; Matthews & Haaland, 1979; Talland & Schwab, 1964); micrographia; decreased output on verbal fluency tasks, without dysarthria or aphasia, suggesting a central problem of impaired initiative or spontaneity (M. L. Albert, 1978); general decrease of verbal memory; relatively intact for tests of apraxia, object naming, and vocabulary; in general may perform at a lower level on timed tests of the WAIS-R than on the untimed Verbal Scale subtests; attention, concentration, and immediate memory may remain intact (Walker et al., 1982); depression is common and should be taken into consideration when evaluating performance on tests, attention, memory, and calculations (Mayeux et al., 1981); irritability, suspiciousness, and egocentricity occur frequently (Lishman, 1978); neuropsychological defi-

P

cits: general intelligence as measured by the WAIS-R is relatively intact, particularly in terms of verbal intelligence; dyskinesia appears prominently on the motor tests in the Halstead-Reitan Battery: tremor in drawing, micrographia, poor complex psychomotor task (Tactual Performance Test), and impairment of primary motor ability (Finger Oscillation Test), impairment on the Category Test suggesting impairment of abstraction, reasoning, and logical analysis skills which may interfere with activities of daily living; a person who is not able to understand complex situations or relationships between events and circumstances, and is not able to draw reasonable conclusion on the basis of readily available observations is not likely to be able to adjust to the requirements of the environment in which he/she lives; neuropsychological deficits are not likely to be improved with medication that may improve some of the physical manifestations (Reitan & Wolfson, 1985).

PARKINSONIAN TREMOR: coarse, rhythmic tremor, most often localized in one or both hands; characteristically occurs when limb is in repose, and willed movement temporarily suppresses it; handwriting is often micrographic.

PAROXYSM: a sudden recurrence or intensification of symptoms; a spasm or seizure.

PAROXYSMAL DISORDERS: epilepsy; narcolepsy; cataplexy; hysterical convulsions; anxiety attacks; vasovagal attacks; migraine; aural vertigo; hypoglycemia (Brain, 1985).

PAROXYSMAL SLEEP: narcolepsy.

PARTIAL SEIZURES: (complex) usually originate in the temporal lobe, but sometimes in the frontal lobe; characterized by three common manifestations: 1. subjective feelings such as forced, repetitive thoughts, alterations in mood, feelings of déjà vu, or hallucinations; 2. automatisms, repetitive stereotyped movements such as lip smacking or chewing, or the repetition of acts such as undoing buttons and the like; 3. postural changes, or frozen postures.

PASAT: Paced Auditory Serial Addition Test.

PASSED POINTING: overshooting the intended mark; lesion of one cerebellar hemisphere, especially the anterior lobe; see also ataxia, overshooting, cerebellar lesions.

PASSIVE: as mental and physical state characterized by inactivity and submissiveness.

PATTERN DISCRIMINATION: visual cortex.

PATHOGNOMONIC: specifically distinctive or characteristic of a disease or pathologic condition; a sign or symptom on which a diagnosis can be made.

PAUSES IN SPEECH/WORD FINDING PROBLEMS/NAMING PROBLEMS: see amnestic a., dysnomic a., blocking.

p.c.: after meals.

P

PEABODY INDIVIDUAL ACHIEVEMENT TEST (PIAT): the wide coverage of achievement levels makes this test a valuable instrument for measuring residual intellectual competency of brain-injured adults; tests verbal conceptual functions, primarily; a variety of visuoperceptual functions also enter into the performance; useful with physically handicapped patients.

PEABODY PICTURE VOCABULARY TEST (PPVT): sensitive to dominant hemisphere disease.

PEDANT see sleep pedant.

PEDUNCLE: a stem-like connecting part.

PERCEPTION: the processes used in acquiring, through the senses, a knowledge of the environment or one's own body as a result of the activity of cells in the various sensory regions of the neocortex beyond the primary sensory cortex; sensory information is relayed to the frontal and anterior temporal lobes in the form of a perception which project back upon the sensory systems (feedback loops); perceptual feedback loops can be influenced by previous experience, cognitive set, ongoing behavior, etc.; receptive function; integration of sensory impressions into psychologically meaningful data; includes awareness, recognition, discrimination, patterning, orientation; left parietal tertiary zones, Brodmann's areas 39 & 40.

PERCEPTUAL DISRUPTION: may be directly due to either absence of sensory input as in blindness or deafness or by a lesion of the secondary and tertiary sensory zones which produces an agnosia; may be indirect as a result of higher-level control factors involved in perception.

PERCEPTUAL MAZE TEST: (Elithorn et al., 1964) sensitive to brain-damage particularly right-hemisphere lesions; frontal-lobe lesioned patients may disregard the rules (Walsh, 1978).

PERCEPTUAL SPEED TASK: (Moran & Mefford, 1959) a paper and pencil cancellation task of vigilance and shift of set.

PERFORMANCE EFFECTIVENESS: performance is as effective as the performer's ability to monitor, self-correct, and regulate the intensity, tempo, and other qualitative aspect of delivery. Brain-damaged patients often perform erratically and unsuccessfully since abilities for self-correction and self-monitoring are vulnerable to many different kinds of brain-damage. Some patients cannot correct their mistakes because they do not perceive them. Patients with pathological inertia may perceive their errors, identify them, but not correct them. Defective self-monitoring can spoil any kind of performance (Lezak, 1983).

PERFUSION: the act of pouring over or through, especially the passage of a fluid through the vessels of a specific organ; a liquid poured over or through an organ or tissue.

PERIAQUEDUCTAL GRAY (CENTRAL GRAY): part of tegmentum

P

in midbrain; see also central gray.

PERILYMPH: the fluid contained within the space separating the membranous from the osseous labyrinth of the ear; it is entirely separate from the endolymph.

PERINATAL INJURY: pertaining to or occurring in the period shortly before and after birth; in medical statistics generally considered to begin with completion of 28 weeks of gestation and variously defined as ending one to four weeks after birth.

PERIPHERAL NERVOUS SYSTEM: the part of the nervous system that lies outside of the CNS (e.g., outside of the brain and spinal cord).

PERISTALSIS: the wormlike movement by which the alimentary canal or other tubular organs provided with both longitudinal and circular muscle fibers propel their contents; consists of a wave of contraction passing along the tube for variable distances.

PERISYLVANIAN LESIONS, LEFT: causes global aphasia.

PERLA: pupil equal, react to light, and accommodation.

PERSEVERANCE: problems in perseverance may compromise any kind of mental or motor activity. Inability to persevere can result from distractibility, or it may reflect impaired self-control usually associated with frontal-lobe damage. In the former case, ongoing behavior is uninterrupted by some external disturbance; in the latter, dissolution of ongoing activity seems to come from within the patient as he loses interest, slows down, or gives up. Motor impersistence tends to occur in those patients with right hemisphere or bilateral cortical damage who display fairly severe mental impairment (Joynt et al., 1962; Joynt & Goldstein, 1975); perseveration is involuntary while perseverance implies a voluntary control of the act, thus, perseveration tests measure any lag in the mental processes (Lezak, 1983).

PERSEVERANCE TEST: (Tow, 1955) a seated patient is told to hold a leg a little above a chair in front of him as long as possible while performing a writing task; impersistence will be demonstrated by the leg slowly descending to the ground.

PERSEVERATION: continuance of any activity after cessation of the causative stimulus; persistent repetition of words, ideas, or subjects so that, once an individual begins speaking about a subject or uses a particular word, it continually recurs; commonly seen in Organic Mental Disorders and Schizophrenia; controlled by Brodmann's area 9, left.

PERSISTENT VEGETATIVE STATE: clinically similar to appallic state.

PERSONAL AND CURRENT INFORMATION SUBTEST: (WMS) most persons who are not severely brain-damage are able to give information such as their own birthdate, etc.; this subtest of the

Wechsler Memory Scale discriminates poorly for mild to moderate memory deficits (Lezak, 1983).

PERSONAL ORIENTATION TEST: (Semmes et al., 1963; Weinstein, 1964); a test for autotopagnosia (body image agnosia); verbal instructions sensitive to left-hemisphere lesions; left-posterior lesioned patients may also have a global aphasic disorder or an inability to comprehend how single parts relate to a whole structure (De Renzi & Scotti, 1970); right-hemisphere lesioned patients may ignore the left side of body (Raghaven, 1961); disturbances in scanning, perceptual shifting, and postural mechanisms may be a result of frontal-lobe lesions (Teuber, 1964); Parkinsonian patients (subcortical lesions) may demonstrate body disorientation (Bowen, 1976).

PERSONALITY: deeply ingrained behavior patterns which include the way one relates to, perceives, and thinks about the environment and oneself; personality traits are prominent aspects of personality and do not imply pathology; personality disorder implies inflexible and maladaptive patterns of sufficient severity to cause significant impairment in functioning.

PERSONALITY AND AFFECT CHANGES: Brodmann's areas 21 & 38; amygdala; frontal-lobe dysfunction.

PERSONALITY CHANGES: Many movement disorders appear to have associated changes in personality. Parkinsonian patients may be depressed; hypothesized to be associated with the caudate nucleus which is anatomically close to the frontal lobe (Pincus & Tucker, 1974); Huntington'a chorea may produce depression, bipolar-like symptoms, or delusionary-hallucinatory state; presenile dementias may produce numerous adverse personality changes (Malamud, 1975); temporal-lobe and psychomotor epileptic patients may experience personality changes after several years of seizures; moderate to severe head injuries cause major personality changes (Brooks et al., 1979; McKinlay et al., 1981; Panting & Merry, 1972), and are rarely able to form or maintain close relationships (Weddell et al., 1980) so that those who have not been rendered euphoric or apathetic by their injuries, are often lonely and depressed as well (Lezak et al., 1980; Oddy & Humphrey, 1980); changes may include emotional dulling, disinhibition, reduced anxiety, euphoria, decreased social sensitivity, depression, hypersensitivity, hypo-/hyper-sexuality, irritability, anxiety, restlessness, low frustration tolerance, and apathy.

PERSONALITY TESTS - OBJECTIVE: Minnesota Multiphasic Personality Inventory (MMPI).

PERSONALITY TESTS - PROJECTIVE: Rorschach Technique; Thematic Apperception Test; Drawing Tests.

PET: Positron emission computerized tomography.

P

PETIT MAL SEIZURE: brief seizure with minimal motor accompaniment; brief loss of consciousness/awareness (few seconds to 10 sec., at the most); few (3-per-second) blinks or jerks of eyelids and sometimes arms; causes: (typical) thalamic lesion, (atypical) mesial frontal-lobe lesion; also called absence attack; loss of awareness during which there is no motor activity except blinking and/or turning the head, rolling the eyes, etc.; often with loss of memory of what was occurring just prior to the attack; attacks start in infancy or childhood and may cease or be replace by grand mal seizures in adolescence; dazed appearance with eyes staring; facial pallor; usually a result of wave-and-spike dysrhythmia in both frontal lobes; site of origin thought to be the diencephalon (Brain, 1985).

PHARYNX-LOWER-PARALYSIS OR ANESTHESIA: Vagus nerve (X).

PHARYNX-UPPER-PARALYSIS OR ANESTHESIA: Glossopharyngeal nerve (IX).

PHENOTHIAZINE DRUG REACTION: see extrapyramidal reaction; oculargyral crisis.

PHENYLKETONURIA: see PKU.

PHOBIA: a persistent, irrational fear of a specific object, activity, or situation that results in a desire to avoid the dreaded object, activity, or situation.

PHONALOGICAL DEFICITS IN APHASIA: 1. phoneme substitution errors; 2. simplification errors in which a phoneme or syllable is lost; 3. addition errors (extra phoneme or syllable is added); 4. environmental errors in which a particular phoneme occurs that can be accounted for by the influence of surrounding phonemes (Blumstein, 1981).

PHONATION: function of larynx, changes in size and shape of the glottis and in length and tension of the vocal cords controlled by the laryngeal muscles; vibrations transmitted to the column of air passing over the vocal cords; sounds modified as air passes through the nasopharynx and mouth which act as resonators.

PHONEMATIC SYSTEM OF LANGUAGE: (Luria, 1973b) the secondary association areas secure the precise differentiation of separate sounds; *pathology*: sounds are perceived only as undifferentiated noise in severe cases or closely related different letters or sounds that are perceived as the same, e.g., b-p; z-x; d-t; leads to the disintegration of writing capcity and to reading disorders.

PHONEMES: basic units of speech in a given language which are combined to form a spoken word.

PHONEMIC HEARING DEFICIT: left temporal-lobe lesion; posterior part of Brodmann's area 22 near Wernicke's area.

PHONETIC DISCRIMINATION IMPAIRMENT: damage to the precentral and post central gyri containing the motor and sensory representations of the face; produce ineffective use of the phonetic elements of language and poor performance on the word fluency test (worse than frontal-lobe patients); slight residual expressive dysphasia; poor spelling; very low design fluency; normal facial control of expression (Taylor, 1979).

PHYSIOLOGICALLY ZERO: the normal skin temperature.

PHYSOSTIGMINE: constricts pupils by inhibiting cholinesterase activity at the neuromuscular junction; may be implicated in depression.

PIA MATER: the innermost of the three membranes covering the brain and spinal cord, extending into the depths of the fissures and sulci; consists of reticular, elastic, and collagenous fibers.

PICK'S DISEASE: relatively rare disease; inherited in a dominant way, a pre-senile dementia; also called circumscribed cortical atrophy (Walton, 1977); similar to Alzheimer's disease; cellular degeneration and atrophy confined to frontal and temporal cortex; symptoms included silliness, social disinhibition, and impulsivity with apathy or impaired capacity for sustained motivation (Roth, 1978; Walton, 1977); personality disturbances precede memory loss (Berry, 1975); resembles frontal-lobe syndrome: reduced personal cleanliness, reduced memory function, paranoia, flippancy and arrogance, social irresponsibility/ inappropriateness, agitation, inattentiveness, concreteness; see also pre-senile dementia, Alzheimer's disease; differential clinicial diagnosis from Alzheimer's disease can only be made at autopsy; atrophy of the frontal-orbital area, anterior part of superior temporal gyrus, and the inferior and middle temporal gyri; atrophy of the parietal lobe has also been found; atrophy of the subcortical nuclei: globus pallidus, caudate nucleus, putamen, and thalamus (Reitan & Wolfson, 1985).

PICKWICKIAN SYNDROME: obesity, dyspnea, hypercapnea, and drowsiness; sometimes sleep apnea; see also hypoventilation syndrome.

PICTORIAL SIMILARITIES AND DIFFERENCES I: Stanford-Binet subtest, age level IV-6; test of conceptual functioning.

PICTORIAL SIMILARITIES AND DIFFERENCES II: Stanford-Binet subtest, age level V; test of conceptual functioning.

PICTORIAL TEST OF INTELLIGENCE (PTI): children's test; requires no verbal or fine motor response from the patient; untimed; sometimes appropriate for severely brain-damaged adults to get a rough estimate of current abilities.

PICTORIAL WORD LEARNING TEST: an alternative word learning test that does not require auditory input; most people recall two or three more pictures than words on the first trial and reach their ceiling (14 or 15) by the fourth trial; brain-injured patients may learn more words on the pictorial than the auditory presentation and retain more (O'Brien & Lezak, 1981); left-sided damaged patients

P

tend to retain pictorial information better whereas auditory presentation benefits patients with right-sided damage (Davies et al., 1983).

PICTURE ABSURDITIES subtest: (Stanford-Binet) may be used to assess impairments in the ability to evaluate and integrate all elements of a problem; test of reasoning and judgment.

PICTURE ARRANGEMENT SUBTEST: (WAIS-R) tends to reflect social sophistication; nonverbal counterpart of Comprehension subtest; tests sequential thinking, including the ability to see relationships between events, establish priorities, and order activities chronologically; vulnerable to brain injury in general; right-hemisphere lesions have a more depressing effect on these scores than left-hemisphere lesions (McFie, 1975), particularly right temporal-lobe damage (Dodrill & Wilkus, 1976); Long & Brown, 1979; Piercy, 1964); frontal-lobe damaged patients may shift the cards only a little, if at all, and to present this response (or nonresponse) as the solution (McFie, 1975; Walsh, 1978). Walsh (1979) suggests that this behavior is akin to the tendency of patients with frontal-lobe lesions to make hypotheses impulsively and uncritically based on first impressions or on whatever detail catches their eye without analyzing the entire situation; may be used to test reasoning (logical thinking, comprehension of relationships, and practical judgment) (Lezak, 1983).

PICTURE COMPLETION SUBTEST (WAIS-R): may be used to screen for perceptual recognition deficits; does not discriminate well between superior and very superior ability levels (Lezak, 1983); basically tests visual recognition; tests remote memory and general information; reasoning components involving judgments about both practical and conceptual relevances (Saunders, 1960b); resilience to the effects of brain-damage; does not differentiate laterally (Lezak, 1983).

PICTURE MATRIX MEMORY TASK: (Deutsch et al., 1980); a visual neglect/inattention test.

PICTURE-NAMING TESTS: can give information about the patient's ability to use words; open-ended vocabulary questions can be evaluated for conceptual level and complexity of verbalization; descriptions of activities and story telling can demonstrate how expressive deficits interfere with effective communication (Lezak, 1983).

PILOERECTION: erection of the hair.

PINEAL GLAND (EPIPHYSIS CEREBRI): secretes melatonin hormone.

PKU: phenylketonuria; an inborn error of metabolism attributable to a deficiency of or a defect in phenylalanine hydrocylase, the enzyme that catalyzes the conversion of phenylalanine to tyrosine; accumulation of phenylalanine and its metabolic products in the body's fluids results in mental retardation, neurologic manifestations such as hyperkinesia, epilepsy, and microcephaly, light pigmentation, eczema, and a mousy odor unless treated by administration of a diet low in phenylalanine; transmitted as an autosomal recessive trait.

PLANNING: planning involves the ability to conceptualize change from present circumstances, and view the environment objectively (abstractly), be able to conceive of alternatives, weigh and make choices, and evolve a conceptual framework or structure that will give direction to the carrying out of a plan; requires a capacity for sustained attention (Lezak, 1983).

PLANNING TESTS: Bender-Gestalt; Thematic Apperception Test; WAIS-R Block Design subtest; Sentence Building (Stanford-Binet SA I, 1960 Revision); Complex Figure Test; Osterreith Complex Figure Test; Porteus Maze Test.

PLASTICITY - BRAIN: (Luria's theory); the brain is able to reorganize actions within each level of functioning and also to shift these actions from one level to another; also refers to rehabilitative treatment that may surpass what can be expected from the natural recovery process particularly when residual capacities are capitalized upon and areas of permanently impaired function are detoured (Goldstein, 1984).

PLATYSMA MUSCLE: a plate-like muscle that originates from the fascia of the cervical region and inserts in the mandible and the skin around the mouth; enervated by the cervical branch of the facial nerve, and acts to wrinkle the skin of the neck and to depress the jaw.

PLEASURE CENTER: nucleus in ventral tegmental reticular formation; see also tegmentum.

-PLEGIA: a word termination meaning paralysis or severe loss of motor function.

PMH: past medical history.

PMS: premenstral syndrome.

PNEUMOENCEPHALOGRAPHY: x-rays taken after the cerebrospinal fluid is replaced by air introduced by a lumbar puncture; allows location of blockages in the ventricles, displacements in the position of the ventricles, or enlargements of the ventricles.

PNS: parasympathetic nervous system.

p. o.: by mouth; orally.

POINT DIGIT SPAN: (Smith, 1975); digit series are pointed out on a card to test verbal span of patients who cannot speak; when both verbal and point digit span are given, a poorer performance on the point test suggests problems in integrating visual and verbal processes.

POISONED FOOD PROBLEMS: (Arenberg, 1968) may be used to test reasoning (logical thinking and practical judgments).

POLARIZATION: basic activity in neuronal conduction within axons: unequal distribution of positive or negative ions on either side of the

P

semipermeable cell membrane of axon.

POLIOMYELITIS: acute infectious disease due to a virus with a predilection for the cells of the anterior horns of the grey matter of the spinal cord and the motor nuclei of the brainstem; muscular paralysis and subsequent atrophy; usual route of infection in man is thought to be the alimentary tract; may be transmitted by healthy carriers; *early symptoms*: fever, malaise, headache, drowsiness or insomnia, sweating, flushing, faucial congestion, and often gastrointestinal disturbances (one or two days); may either remit for 48 hours or merge into second phase of severe headache, pain in back and limbs, hyperesthesia, delirium, cervical rigidity, and Kernig's sign; *paralytic stage*: muscular fasciculation, severe pain; maximum damage to muscles in 24 hours or progression in an ascending form which gradually spreads upwards from the legs with possible respiratory paralysis; improvement usually begins at the end of the first week after the onset of paralysis (Brain, 1985).

POLYCYTHEMIA: an increase in the total red cell mass of the body.

POLYNEURITIS: inflammation of many nerves at once; multiple or disseminated neuritis.

POLYNEUROPATHY: sensory changes accompanied by varying degrees of motor and reflex loss; impairment usually symmetric; most severe over the feet and legs; less severe over the hands.

PONS: part of the lower hindbrain; organ which connects the cerebrum, cerebellum, and oblongata immediately rostral to the medulla; broad transverse band of white fibers arching across the upper part of the medulla oblongata, contracting to a cord to enter the cerebellum; works together with the cerebellum to correlate postural and kinesthetic information; refining and regulating motor impulses relayed from the cerebrum at the top of the brainstem; contains major pathways for fibers running between the cerebral cortex and the cerebellum; subserves both visceral and motor reflexes and contains nuclei which mediate two qualitatively different kinds of sleep.

PONS INFARCT: multiple cranial nerve palsies, dysphagia, vertigo, nystagmus, facial paralysis, diplopia, and gaze palsies; may result in a state of akinetic mutism; cerebellar signs include dysyneriga, dysmetria, and dysdiadochokinesia of the same side as the lesion are common with infarction of the lateral and tegmental parts of the pons (Reitan & Wolfson, 1985).

PONTINE GLIOMA: tumor that often starts in the region of the 6th nerve nucleus and may cause any combination of a 6th and 7th nerve palsy; minimal motor signs, brisk reflexes and extensor plantar responses often present; hemiplegia is not an early symptom.

PONTINE LESIONS: found in conjunction with basilar artery thrombosis, multiple sclerosis, pontine gliomas, and Wernicke's encephalopathy; *dorsolateral infarction*: Horner's syndrome on the side of the lesion coupled with loss of pain and temperature sensation in the limbs on the opposite side of the body; below mid-pontine levels there is an increasing likelihood of finding loss of sensation over the face on the same side because of damage to the 5th nerve fibers; cerebellar involvement on the same side; *mid-pontine infarction*: lateral gaze center may be affected with loss of conjugate lateral gaze towards the side of the lesion; 6th nerve spared; *lower pontine infarction*: (near the 6th nerve nucleus) causes homolateral paralysis of the lateral rectus muscle and failure of adduction of the opposite eye; causes limitation of conjugate lateral gaze or sixth nerve palsy; the vestibular and cochlear nuclei may be damaged causing severe vestibular symptoms, nystagmus, and deafness combined with loss of pain and temperature sensation over the face on the side of the lesion and loss of the same modalities on the opposite side of the body; *paramedian infarction*: damage to the fascicles of the 6th and 7th nerve and the pyramidal pathways; a complete hemiplegia may result (Millard-Gubler syndrome) or a partial hemiplegia, a 6th nerve palsy, and weakness of the opposite arm with conjugate gaze intact.

PORCH INDEX OF COMMUNICATIVE ABILITY: (Porch, 1967) provides a sensitive measure of small changes in patient performance; malingerers may have higher scores than aphasics on the difficult end of the profile curve and lower scores on the easier end (Porch, 1977); should be administered by trained PICA testers.

PORENCEPHALY: symmetrical cavities in the cortex, where cortex and white matter should be.

PORTEUS MAZE: (Porteus, 1959, 1965) test of frontal-lobe dysfunction involving ability to plan and use foresight.

PORTLAND ADAPTABILITY INVENTORY: (Lezak et al., 1980); a set of three scales designed to provide a systematic record of personal and social maladaptations over time of posttraumatic head-injured patients: Temperament and Emotionality; Activities and Social Behavior; Physical Capabilities; answers can be gleaned from the patient, family, clinical observations, medical records, and social history.

POSITRON EMISSION COMPUTERIZED TOMOGRAPHY: (PET scan) a method of scanning the brain using injected or inhaled radionuclides; used for metabolic studies of regional blood flow, oxygen extraction, or utilization by glucose uptake (Brain, 1985).

POSTCENTRAL ANTERIOR PARIETAL INFARCTION: errors in positioning of the oral cavity for individual sounds, syllables, and whole words; acustic features of the utterance is often distorted; may sound like literal paraphasias.

POSTCENTRAL GYRUS: ridge or convolution immediately after the

P

central sulcus of the cerebral cortex; also known as the retrorolandic area, primary somesthetic area, and primary sensory projection area.

POST-CEREBRAL ARTERY CVA, MAIN BRANCH: confusion, memory deficit, sensory deficit, and a visual field defect due to thalamo-geniculate artery occlusion.

POST-CONCUSSIONAL SYNDROME: impaired learning capacity after the acute amnestic stage.

POST-ICTAL: following a seizure; depression following a grand mal seizure in which the patient is confused.

POSTERIOR ASSOCIATION CORTEX: see parieto-temporo-occipital region.

POSTERIOR CEREBRAL ARTERY OCCLUSIONS: *main branch*: variable effects because there are connections between this vessel and the middle cerebral arteries; variable degrees of confusion and memory deficit; sensory deficits and a field defect due to thalamo-geniculate artery occlusion; *perforating vessel*: occlusion of one of the thalamo-geniculate vessels involves the posterior limb of the internal capsule, part of the thalamus, and the visual radiation resulting in hemianesthesia with loss of all sensory modalities, and complete hemianopia; may be a residual Dejerine-Roussy syndrome (thalamic pain); if the branches to the upper brainstem are affected hemiballismus may occur; *terminal branch*: calcarine artery causes a macular sparing hemianopia; sudden and permanent onset of homonymous visual field losses without corresponding evidence of unilateral motor dysfunction; supplies the upper end of the midbrain, cerebral peduncles, portions of the thalamus, the subthalamic area, and parts of the hypothalamus in addition to the occipital lobes; a number of other symptoms suggesting midbrain involvement may also be present; aphasic manifestation may be associated with occlusion of the left side; impairment in dealing with simple spatial configurations, of both an expressive and receptive nature, may present with a right-sided lesion (Reitan & Wolfson, 1985).

POSTERIOR COLUMN SYNDROME: loss of vibratory and position sense below the lesion; senses of pain, temperature, and touch affected relatively little or not at all; paresthesias of tingling and pins and needles; hyperpathia.

POSTERIOR COMMISSURE: large fiber bundle that crosses from one side of the cerebrum to the other just dorsal to the point where the aqueduct opens into the third ventricle.

POSTERIOR FOSSA TUMORS: rare in adulthood; may produce intermittent brainstem symptoms, mimicking multiple sclerosis, transient ischemic attacks, or transient 6th nerve palsies; ataxia and pyramidal signs may be found; vertical nystagmus due to extrinsic compression of the brainstem; tumors in the region of the foramen magnum may produce recurrent episodes of tetraparesis and ultimately tetraplegia.

POSTERIOR PARIETAL ARTERY (OCCLUSION): produces complete aphasia with loss of comprehension and loss of speech.

POSTERIOR PITUITARY GLAND: secretes oxytocin and antidiuretic (ADH) hormone.

POSTERIOR PARIETAL ARTERY OCCLUSION: produces complete aphasia with loss of comprehension and loss of speech.

POSTHEMIPLEGIC CHOREA: see athetosis.

POSTTRAUMATIC AMNESIA: (PTA) period of clouded consciousness which precedes the attainment of full orientation and continuous awareness in persons recovering from head injuries; characterized primarily by deficit or failure in mnestic processes; both retrograde and anterograde amnesia; most often an intractable amnesia for the traumatic event.

POSTTRAUMATIC AMNESIA QUESTIONNAIRE: (Artioli i Fortuny et al., 1980) a picture and person recognition test which the authors found to be as accurate as usual orientation and memory tests to establish the remission of posttraumatic amnesia.

POST-TRAUMATIC EPILEPSY: epilepsy develops in about 60% of persons who sustain laceration of the brain resulting from a depressed skull fracture or a severe penetrating head injury (Ommaya, 1972); lesions involving the motor area are more likely to cause seizures than lesions near the frontal or occipital poles (Reitan & Wolfson, 1985).

POSTTRAUMATIC SYNDROME: also known as postconcussion syndrome, posttraumatic neurosis; may result from a relatively mild closed-head injury; symptoms may include neurasthenic symptoms, epileptiform attacks, vertigo, headache, forgetfulness, loss of interest, word-finding disturbances, concentration disturbances, loss of initiative, change in sleep pattern, emotional lability, irritability, a tendency to fatigue, disturbance of equilibrium; neurological examination is frequently negative (Reitan & Wolfson, 1985).

POSTURAL HYPOTENSION: see orthostatic hypotension.

POSTURAL REFLEXES: under the control of vision, the labyrinths, or balance receptors, of the middle ear, and proprioception, or sensation, from muscles and joints; see hindbrain functioning, decerebrate rigidity, vestibular system.

POVERTY OF CONTENT OF SPEECH: speech that is adequate in amount but conveys little information because of vagueness, empty repetitions, or use of sterotyped or obscure phrases.

PPD: primary degenerative dementia; Alzheimer's Disease or purified protein derivative (of tuberculin).

PPVT: Peabody Picture Vocabulary Test.

PRACTIC FUNCTIONS: see apraxia-motor tests: symbolic apraxia,

P

symbolic gestures, use of objects tests, manual dexterity, motor functions.

PRAECOX: an obsolescent term for schizophrenia commonly used in Europe to denote process schizophrenia as opposed to reactive schizophrenia.

PRAXIS: the motor integration employed in the execution of complex learned movements (Strub & Black, 1977).

PRE-ICTAL: before a seizure.

PRECENTRAL GYRUS: ridge or convolution immediately forward of the central sulcus; also called primary motor cortex, Brodmann's area 4, motor strip, motor homunculus, Jackson's strip, area pyramidalis, somatomotor strip, gyrus precentralis, preorlandic area.

PREFRONTAL AREA LESIONS (Brodmann's areas 9 to 13): lack of initiative and spontaneity in conjunction with diminished speech; motor inactivity (apathetic-akinetic-abulic states); necessary daily activities are neglected; interpersonal social reations are reduced and shallow; change of personality, usually expressed as lack of concern over the consequences of any action, which may take the form of childish excitement, inapropriate joking and punning, instability and superficiality of emotion, or irritability; may at times assume a pseudopsychopathic form; slight impairment of intelligence, usually described as lack of concentration, vacillation of attention, inability to carry out planned activity or to form the intention to perform and activity, difficulty in changing from one activity to another, or slight loss of recent memory; motor abnormalities such as decomposition of gait and upright stance, wide base, flexed posture, and small shuffling steps, culminating in an inability to stand (truncal ataxia of Bruns), abnormal postures, reflex grasping or sucking, and incontinence of sphincters.

PREFRONTAL CORTEX: old name: frontal granular cortex; transcortical and extracortical connections: receives afferents from the visual, auditory, and somatosensory areas by way of the parietal cortex; receives fibers from the caudate nucleus, the dorsomedial thalamus, the amygdala, and the hypothalamus; sends projections to the parietal and temporal association cortex and cingulate cortex, basal ganglia, dorsomedial thalamus, amygdala, hippocampus, hypothalamus, and other lower brainstem structures; tertiary zones of the frontal unit; formation of intentions; integrated area of function (the superstructure above all other parts of the cerebral cortex (Luria, 1977)).

PREMORBID: symptoms presenting just prior to an acute state.

PREMOTOR AREA LESION: (Brodmann's area 6) characterized by prominent grasp and sucking reflexes; interferes with the mechanism for turning the head and eyes contralaterally.

PREOCCUPATION: compulsion to dwell upon specific ideas, complaints, somatic concerns, etc., to the exclusion of being able to pursue other thoughts or actions without relating them to the subject of the preoccupation.

PREORLANDIC AREA: see precentral gyrus.

PREPAROXYSMAL STATE: before a sudden recurrence or intensification of symptoms, spasm, or seizure.

PRESENILE: pertaining to a condition resembling senility but occurring in early or middle age.

PRESENILE DEMENTIA: see Alzheimer's disease, Pick's disease.

PRESS TEST: (Baehr & Corsini, 1980) a paper and pencil form of the Stroop Test.

PRESSURE AND TOUCH: impulses from the pressure and touch receptors (Pacinian corpuscles) on the skin surface are projected in such a way that stimulation of neighboring areas on the body produces neural activity in neighboring areas on the cortex; the more sensitive to touch a particular part of the body is, the more densely packed is the cortical area devoted to coding stimuli originating from the receptor area; a disproportionate amount of the cortex is devoted to sensory input from lips, tongue, and hands; a column of cells extends downward through the cortex from each encoding area which responds to the same pressure/touch stimulus; the Pacinian corpuscles undergo mechanical deformation to transduce pressure into neural impulses.

PRESYNAPTIC MEMBRANE: the layer separating the neuroplasm of an axon from that part of the nerve cell with which it makes synapsis.

PRESSURED SPEECH: speech that is increased in amount, accelerated and difficult or impossible to interrupt; usually loud and emphatic; most often seen in manic episodes but may also occur in Organic Mental Disorders, Major Depression, Schizophrenia, and acute stress reactions.

PRIMACY EFFECT: better recall for the words at the beginning of the list than most of the other words.

PRIMARY CORTICAL ZONE - FRONTAL (LURIA): motor strip; Brodmann's area 4.

PRIMARY INSOMNIA: life-long disturbance of restful sleep with no usual symptoms of neurosis, depression or other psychiatric or medical diseases; see also sleep pedants, sleep hypochondriacs.

PRIMARY MOTOR CORTEX: precentral gyrus.

PRIMARY MOTOR PROJECTION AREA: see precentral gyrus.

PRIMARY PROJECTION AREAS OF CORTEX: highly specific neuronal structure of the cortex projecting a particular receptor system or efferent system; lesions of these areas will lead to a defect of the specific function of a particular organ.

PRIMARY SENSORY PROJECTION AREA: see post central gyrus.

P

PRIMARY VISUAL AREA LESION: blind spot in part or all of the visual field.

PRIMARY ZONES - SENSORY (LURIA): projection areas of vision (Brodmann's area 17); audition (Brodmann's area 41); body senses (Brodmann's areas 1 - 3).

PRIMITIVE REFLEXES: snout and grasp reflexes caused by mesial frontal-lobe damage.

PRN: as necessary; whenever necessary.

PROACTIVE INTERFERENCE: confusion of one item of a test with another.

PROBLEM OF FACT TEST: Stanford-Binet subtest, age XIII a story and picture test which requires attention to situational cues to interpret and tell a story about the picture; a test of goal formulation; sensitive to frontal-lobe lesions; may be used to test reasoning (logical thinking, comprehension of relationships, and practical judgment).

PROBLEM SITUATIONS I AND II: Stanford-Binet subtest, ages VIII and XI; may be used to test reasoning (logical thinking, comprehension of relationships, and practical judgment).

PRODROME: a premonitory symptom or precursor; a symptom indicating the onset of a disease.

PROGESTERONE HORMONE: prepares the uterus for implantation of a fertilized egg; acts back on the hypothalamus to inhibit the FSH releasing factor.

PROGRESSIVE SUPRANUCLEAR PALSY: Richardson-Steele-Olszewski syndrome; disease of the elderly characterized by gait disturbance, memory and personality deterioration, supranuclear ophthalmoplegia, pseudobulbar palsy, and truncal dystonia; vertical eye movements more restricted than horizontal eye movements; neuronal loss and gliosis in the periaquiductal grey matter with widespread neuronal loss and neurofibrillary degeneration in the basal ganglia; cause unknown (Brain, 1985).

PROJECTION: a mental mechanism whereby repressed mental processes are ascribed to the external world and so are not recognized as being of personal origin.

PROJECTION FIBERS: include ascending fibers from lower centers to the neocortex and descending fibers from the neocortex to the brainstem and spinal cord; white matter.

PROJECTIONS FROM DORSAL THALAMUS: lateral geniculate body projects to Brodmann's area 17, the medial geniculate body projects to Brodmann's area 41, and the ventral lateral posterior nuclei project to Brodmann's areas 1,2, & 3; a large area of the posterior secondary and tertiary cortex sends projections from the pulvinar; some of the subcortical motor nuclei (globus pallidus, substantia nigra, and dentate nucleus) project to the anterior and lateral ventral nuclei, and these areas project to the primary motor (Brodmann's area 4) and the secondary motor (Brodmann's area 6); the dorsomedial nucleus receives projections from the amygdaloid complex, temporal neocortex, and caudate nucleus, and projects to to the remainder of the frontal lobe.

PROJECTIONS TO DORSAL THALAMUS: lateral geniculate body receives visual system projections; medial geniculate body receives auditory system projections; ventral lateral posterior nuclei receive touch, pain, pressure, and temperature projections from body.

PROJECTIVE TEST RESPONSE TENDENCIES: Lezak (1983) has isolated nine characteristic projective test responses which may show up in the protocols of brain-injured patients: 1. Constriction; 2. Stimulus-boundedness; 3. Structure-seeking; 4. Response rigidity; 5. Fragmentation; 6. Simplification; 7. Conceptual confusion and spatial disorientation; 8. Confabulated responses (of the Rorschach response definition); 9. Hesitancy and doubt; see Lezak pp. 600-601 for further elaboration.

PRONATION SIGN: see Babinski's signs.

PROPRIOCEPTION DISORDER: see sensory ataxia.

PROPRIOCEPTIVE SENSATION: deep sensation.

PROSENCEPHALON: primitive division of the brain; includes the telencephalon structures (neocortex, basal ganglia, limbic system, olfactory bulb, lateral ventricals) and the thalamus of the diencephalon; see also forebrain.

PROSODY: variation in stress, pitch, and rhythm of speech by which different shades of meaning are conveyed.

PROSOPAGNOSIA: a type of visual agnosia in which patients are unable to identify familiar faces but will recognize the person by voice; probably a combination of a disturbance of fine visual discrimination and failure of memory for the discrete category of human faces; lesion usually in the bilateral occipitotemporal areas; in particular, right inferior temporo-occipital region, visual agnosia for faces; inability to recognize faces although able to recognize objects, forms, and colors; able to differentiate one face from another, cannot recognize previously known faces by relying only on the visual perception of them; may not be able to recognize their own faces in the mirror.

PROVERBS TESTS: WAIS, WAIS-R, Stanford-Binet, the mental status examination; proverbs are useful to indicate concrete or abstract interpretations.

PROXIMAL: close to something.

PSEUDOBULBAR PALSY: anarthric or dysarthric (spastic or rigid) and dysphagic; facial expression muscles weakened; no atrophy or fasciculation of paralyzed muscles; jaw jerk and other facial reflexes exaggerated; palatal reflexes retained; poor emotional control (pa-

P

thologic laughter and crying); periodic breathing (Cheyne-Stokes respiration); lability, poorly controlled or uninhibited emotional responses due to diseases of the cerebrum, particularly the cortico-pontine and corticobulbar pathways.

PSEUDODEMENTIA: reduced cognitive performance associated with functional illness such as Major Depressive Disorder or Factitious Disorder; an extreme condition of general apathy simulating dementia, but with no actual defect of intelligence; symptoms include impaired memory, abstract reasoning, and concentration.

PSEUDODEPRESSION: (Blumer & Benson, 1975) in frontal-lobe patients: outward apathy and indifference, loss of initiative, reduced sexual interest, little overt emotion, and little or no verbal output; more likely following left frontal-lobe lesions (Kolb & Whishaw, 1980).

PSEUDOPSYCHOPATHIC: (Blumer & Benson, 1975) in frontal-lobe patients: immature behavior, lack of tact and restraint, coarse language, promiscuous sexual behavior, increased motor activity, and a general lack of social graces; more likely to follow right frontal-lobe lesions (Kolb & Whishaw, 1980).

PSYCHEDELIC DRUGS: mixed group of drugs that alter sensory perception and cognitive processes; three major groups: 1. acetylcholine psychedelics block or facilitate transmission in acetylcholine synapses; atropine; 2. noradrenaline psychedelics may act by stimulating noradrenaline postsynaptic receptors; mescaline and cannabis; 3. serotonin psychedelics may stimulate or block activity of serotonin neurons or may stimulate noradrenaline receptors; LSD and psilocybin.

PSYCHOMOTOR AGITATION: pacing, wringing of hands, and pulling of clothes associated with a feeling of inner tension; the activity is usually nonproductive and repetitious; may be accompanied by shouting or loud complaining.

PSYCHOMOTOR AREA: see precentral gyrus.

PSYCHOMOTOR EPILEPSY: preceded by complex aura of hallucinations or perceptual illusion (unpleasant smell or taste, déjà vu phenomena, or recurrence of a certain thought); may appear partially conscious or in a trance, may resist restraints and become violent; altered perceptions of time and space; may carry out complicated activities without memory (automatisms); may show an abrupt unexplainable behavioral shift bordering on the bizarre.

PSYCHOMOTOR RETARDATION: a generalized slowing down of physical reactions, movements, speech, and cognitive processing.

PSYCHOACTIVE DRUGS: drugs that affect cognitive functions can be classified in a number of ways, among the most useful of which is by their behavioral effects; actions may include intervention in the process of intercellular communication at any of a number of stages by either increasing or decreasing the effectiveness of transmission at the synaptic junction; see also sedative-hypnotics, stimulants, antipsychotic agents, opiates, psychedelics.

PSYCHOSENSORY APHASIA: receptive a.; Wernicke's a.

PSYCHOSIS: cognitive distortion; emotional distortion, distorted reality contact; the patient incorrectly evaluates the accuracy of perceptions and thoughts and makes incorrect inferences about external reality even in the face of contrary evidence; hallucinations and delusions without insight into their pathological nature; disturbance in synthesis and/or degradation of synaptic neurotransmitters especially acetylcholine, dopamine, noradrenaline, and serotonin; may be due to either organic brain syndromes (known neurological disorders) or to nonphysical conditions.

PSYCHOSIS (NONORGANIC): (DSM III-R) some affective disorders, depressions, and mania; specific diagnositic labels include: Pervasive Developmental Disorders, Schizophrenia, Paranoid Disorders, Psychotic Disorders not elsewhere classified, some Organic Mental Disorders, Major Depressive Disorders, and Bipolar Disorders.

PSYCHOSIS (ORGANIC BRAIN SYNDROMES - OBS): mental disorders associated with pathological brain and physical conditions; organic brain syndromes include psychosis associated with alcoholism (Wernickes's disease), intracranial infection, neoplasms, vascular disturbances, endocrine (hormone) disorders, metabolic or nutritional disorders, and drug or poison intoxications, as well as psychosis resulting from diseases producing senility (senile and presenile dementias).

PSYCHOSIS-TREATMENT: varies with the type of disorder; OBS is treated indirectly by treating the neurological disease producing it; nonphysical psychosis is usually treated with antipsychotic drugs.

PSYCHOSOCIAL RATING SCALE: (Horowitz et al., 1970); a 7-subscale test of the psychosocial ramifications of post temporal lobectomy patients; scored on a 6-point continuum of socially desirable traits and behaviors; also see Goodwin Psychosocial Assessment Battery for prediction of psychosocial functioning of post head-trauma patients.

PSYCHOTIC LANGUAGE: rambling, disjointed, neologistic, loosely connected associations between ideas and subjects such as found in schizophrenia, bipolar disorders, advanced organic dementia, fluent jargon aphasia.

PSYCHOTOMIMETIC DRUGS: cause symptoms imitating psychosis.

PSYCHOTROPIC: having a specific effect on the mind; includes all the "mind-altering" drugs such as amphetamines, LSD, etc., as well as tranquilizers.

PTA: posttraumatic amnesia.

P

PTOSIS: drooping eyelid; damage to some portion of the oculomotor nerve (III) third nerve; paralysis of accommodation; a complete lesion of third nerve causes inability to turn the eye upward, downward, or inward, a divergent strabismus, dilated nonreactive pupil; see also Horner's syndrome.

PUERILITY: childishness.

PULSES CHECK LIST: (Granger et al., 1979); a graduated disability check list covering current behavioral functioning of demented patients; yields a disability score.

PULVINAR: the prominent medial portion of the posterior end of the thalamus, which is cushion-like and partly overhangs the superior colliculus; receives fibers from other thalamic nuclei and gives off widespread cortical projections; thought to coordinate the activity of the cortical speech zones by Penfield and Roberts (1959); lesions produce symptoms such as transient post-operative dysphasia, increased verbal response latency, decreases in voice volume, alterations in speaking rate, and slurring or hesitation in speech as well as impaired performance on test of verbal IQ and memory.

PUNCH-DRUNK SYNDROME: believed to result from cumulative effects of cerebral concussion and subsequent cortical atrophy (also known as boxer's syndrome).

PUPIL ENLARGEMENT: see oculomotor nerve (III).

PUPILLARY ESCAPE PHENOMENA: see Marcus Gunn pupil.

PUPILLARY SIZE AND RESPONSE: pupil size is controlled by a ring of constrictor fibers innervated by the parasympathetic nervous system and a ring of radially arranged dilator fibers controlled by the sympathetic nervous system; the SNS controls pupillary dilation (in anxiety state, for example); the PNS nervous system controls constriction of the pupil; pupil size is small in infancy and again in old age (senile miosis).

PUPILS - BILATERAL DILATION: (in the unconscious patient) the final stage of progressive tentorial herniation is shown by progressive dilation of previously unaffected pupils; a sign of irreversible cerebral damage in cardiac arrest; glutethamide, atropine, and amphetamine poisoning may cause bilateral dilation of the pupils.

PUPILS - PIN-POINT: (in the unconscious patient) massive intrapontine hemorrhage which is usually accompanied by deep coma and a spastic tetraparesis with brisk reflexes; opiate ingestions cause pin-point pupils accompanied by depressed reflexes.

PUPILS - UNEQUAL: (in the unconscious patient) suggests a herniated temporal lobe that is stretching the third nerve on that side; usually prompt surgical action is required.

PURDUE PEGBOARD TEST: (Purdue Research Foundation, 1948); a manual dexterity test which is sensitive to brain damage, particularly right-hemisphere damage (Vaughn & Costa, 1962); a brain lesion is likely if the preferred hand score exceeds the nonpreferred hand by 3 or more points; a nonpreferred hand score greater than 3 or more points over the preferred hand suggests a lesion contralateral to the preferred hand; a preferred hand score that is greater than the nonpreferred hand score by 5 or more points suggests an ipsilateral lesion to the preferred hand; may not discriminate well between organic and functional dysfunctions.

PURE WORD BLINDNESS: loss of ability to read and name colors; can not name or point on dictated command to visual letter or word stimuli; understands spoken language; repetition of what is heard, writing to dictation, and conversation are all intact; unaware of difficulty; caused by a lesion of the dominant hemisphere; may be a right homonymous hemianopia, amnestic defect; hemisensory defect on the right due to involvement of the left occipital-lobe, the left fornix and its decussation, and left thalamus; deep lesion in left parietooccipital region may prevent visual information from both occipital lobes reaching the left angular gyrus; no right homonymous hemianopia; lesion of left visual striate cortex (Brodmann's area 17) and visual association areas (Brodmann's areas 18 & 19); connections of right visual cortex and association areas with temporoparietal region disconnected due to interruption of fibers passing through posterior part (splenium) of corpus callosum, which connect the visual association areas of the hemispheres.

PURE WORD DEAFNESS: loss of ability to comprehend spoken language with no physical hearing defect; able to hear and to identify nonverbal sounds; speech remains normal; subcortical lesion sparing Wernicke's area deep in the left temporal-lobe area which disconnects the auditory input from the auditory cortex; may be caused by embolic lesions, bilateral in superior temporal gyrus with damage to the primary auditory cortex in the transverse gyrus of Heschl, or association areas of the superior, posterior part of the temporal lobe; auditory form of Wernicke's aphasia; impaired auditory comprehension and inability to repeat what is said or to write to dictation; no impairment of comprehension of visually presented material.

PURKINJE CELL: see cerebellum and the extrapyramidal system.

PURPOSIVE BEHAVIOR: the translation of an intention or plan into productive, self-serving activity requires the patient to initiate, maintain, switch, and stop sequences of complex behavior in an orderly and integrated manner; disturbances in the programming of activity can thwart the carrying out of reasonable plans regardless of motivation, knowledge, or capacity to perform the activity; patients who have trouble programming activity may display a marked dissociation between their verbalized intentions and plans and their actions; programming difficulties may affect large-scale purposive

P

activities or the regulation and fine-tuning of discrete intentional acts or complex movements; patient who have trouble performing discrete actions also tend to have difficulty carrying out broader purposive activities; inability to perform purposive behavior is most often a frontal-lobe dysfunction.

PURPOSIVE BEHAVIOR TEST: (Lezak, 1982b, 1983) Tinkertoy Test.

PURPOSIVE MOVEMENTS: also called voluntary, instrumental, operant, or appetitive movements.

PURSUIT TEST: (MacQuarrie, 1927, 1953) a subtest of the MacQuarrie Test for Mechanical Ability; a test of visual scanning; sensitive to right-hemisphere lesions.

PUTAMEN: part of the basal ganglia; see chorea or choreoathetosis, Sydenham's chorea, Huntington's chorea, senile chorea, tardive dyskinesia.

PUTATIVE NEUROTRANSMITTERS: the word putative means "supposed;" since no proof that some chemicals in the body labelled neurotransmitters actually are neurotransmitters other than acetylcholine, the scientific supposition is made for adrenaline, dopamine, noradrenaline, serotonin, enkephlins, some amino acids, histamine, prostaglandins, ergothioneine, substance P, and GABA.

PYRAMIDAL SYSTEM: the pyramidal system differs from the extrapyramidal system mainly in the degree of synapsing and in the number of sources from which it draws information; mainly under the control of areas of the cortex; neurons within the tracts of the pyramidal system have their cell bodies along the precentral gyrus, as well as in the prefrontal, parietal, and temporal areas of the cortex; some cell bodies are very large and give rise to very long neurons that stretch for up to two feet without synapsing (Betz cells); most of the fibers in this system cross in the medulla to innervate muscles opposite the side of the brain in which they originated; the pyramidal system derives its name from the area in the medulla where it crosses; tracts pass through an area of the medulla that contains large, pyramid-shaped neural bundles although 20% remain on the same side of the body as the hemisphere from which they originate; crossed neurons descend in the spinal cord in the lateral corticospinal tract; uncrossed neurons descend in the spinal cord in the ventral corticospinal tract; both tracts synapse either directly with alpha motor neurons or with interneurons that synapse with alpha neurons.

PYREXIAL: characterized by fever or a febrile condition; abnormal elevation of the body temperature.

Q

q.: every.
q.AM: every morning.
q.d.: every day.
q.2d.: every 2 days.
q.h.: every hour.
q.2h.: every 2 hours.
q.i.d.: four times a day.
q.I. or q.p.: as much as desired.
q.q.h.: every four hours.
q.I. or q.p.: as much as desired.
q.q.h.: every four hours.
Qq-hor.: every hour.
QUADRANT/QUADRANTIC HEMIANOPIA: hemianopia in one fourth of the visual field in each eye; caused by destruction of a portion of the visual field as a result of a partial lesion of the optic tract, lateral geniculate body, Brodmann's area 17, or lesion of the opposite anterior temporal lobe.
QUADRANTOPSIA/ QUADRANTOPIA: same as quadrantic hemianopia.
QUADRIPLEGIA: paralysis of upper and lower extremities; lesions usually involve the cervical spinal cord.
QUALITATIVE DATA: data from direct observations of patient's behavior or summary statements about the observed behavior (Cronbach, 1970).
QUALITY EXTINCTION TEST: (Schwartz et al., 1977); sensitive to complex discriminations.
QUASI-EMOTIONAL PHENOMENA: rage in the diencephalic animal.

R

R: respiration.
RA: rheumatoid arthritis.
RADICULAR: of or pertaining to a radical, root, or source.
RADIOISOTOPE SCANNING: an intravenous injection of a radioisotope is given and the cranial surface is scanned with a Geiger counter; any alteration in blood supply can be detected, including alterations associated with the growth of a tumor.

R

RAMP MOVEMENTS: slow movements.

RAGE/FEAR REACTIONS: see central gray, tegmentum, amygdala, hypothalamus, periaqueductal gray.

RAMUS/RAMI: general term for a smaller structure given off by a larger one, or into which the larger structure, such as a blood vessel or nerve, divides.

RANDOM LETTER TEST: see recurring letter test.

RAPHÉ: a general term for the line of union of the halves of various symmetrical parts.

RAPHÉ NUCLEUS: part of the reticular formation in the tegmentum; an area in the pons involved in the control of slow-wave sleep; contains high levels of serotonin; mediates defensive-aggressive behavior.

RAPPAPORT DISABILITY RATING SCALE: (Rappaport, et al., 1982) designed to repeatedly evaluate the behavior of severely head-injured patients by ward staff; adapted from the Glasgow Coma Scale (Teasdale & Jennett, 1974), cognitive awareness with respect to toileting, feeding, and grooming (Rappaport et al., 1982), level of functioning in terms of degree of dependence on others (modified from Scranton, Fogel, & Erdman, 1970), and level of employability; yields a disability score.

RAS: reticular activating system.

RATIONAL: arrived at by the process of thinking as opposed to emotion.

RATIONALIZATION: a common mental mechanism wherein one finds plausible "reasons" for doing what one unconsciously wished to do all along.

RAVEN'S COLORED PROGRESSIVE MATRICES: (Raven, 1965) sensitive to right-sided posterior lesions (Costa, 1976; Costa et al., 1969, 1976; Smith, 1972); tests visuoperceptual skills; sensitive to receptive or mixed aphasia and construction disorders (Costa et al., 1969).

RAVEN'S PROGRESSIVE MATRICES: (Raven, 1960) designed to be a culture fair test of general ability; norms available; tests conceptual thinking (reasoning in the visuospatial modality) (Archibald et al., 1967; Colonna & Faglioni, 1966); may be correlated with drawing and constructional tasks; sensitive to unilateral visual neglect (unilateral visuospatial inattention) (Campbell & Oxbury, 1976; Colombo et al., 1976; Costa et al., 1969; De Renzi & Faglioni, 1965).

RBBB: right bundle branch block.

RBC: red blood count; red cell count.

rCBF: regional cerebral blood flow; often seen as simply CBF.

REACTIVE DEPRESSION: an emotional depression produced by an incident or experience that might naturally tend to produce sadness.

READING: (Geschwind model, 1972) comprehension; the percept of a printed or written word is received in the primary visual area

(Brodmann's area 17), transmitted through the visual association areas (Brodmann's areas 18 & 19) to the angular gyrus (Brodmann's area 39) where a visual pattern is elicited, transmitted to Wernicke's area (Brodmann's 22) where the auditory form is elicited completing the comprehension of a written word.

READING COMPREHENSION subtest: (Gates-MacGinitie Reading Test) may be used to test reasoning.

READING DYSFUNCTION: see alexia, dyslexia; angular gyrus.

READING FLUENCY TESTS: Stroop Color/Word Test; Gates-MacGinitie Reading Tests; Diagnositic Screening Procedure for the diagnosis of developmental dyslexia; Minkus completion; New Adult Reading Test; Reading/Everyday Activities in Life.

READING TESTING: bedside: determine educational background prior to testing; test both reading comprehension and reading aloud: both are usually defective, but can occur in isolation; begin with short single words, then phrases, sentences and paragraphs: single word test: refer to objects, phrases and sentences that would require a yes/no answer; have the patient read items aloud and then the examiner points to objects or asks questions about the reading material expecting a yes/no answer; note syllable or word substitutions, omitted words, defects in comprehension (Strub & Black, 1977).

READING/EVERYDAY ACTIVITIES IN LIFE TEST: (Lichtman, 1972) Test of practical reading ability.

REASONING: tertiary zones of left parietal-lobe; Brodmann's area 39.

REASONING TESTS: WAIS-R subtests: Comprehension, Arithmetic, Picture Completion, and Picture Arrangement; Reading Comprehension subtest of the Gates-MacGinitie Reading Test; Bicycle drawing test; Stanford-Binet subtests: Problem Situations I and II at ages VIII and XI, Problems of Fact at age XIII, Verbal Absurdities, Picture Absurdities, Codes (AA & SA II); Paper Cutting (IX, XIII, & AA levels); Poisoned Food Problems; McGill Picture Anomalies Test; Raven's Progressive Matrices.

REASONING TESTS (I & II): (Stanford-Binet subtest) a serial reasoning task.

RECALL: process of remembering by association; retracing of categorized coding.

RECENCY DISCRIMINATION TASK: (Milner, 1971) a recognition of recency task based upon the idea that memories carry "time tags" (Yntema & Trask, 1963); sensitive to left frontotemporal and left temporal lesions; frontal-lobe patients have difficulty with the recency aspect and temporal-lobe patients have difficulty with recognition.

RECENCY EFFECT: short-term retention in patients whose learning ability is defective shows up in a better recall of the words at the end

R

of the list than of those at the beginning, as the presentation of new words in excess of the patient's immediate memory span interferes with retention of the words first heard.

RECENCY/ORDER MEMORY DEFECT: see dorsolateral frontal-lobe lesion.

RECENT MEMORY: a clinical term which refers to memories stored within the last few hours, days, weeks, or months.

RECEPTIVE APHASIA: see Wernicke's aphasia.

RECIPROCAL INHIBITION-SPINAL REFLEX: opposing muscle relaxes in response to the stretch (stretch reflex); allows a joint to move.

RECOGNITION: remembering when a like stimulus triggers awareness.

RECOGNITION - LACK OF: agnosia.

RECOGNITION OF INCOMPLETE STIMULI TESTS: Street Completion Test; Mooney's Closure Test (Closure Faces Test); Gollin figures test.

RECOGNITION OF PICTURED OBJECTS TEST: (Warrington & Taylor, 1973) identification of familiar objects under distorting conditions; sensitive to right posterior lesions.

RECOGNITION OF THE FACIAL EXPRESSION OF EMOTION TEST: (De Kosky et al., 1980; Prigatano & Pribram, 1982) sensitive to right-hemisphere lesions.

RECOVERY FROM BRAIN DAMAGE SEQUENCE: 1. shock or diaschisis; 2. recovery; 3. chronic impairment that reflects the locus and extent of the tissue destroyed.

RECOVERY FROM MOTOR-CORTEX DAMAGE: (Twitchell, 1951) result of CVA: 1. onset of hemiplegia marked by complete flaccidity of the muscles and loss of all reflexes and voluntary movements; 2. return of tendon and stretch reflexes; 3. development of rigidity; 4. grasping facilitated by, or occurring as a part of proprioception (part of postural reflexes of turning, righting, etc.); 5. development of voluntary grasping (involving recovery of movement in the sequence of shoulder, elbow, wrist, and hand, first in the flexor musculature, than in the extensor musculature); 6. facilitation of grasping by tactual stimulation of the hand, and finally; 7. grasping occurring predominantly under voluntary control.

RECEPTIVE FUNCTIONS: sensation; perception (visual, auditory, or tactile).

RECURRING FIGURES TEST: (Kimura, 1963) sensitive to right-hemisphere lesions.

RED NUCLEUS: part of the reticular formation in the tegmentum; exptrapyramidal motor system; the red nucleus of one hemisphere controls distal musculature of the contralateral part of the body; participates importantly with other brain structures.

R

REDUPLICATION PARAMNESIA: distortion of memory involving geographic locations.

REDUPLICATION - OF BODY PARTS: (in hemiplegia) denial by unilaterally paralysed patient that the limb belongs to patient; rehabilitation prognosis is poor because the patient is unaware of his weakness and falls repeatedly.

REFLEX: an automatic response to a stimulus, such as the knee jerk; unlearned and usually unmodifiable.

REFLEX EPILEPSY: convulsion excited by some form of external stimulation such as a touch on skin, sudden loud noise, flickering light; *types*: acousticomotor epilepsy (loud noise); musicogenic (music); photic (visual stimulus such as flickering light); may be self-induced (Brain, 1985); may be focal or generalized.

REFLEXIVE BEHAVIORS: also called automatic, consumatory, or respondent behaviors.

REFRACTORY PERIOD: the period of time after a neuron fires during which it recovers its resting potential.

REGIONAL BLOOD FLOW: blood flow is assumed to increase in the neocortex in areas where neurons increase their activity, presumably because neurons in the area have a more active metabolism; to examine blood flow: xenon is injected into an artery while special detectors on the skull monotor its concentration.

REGISTRATION: selection and recording process by which perceptions enter the memory system.

REHAB.: rehabilitation.

REHEARSAL: repetitive process that serves to lengthen the duration of a memory trace; a form of attention.

RELATIVE HEMIANOPIA: hemianopia to form or color in half of the visual field, the perception of light being retained.

RELATIVES' ASSESSMENT OF PATIENT'S FUNCTIONING: (Heaton et al., 1981) Relatives Assessment of Patient Functioning Inventory; an 8-category test that documents the relatives assessments of disability level of a patient which can be compared with the patient's evaluations thereby illuminating the patient's misperceptions regarding his disability used in conjunction with Patient's Assessment of Own Functioning Inventory (listed under Function Levels — Self Rating).

RELIABILITY (STATISTICAL): the degree to which a test score, item score, etc., evaluates accurately over repeated testing.

RELIGIOSITY: an overly religious orientation, often personalized or misinterpreted; frequently seen in schizophrenia, bipolar disorders, or temporal-lobe epilepsy.

REM: rapid eye movement during paradoxical sleep; coincides with dreaming.

REM SLEEP: the stage of sleep in which dreaming is associated with

R

mild involuntary muscle jerks and rapid eye movements; usually occurs three to four times each night at intervals of 80 to 120 minutes, each occurrence lasting from 5 minutes to more than an hour; in adults, about 20% is REM sleep.

REM-REBOUND: when deprived of REM sleep for a long time, the subject will compensate by having about 60% more REM sleep than normal when permitted to sleep undisturbed; usually occurs on the second night following sleep deprivation.

REMEMBERING: information retrieval from memory storage.

REMINDING: the differentiation of retention, storage, and retrieval can be facilitated by selective reminding and restricted reminding; *selective reminding*: the subject recalls as many words as he can in any order from a list just read; the examiner repeats all the words the patient omitted in that trial; the reminding and recall trials continue until the patient recites the whole list; this technique facilitates learning by focusing attention on unlearned items only; *restricted reminding*: following the first reading of the word list, the examiner repeats those words the subject did not recall and tells him to recall as many words as he can; all subsequent reminding is limited to words not recalled on any trial; recall trials and reminding continue until each word has been recalled at least once; the first recall tests immediate retention span; spontaneous recall is demonstrated by recall of word previously named; retrieval problems become evident when a once-named word is recalled only sporadically thereafter.

REMOTE MEMORY: older memories dating from early childhood.

RENSHAW CELLS: interneurons that protect muscles from overcontraction by inhibiting firing in the alpha motor neurons.

REPETITION: a test in which the patient is asked to repeat something after the examiner gives a word, name, or paragraph; the examiner listens for paraphasias, grammatical errors, omissions and additions, as well as failures to approximate; a complex process which can be affected by impaired auditory processing, disturbed speech production, or disconnection between the receptive and expressive language centers.

REPETITION DISORDERS: Many aphasics can repeat aurally presented material, others cannot, even though other language functions may appear intact. Disorders of repetition may result either from deficits in comprehension or articulation (associated with aphasic symptoms) or from a selective dissociation between auditory-input and speech-output systems. In selective dissociation, the disorder of repetition may be the only significant language disturbances, and may go unnoticed except through special testing; repetition is poor in conduction aphasia as a result of an arcuate fasciculus lesion.

REPRESSION: a mental mechanism by which ideas that would be painful to the consciousness are forced into the unconscious.

RESERPINE: reduces dopamine levels by destroying storage granules within the synapse.

RESIDUAL: the phase of an illness that occurs after remission of the florid symptoms or the full syndrome.

RESPIRATORY ARREST: if more than six minutes, the patient who recovers usually shows evidence of anoxic encephalopathy (Gilroy & Meyer, 1979).

RESPONDENT BEHAVIORS: also called automatic, reflexive, consumatory behaviors.

RESPONSE INHIBITION IMPAIRMENT: Brodmann's areas 9 and 10 (Milner, 1964; Perret, 1974).

RESTING POTENTIAL: the state of a neuron when it is available to transmit a neural impulse (as opposed to the refractory period).

RESTLESS LEGS SYNDROME: (Ekbom's syndrome) leg movements called dyslisi; may be due to iron deficiency or ischemia causing hyperexcitability of spinal cord motor neurons (Brain, 1985).

RESTLESSNESS: see akathesia.

RESTRICTED REMINDING: see under reminding.

RETICULAR ACTIVATING SYSTEM: consists of a complex network of nuclei and fiber tracts that stretch from the diencephalon through the hindbrain. These nuclei and fiber tracts have two distinguishing features: 1. no clearly defined sensory or motor functions; 2. each sends fibers to a number of areas of the forebrain, brainstem, and spinal cord; surrounds central gray; part of tegmentum in midbrain; contains the red nucleus, Raphè nucleus and ascending reticular activating system (ARAS); mottled grey and white, or netlike, appearance; runs through the medulla oblongata from the upper spinal cord to the diencephalon; connected to the lateral edge of the posterior gray horn of the cord; control sleeping and waking; mediate important and complex postural reflexes; contribute to the smoothness of muscle activity and maintain muscle tone; the RAS does not relay specific signals to the cortex; it puts the cortex into a state of diffuse arousal whereby specific cortical areas are prepared to react to specific sensory signals; the descending influence on the spinal cord is primarily one of regulating tension in the muscles; lesions give rise to global disorders of consciousness such as drowsiness, somnolence, stupor, and coma; also known as the reticular formation.

RETICULAR FORMATION: see reticular activating system.

RETRIEVAL PROBLEMS: words are remembered only sporadically from repeated memory test lists.

RETROACTIVE INHIBITION: see retrograde interference.

RETROGRADE AMNESIA: defect in the recall and reproduction of memories formed some days, weeks, or months before the onset of

R

the amnesia; usually lasts for a matter of seconds in minor injuries; may be prolonged when there is selective bitemporal brain-damage.

RETROGRADE INTERFERENCE: the disruptive effect on recall of prevously acquired information produced by newly acquired information.

REUPTAKE: see neurotransmitter inactivation or reuptake.

REVERBERATING NEURAL CIRCUITS: self-contained neural networks that sustain a nerve impulse by channeling it repeatedly through the same network (Rosenzweig & Leiman, 1968).

REVERSING SERIAL ORDER: digits or words backwards requires ability to simultaneously track the forward order while reciting the backwards order; sensitive to brain-damage or acute episodes of functional disorders (schizophrenia and affective disorders).

REVISED WECHSLER MEMORY SCALE: (Russell, 1975) memory test made up of the Logical Memory and Visual Reproduction subtests from the original WMS with delayed recall factors; this test and scoring method is reported to be a more reliable measure than the original WMS.

REY AUDITORY-VERBAL LEARNING TEST: see auditory-verbal learning test; immediate memory span for digits and the number of words recalled on trial I will be within one or two points of each other; larger differences usually favor the digit span and seem to occur in patients with intact immediate memory and concentration who become confused by too much stimulation suggesting difficulty with complex material or situations, doing better with simplified, highly structured tasks; when the difference favors the more difficult word list retention task, the lower digit span score is usually due to inattention, lack of motivation, or anxiety at the time digit span was given; when proactive inhibition is very pronounce, intrusion words from list A may show up in the list B recall; most brain-damaged patients show a learning curve over the five trials; if there is any learning curve (3-4 words on trial I to 8-9 on trial V), then there is some ability to learn providing some of the gain is maintained on the delayed recall trial (VI); such a patient may benefit from psychotherapy or personal counseling and may profit from rehabilitation training and perhaps formal schooling since he can learn, although at a slower rate than normal.

REY COMPLEX FIGURE TEST: test of the nonverbal memory function of the right temporal lobe; see Complex Figure Test.

REY-OSTERRIETH COMPLEX FIGURE TEST: see Complex Figure Test.

Rh.: Rhesus factor (blood group)

RHINENCEPHALON: limbic system or lobe; literally the "smell brain;" also called the nose brain; the oldest part of the cerebral hemispheres.

R

RHOMBENCEPHALON: primitive division; hindbrain; 2 parts: metencephalon and myelencephalon; includes cerebellum, pons, medulla oblongata, and 4th ventricle.

RICHARDSON-STEELE-OLSZEWSKI SYNDROME: see progressive supranuclear palsy.

RIBONUCLEIC ACID: (RNA) a nucleic acid originally isolated from yeast, but later found in all living cells.

RICKETTSIAL DISEASES: a group of microorganisms, parasitic in arthropods, that almost always invade the human nervous system and cause particular damage to the endothelium of small blood vessels, which become swollen and thrombosed; residual degenerative changes of nerve cells and glial scars are common; include epidemic typhus (louse vector), scrub typhus (mite vector), murine typhus (rat flea vector), and Rocky Mountain spotted fever (tick vector), cat-scratch disease; see Reitan & Wolfson (1985) for further discussion.

RIGHT HEMIPARESIS: weakness or paralysis which usually accompanies Broca's aphasia.

RIGHT HEMISENSORY SYNDROME: usually accompanies Broca's aphasia.

RIGHT HEMISPHERE: controls left motor and sensory functions; controls spatial functions (ability to draw, copy, remember forms, or construct objects), direction finding, musical perception, nonverbal visual-spatial transformations including processing and storage of visual information, tactile and visual recognition of shapes and forms, perception of directional orientation and perspective, copying and drawing geometric representations of designs and pictures, native musical ability; stores information as visual, spatial and auditory configurations (Kimura, 1973); reconstructs perceptual wholes from fragmented or incomplete sensory data (closure function); organizes data on the basis of structural similarities; gives rise to intuition (non-verbal perceptiveness), inspirational hunches, and uncritical imagination (Levy-Agresti & Sperry, 1968); synthesizes activity such as depth perception, perspective, and perceptual constancy operations; stores simple configural concepts in order to identify and remember faces, musical passages, and cognitive maps.

RIGHT HEMISPHERE LESIONS: cause groups of movement deficits (constructional apraxias); for example, reduced efficiency or inability to assembling pieces of jigsaw puzzle together to form a picture, to draw a clock face, map, etc., to copy a design with sticks of various lengths, to build bridges, towers, etc. with blocks, to copy designs with different colored blocks; all constructions that require objects be ordered in extrapersonal space may be affected; lesions have a stronger effect upon attention than do left-hemisphere lesions (Strub & Black, 1977).

R

RIGHT PARIETAL-LOBE SENSITIVE TESTS: Mooney Faces Test; Rey-Osterrieth Complex Figures; Block Design (WAIS-R), WAIS-R Object Assembly, Facial Recognition Test (Benton & Van Allen, 1968; Benton & Hamsher, 1983), Bender-Gestalt, Background Interference Procedure with the Bender-Gestalt Test (BIP)(Canter, 1966,1968), Cube Construction Test; Visual Retention Test (Metric Figures) (Warrington & James, 1967a).

RIGHT-LEFT CONFUSION: lesion(s) in Brodmann's areas 7 and 40, left (Semmes 1960; Benton, 1959); see also Gerstmann's syndrome.

RIGHT-LEFT DIFFERENTIATION: sensitive to left parietal-lobe damage usually; sometimes this deficit may be due to left frontal-lobe damage.

RIGHT-LEFT ORIENTATION TESTS: Show Me Test, Standardized Road-Map Test of Direction Sense.

RIGID DYSARTHRIA: see paretic dysarthria.

RIGIDITY: muscles continuously or intermittently firm, tense, and prominent; resistance to passive movement is intense and even, like that noted in bending a lead pipe or in stretching a strand of toffee.

RINDS: reversible ischemic neurological deficits.

RLE: right lower extremity.

RLQ: right lower quadrant.

RNA: ribonucleic acid.

R/O; RO: rule out.

ROAD-MAP TEST: see Standardized Road-Map Test of Direction sense.

ROENTGENOGRAPHY: x-ray.

ROLAND, FISSURE OF: see central sulcus.

ROLANDIC AREA: precentral gyrus.

ROLANDIC INFARCTION: poor articulation, lowered volume, and pitch of speech, and a nasal quality to the voice; paresthesia of speech musculature.

ROM: range of motion.

ROMBERG'S SIGN: increased swaying or falling when patient stands with feet together and eyes closed; clinical test for damage to labyrinthine receptors.

RORSCHACH (scoring): (sign system for brain-damage - Piotrowski, 1937); 5+ "signs" suggest cortical brain disease; does not differentiate chronic schizophrenics from organic patients (Goldfried et al., 1971; Suinn, 1969); Piotrowski's (1937) 10 signs of organicity: 1. R less than 15 responses; 2. T average time per response is greater than 1 minute; 3. M 0 to 1 movement response; 4. Cn color naming; 5. F% 70% or less good form responses; 6. P% 25% or less popular responses; 7. Rpt (Repetition) perseveration over several inkblots; 8. Imp (Impotency) patient recognizes inappropriate response, but does not change it; 9. Plx (Perplexity) hesitancy and doubt about perceptions;

10. AP (automatic phrase) repetative expression, indiscriminately used. Plx, Imp, Rpt, and AP are particularly sensitive to mild and moderate brain dysfunction(Baker,1956); right-hemisphere lesioned patients tend to be uncritically free in the use of determinants and overexpansive; left-hemisphere lesioned patients may display perplexity, may reject cards, and may give unelaborated form-dependent responses (Hall & Hall, 1968); head-trauma patients tend to give few responses that may be repetitive and concrete (Dailey, 1956; Klebanoff et al., 1954; Vigouroux et al., 1971); brain-damaged patients may show difficulties in synthesizing discrete elements into a coherent whole, breaking down a perceptual whole into its component parts, clarifying figure ground relationships, and identifying relevant and irrelevant details; only brain-damaged patients attempt to clarify visual confusion by covering parts of the blot with the hand (Lezak,, 1983); may not be able to process and integrate multiple stimuli resulting in a narrowed perceptual field and simplified percepts; below average color and shading responses; perplexity and slowed reaction times; malingerers may give sparse, constricted responses with slow reaction time contrasted with more appropriate performances on intelligence tests; fewer responses with frontal-lobe damage; see Lezak (1983) for a more complete discussion of Rorschach interpretation for brain-damage, aging, and psychoses; see Exner (1986) for general interpretations.

ROSTRAL: toward the head; up; above.

ROUTE FINDING TEST: Extrapersonal Orientation Test (Weinstein et al., 1956); test of ability to find way around familiar places or to learn new routes; sensitive to brain-damage; parietal-lobe patients have the most impairment (Semmes et al., 1963; Teuber, 1964); patient may also be aphasic (Weinstein, 1964); Parkinsonian patients may score lower than normals (Bowen, 1976); particularly sensitive to left-sided lesions.

Rt.: right.

RUB: a scraping or grating noise heard with the heart beat, usually a to-and-fro sound, associated with an inflamed pericardium (heart).

RUBIN VASE ILLUSION: test of perceptual fluctuation/ reversals; most often scored by the "rate of apparent change" (Cohen, 1959); brain-injured patients show fewer reversals; right-hemisphere lesioned patients show fewer reversals than left; frontal-lobe lesioned patients (bilateral lesions) may see more reversals, but reversal rate slowest (Teuber, 1964; Yacorzynski, 1965); no right-left lesion differential with frontal-lobe lesions.

RUBROSPINAL MOTOR TRACT: (lateral system) connects with interneurons in the dorsolateral portion of the intermediate zone of the spinal cord.

RUBROSPINAL SYSTEM LESION: severe disruption of the independ-

S

ent use of the limbs in reaching and grasping, but spares their ability to participate in whole body movements.

RUE: right upper extremity.

RUFFINI ENDINGS: endings of sensory neurons in skin areas that are receptive to warmth.

RULE-BREAKING BEHAVIOR: an inability to follow instructions or commands; common with frontal-lobe lesioned patients; a dysfunction of the executive functions.

RUQ: right upper quadrant.

Rx: symbol for prescription or treatment.

S

s̄: without.

7/24 TEST: (Barbizet & Cany, 1968) nonverbal memory test of visuospatial recall without requiring either good eyesight or good motor control.

S: Sacral.

SACCULE: vestibular sac that signals when the head is oriented in the normal position; communicates with the cochlear duct.

SAGGITAL: midline plane.

SAME SIDE: ipsilateral.

SANDOZ CLINICAL ASSESSMENT — GERIATRIC: (Shader et al., 1974); a 19 - item assessment of dementia or depression; needs to be administered by a "skilled clinician" because some of the items require professional judgment as to level of impairment.

SANGER-BROWN ATAXIA: spinocerebellar ataxia; hereditary; degeneration of the spinocerebellar tracts.

SATIETY: a state or condition of sufficiency or satisfaction, as full gratification of appetite or thirst, with abolition of the desire to ingest food or liquids; see also hypothalamus functions.

SAVINGS: (to evaluate forgetting) (Ingham, 1952) the "savings" method provides an indirect means of measuring the amount of material retained after it has been learned; patient is taught the same material on two or more occasions, which are usually separated by hours, days or weeks; the number of trials the patient takes to reach criterion is counted each time; reductions in the number of trials needed for criterion learning at a later session is interpreted as indicating retention from the previous set of learning trials (see Brooks, 1972 and Snow, 1979 for "forgetting" formulae).

SCALA: a stairlike structure; applied especially to various passages of cochlea.

SCALA MEDIA: cochlear duct; a spirally arranged membranous tube in the bony canal of the cochlea along its outer wall, lying between the scala tympani below and the scala vestibuli above; also called cochlear canal.

SCALA TYMPANI: the perilymph-filled part of the cochlea that is continuous with the scala vestibuli; separated from other cochlear structures by the spiral lamina and the cochlear duct.

SCALA VESTIBULI: the perilymph-filled part of the cochlea that begins in the vestibule; separated from other cochlear structures by the spiral lamina and the cochlear duct.

SCANNING DEFECTS: see visual scanning defects.

SCATTER: variability in the pattern of successes and failures in a test performance.

SCENE RECALL TEST: (Bisiach & Luzzatti, 1978); spatial inattention/ unilateral visuospatial inattention test.

SCHIZOPHRENIA BRAIN IMPAIRMENT THEORIES: frontal- and temporal-lobe functioning poor and normal on parietal-lobe functions (Kolb & Whishaw, 1980); more impaired performance on tests of left-hemisphere function (Flor-Henry, 1975); poor performance on perceptual and cognitive tests which demand complex information processing, maintenance of attention, and exercise of rapid psychomotor speed (Heaton & Crowley, 1981); the Halstead-Reitan test battery does not discriminate between schizophrenia and brain-damage (Watson et al., 1968); Purisch, Golden, & Hemmeke (1978) found that schizophrenics performed significantly better than brain-injured patients on all the subscales of the Luria-Nebraska Test except Rhythm, Impressive (Receptive) Speech, Memory, and Intellectual Processes; however, the schizophrenic's performance was not distinguishable from normals; rCBF and PET scale studies show an "at rest" hyper posterior blood flow and glucose uptake posterior to the Sylvian and Rolandic fissures rather than the opposite normal blood flow and glucose uptake (Buchsbaum & Ingvar, 1982); for more extensive discussion of current theories and findings refer to Grant & Adams (1986).

SCHWANN CELLS: large nucleated masses of protoplasm lining the inner surface of the neurilemma; insulate and speed transmission of peripheral nervous system impulses.

SCISSORS GAIT: see paraplegic gait.

SCOTOMAS: small areas of blindness caused by lesions of parts of the visual projection fibers or primary projection areas; an area of depressed vision within the visual field, surrounded by an area of less depressed or of normal vision; may go unnoticed because of nystagmus and spontaneous filling in.

SDAT: senile dementia of the Alzheimer's type.

SDMT: Symbol Digit Modalities Test.

S

SEASHORE RHYTHM TEST: subtest of the Halstead-Reitan battery; subtest of the Seashore Test of Musical Talent (Seashore et al., 1960); patients with right temporal brain-damage tend to do poorly; rhythm pattern recognition may be depressed by diffuse cerebral dysfunction (Beniak, 1977).

SECONDARY CORTICAL ZONES: *frontal*: premotor area; Brodmann's area 6: motor programs are prepared in the secondary zone for execution by the primary zone; *sensory*: projection areas of the primary zones; secondary zones maintain the modality of functional sensation, but have a less fixed topographic organization.

SECONDARY GAIN: financial or emotional benefits derived from malingering or symptom exacerbation.

SECONDARY VISUAL AREA LESION: perceptual deficit in vision causing inability to recognize the object; Brodmann's areas 18 and 19.

SEDATIVE-HYPNOTIC DRUGS: reduce anxiety at low doses; medium doses produce sedation; high doses produce anesthesia or coma; include barbiturates, benzodiazepines, and alcohol; may depress the noradrenaline synapses at low doses and may block neurotransmission in many systems and produce anesthesia or coma in high doses.

SEESAW NYSTAGMUS: one eye moving up, the other down; usually due to bitemporal hemianopia.

SEIZURES: uncontrolled electrochemical activity in the brain usually producing uncontrollable movement effects and changes of consciousness; recurrent seizures: epilepsy; see also major motor s., petit mal s., Jacksonian s., psychomotor s., temporal-lobe epilepsy, aura, automatism.

SEIZURE NEURONAL PATH: excitatory activity goes from the foci to adjacent cortical areas, to thalamic nuclei, and to brainstem nuclei; excitatory activity feed-back from thalamus to original focus and forebrain; propagation to spinal neurons via corticospinal and reticulospinal path, diencephalocortical inhibition begins and intermittently interrupts seizure discharge which causes the change from tonic to clonic phases.

SEIZURE-SOMATOSENSORY: numbness, tingling, feeling, crawling (formication), buzzing, electricity, or vibration; onset in the lips, fingers, and toes; spreads to adjacent parts; follows pattern of sensory arrangements in postcentral convolution; either focal or marching on one side: lesion in parietal lobe, or near striate cortex of occipital lobe causing lights, darkness, color-stars, or moving lights.

SELECTIVE REMINDING: see reminding.

SELF-CORRECTION TESTS: see self-regulatory tests.

SELF-REGULATION AND CAPACITY TO SHIFT: The ability to

regulate one's own behavior can be demonstrated on tests of flexibility that require the subject to shift a course of thought or action according to the demands of the situation. The capacity for flexibility in behavior extends through perceptual, cognitive, and response dimensions. Defects in mental flexibility show up perceptually in defective scanning and inability to change perceptual set easily. Conceptual inflexibility appears in concrete or rigid approaches to understanding and problem solving, and also as stimulus-bound behaviors. It may appear as inability to shift perceptual organization, train of thought, or ongoing behavior to meet the varying needs of the moment. Inflexibility of response results in perseverative, stereotyped, nonadaptive behavior, and difficulties in regulating and modulating motor acts. In each of these problems there is an inability to shift behavior readily, to conform behavior to rapidly changing demands on the person. This disturbance in the programming of behavior appears in many different contexts and forms and is associated with lesions of the frontal lobes (Luria, 1966; Luria & Homskaya, 1964). Its particular manifestation depends, at least in part, on the site of lesion.

SELF-REGULATORY TESTS: (flexibility and the capacity to shift): Bender-Gestalt Test; Luria-type tests; Line Tracing Task; Tracing, Tapping, and Dotting (subtests of MacQuarrie Test for Mechanical Ability); Stroop Color/Word Test; Motor Impersistence Tests; Benton Visual Retention test; writing to command; copying letters, numbers, or words; difficulty in reversing motor sets; Uses of Objects Test; Design Fluency Test; Tests for perseveration and perseverance.

SEMANTIC APHASIA: see Wernicke's aphasia.

SEMICIRCULAR CANALS: three long canals of the bony labyrinth of the ear (lateral, anterior, and posterior), forming loops and opening into the vestibule by five openings.

SEMI-COMA: see stupor.

SEMMES BODY-PLACING TEST: simple, easily administered test of personal spatial orientation; left frontal-lobe patients do more poorly on this test than other patient groups, although left parietal-lobe patients often are impaired; should be administered in conjunction with a left-right differentiation test which may help to differentiate between left-frontal and left-parietal lesioned patients; the parietal-lobe lesioned patients are likely to perform left-right discrimination tasks at chance level whereas the frontal-lobe patients will score above chance levels.

SEMMES LOCOMOTOR MAP: test of spatial relations.

SENILE CHOREA: benign, usually mild, disorder of the elderly, marked by choreoform movements unassociated with mental disturbance; lesion(s) in the putamen, or striatum caudate nucleus.

S

SENILE GAIT: slightly flexed posture, marche à petits pas; speed, balance, and all graceful, adaptive movements lost; probably caused by a combination of frontal-lobe and basal-ganglionic defects.

SENILE PUPILLARY RESPONSE: see pupillary size and response.

SENSATION: the result of activity of receptors and their associated afferent pathways to the corresponding primary sensory neocortical areas; in the neocortex sensory information is transformed into a percept by such factors as experience and context; the percept may differ in a number of ways from the sensory information sent to the neocortex.

SENSATION, DEEP: proprioceptive sensation.

SENSATION, SUPERFICIAL: cutaneous, exteroceptive.

SENSE OF DIRECTION TEST: (Gooddy & Reinhold, 1963) a test of spatial orientation; sensitive to right posterior lesions, primarily.

SENSORINEURAL DEAFNESS: nerve deafness due to disease of the cochlea or of the cochlear division of the eighth cranial nerve.

SENSORY ANESTHESIA: loss of all forms of sensation.

SENSORY APHASIA: see Wernicke's aphasia; receptive aphasia.

SENSORY APRAXIA: see ideational apraxia.

SENSORY ATAXIA: ataxia due to impairment of proprioception (joint position sense); interruption of afferent nerve fibers in peripheral nerves, posterior roots, posterior columns of spinal cords, or medial lemnisci; sometimes caused by lesions of both parietal lobes; patient is unable to determine limb position resulting in poorly judged movements; gait is uncertain, irregular, stomping, and wide-base; patient watches feet and floor; postive Romberg's sign; incoordination becomes aggravated when the eyes are closed; may be caused by tabes dorsalis, Friedreich's ataxia, subacute combined degeneration, syphilitic meningomyelitis, chronic polyneuritis, or multiple sclerosis.

SENSORY CORTEX UNITS (LURIA): *primary zones*: projection areas of vision (Brodmann's area 17); audition (Brodmann's area 41); body senses (Brodmann's areas 1, 2, & 3); *secondary zones*: projection areas of the primary zones; vision (Brodmann's areas 18 & 19); secondary zones maintain the modality of functional sensation, but have a less fixed topographic organization; *tertiary zones*: lie on the boundary of the occipital, temporal and parietal cortex (Brodmann's areas 5, 7, 21, 22, 37, 39,& 40; function of the tertiary zones is to integrate the excitation arriving from the different sensory systems and this sensory input is translated into symbolic processes and abstract thinking.

SENSORY-MOTOR TESTS: tests of somatosensory system of fine touch and pressure, deep muscle and joint senses, pain, and temperature, as well as the motor system laterality; blindfolded subjects perform various tasks with each hand; difference in efficiency of performance by the two hands can be taken to imply functional asymmetry in the cerebral organization of the system.

SENSORY SEIZURES: parietal lobe, post-rolandic convolution foci; feelings of numbness, tingling. and sensation of crawling.

SENSORY SYSTEMS LESIONS: lesions in the primary visual, somatosensory, and auditory systems produce serious deficits in sensory discrimination by significantly reducing acuity; secondary zone lesions: acutity is preserved but, although intellectual functioning is not disturbed, there is an inability to recognize objects or patterns; there is tentative evidence of specific neurological substrates of illusions, hallucinations, and dreaming.

SENSORY SYSTEMS ORGANIZATION: arranged hierarchically from the receptors at the bottom to the neocortex at the top, with complexity increasing at each higher level; function is lateralized at the highest levels.

SENTENCE BUILDING TEST: (Terman & Merrill, 1973) Stanford-Binet, SA I, 1960 Revision; test of frontal-lobe planning ability; demonstrates the ability to organize thoughts into a sensible and linguistically acceptable construct; tests verbal and sequential organizing abilities, use of syntax, spelling, punctuation, and graphomotor behavior; sensitive to slight impairments of verbal functions; does not differentiate between nonaphasic patients with left-hemisphere lesioned patients and those with right-hemisphere lesions (Miceli et al., 1977, 1981).

SENTENCE RECALL/MEMORY TEST: tests to what extent meaning contributes to the patient's span of immediate memory; normal adults can correctly recall sentences of 24 to 25 syllables (Williams, 1965); sensitive to left-hemisphere lesions; aphasic patients are more likely to misuse or omit function words rather than content words (Caramazza et al., 1978).

SENTENCE REPETITION TESTS: Stanford-Binet subtests age levels IV, XI, and XIII; subtest of the Multilingual Aphasia Exam (Benton & Hamsher, 1978); provides a measure of span for meaningful verbal material ranging from abnormally short to the expected normal adult length of 24 syllables; also tests for sensitivity to syntactical variations in what the patient hears; useful to detect mild linguistic deficits of patients whose communication abilities may seem intact.

SENTENCE STRUCTURE: (poor or lacking) see agrammatism.

SEPTUM: a general term referring to a dividing wall or partition; plural: septa.

SEPTAL REGION OF THE BRAIN: a triangular double membrane separating the anterior horn of the lateral ventricles of the brain; situated in the median plane; bounded by the corpus callosum and the body and columns of the fornix.

S

SEPSIS: the presence in the blood or other tissues of pathogenic microorganisms or their toxins.

SEPTICEMIA: pathogenic bacteria and associate toxins in the blood system.

SEQUELA: any lesion or affection following or caused by an attack of disease; plural: sequelae.

SEQUENCE RECALL TESTS: Block-tapping, Knox Curb Imitation Test, Learning Logical and Sequential Order Test, Learning a Code.

SEQUENTIAL CONCEPT FORMATION TEST: (Talland, 1965a) a test conceptually similar to maze learning and tests short-term memory storage capacity.

SEQUENTIAL MATCHING MEMORY TASK: (Collier & Levy, undated) requires sustained attention over a long period of time, perceptual and response flexibility; discriminates between epileptic, post-lobotomy, and paranoid schizophrenic patients.

SEQUIN-GODDARD FORMBOARD TEST: (Halstead-Reitan subtest) a tactile memory test; also a drawing recall test; may be used to test tactile learning in blind patients (Lezak, 1983); performance deficits are probably due to parietal-lobe dysfunction in Brodmann's areas 5 & 7; the memory and cross-modal matching is probably sensitive to lesions in the tertiary zone (Brodmann's areas 37 & 40).

SERIAL DIGIT LEARNING TEST: (Benton et al., 1983; Hamsher et al., 1980) sensitive to the mental changes that accompany normal aging of persons over 65 and bilateral brain damage.

SERIAL SEVENS: a commonly used mental tracking task used by psychiatrists and neurologists (Strub & Black, 1977); sensitive to brain-damage (Luria, 1966; Ruesch & Moore, 1943) and acute functional and affective disorders; normal women over 45 with no college background more error-prone than men (Smith, 1967).

SERIAL TESTING (WAIS-R): Mandleberg & Brooks (1975) concluded that practice did not affect the three-year WAIS scores given to head-injured patients.

SERIAL WORD-LEARNING TEST: (Vowels, 1979) tests the ability to maintain the order of learned material; used to study the ability to use sequential organization as an aid to learning (Weingartner, 1968); unilateral temporal-lobectomy patients (either side) do not benefit from organization into semantic categories or logical associations.

SEROTONIN: a vasoconstrictor found in blood serum and many body tissues, including the intestinal mucosa, pineal body, and CNS; enzymatically formed from tryptophan by hydroxylation and decarboxylation; also see thrombocytin, thrombolonin.

SEVENTH CRANIAL NERVE: facialis nerve; facial motor nerve, primarily, but is also parasympathetic, general sensory, and special sensory; supplies the frontalis muscle and all the muscles of facial expression and the tensor tympani (ear), also supplies the platysma muscle over the front of the neck and cheek; 2 roots: a large motor root, which supplies the muscles of facial expression, and a smaller root, the nervus intermedius which supplies the lacrimal, nasal, platine, submandibular, sublingual glands, and anterior two-thirds of tongue; originates on the inferior border of the pons, between olive and inferior cerebellar peduncle.

SEVENTH CRANIAL NERVE LESIONS: upper 7th nerve motor neuron affects only the lower face; a lower 7th nerve neuron affects the entire face; weakness of eye closure because the bottom lid is paralyzed and cannot wrinkle to meet the upper lid nor can the upper lid be wrinkled (ptosis is not a feature of a seventh nerve palsy); there is a difference between an upper and lower neuron lesion of the 7th nerve: the difference is based on the supranuclear innervation of the 7th cranial nerve nucleus; the cerebral hemisphere exerts much more control over the opposite lower face; the part most concerned with facial expression; forehead and eye closure mechanisms are mainly concerned with reflex eye closure and have a dual consensual type of innervation (i.e., both eyes shut simultaneously if either eye is threatened); a unilateral lesion of the fibers from the left hemisphere (as occurs in a typical CVA) will lead to readily detectable weakness in the lower face while eye closure and forehead movement remains intact because the other hemisphere pathways provide adequate cross innervation; in a lower motor neuron lesion of either the nucleus or the main 7th nerve trunk, all muscles innervated by the 7th nerve will be affected, leading to complete loss of control of the face on that side.

SEXUAL BEHAVIOR — FRONTAL-LOBE LESIONS: global frontal-lobe lesions may produce abnormal sexual behavior such as public masterbation, by reducing inhibitions; dorsolateral frontal-lobe lesions reduce interest in sexual behavior, but patient can perform sexually if led through the activity step by step.

SEXUAL FUNCTIONING: control is located in the hypothalamus which mediates the medial forebrain bundle.

SHAM RAGE: undirected and excessive rage; in animals: lashing of tail, arching the trunk, making limb movements, displaying claws, snarling, and biting; sympathetic signs of rage are present, including erection of the tail hair, sweating of the toe pads, dilation of the pupils, micturation, high blood pressure, high heart rate, and increases in adrenalin and blood sugar; similar sham emotional attacks can occur in humans who have suffered hypothalamic lesions — unchecked rage or who laugh until they die; found in the diencephalic animal; also called quasi-emotional phenomena.

SHIPLEY INSTITUTE OF LIVING SCALE: (Shipley, 1940, 1946) a neuropsychological paper and pencil screening test; does not dis-

S

criminate well between organic and functional disorders (Aita, Armitage et al., 1947; Parker, 1957).

SHORT PORTABLE MENTAL STATUS QUESTIONNAIRE: (Pfeiffer, 1975); a brief test for dementia.

SHORT-TERM MEMORY: (STM) lasts from one hour to two days; appears to be organized in terms of contiguity or of sensory properties (Broadbent, 1979).

SHORT-TERM MEMORY DYSFUNCTION: left parietal-temporal lobe dysfunction disturbs short-term, or working, memory; lesions seriously impair the ability to recall strings of digits; if there is no primary sensory defect, or agnosia, then a person with this lesion should be able to remember the digits with repeated practice, provided the mechanisms involved in long-term storage (medial temporal lobes) are intact; *left-sided lesion*: impaired short-term memory for verbal material; *right-sided lesion*: impaired short-term memory for spatial location of particular sensory inputs; possibly Brodmann's area 7 is involved (Hécaen & Albert 1978).

SHORT-TERM MEMORY vs LONG-TERM MEMORY: (Kolb & Whishaw theory 1980) may be parallel processes in which material is stored separately in both; the parietal lobe appears to be involved in short-term memory and the temporal lobe in long-term memory.

SHOW ME TEST: (Smith, undated) part of the Michigan Neuropsychological Test Battery; a test for right-left orientation and autotopagnosia.

SHUFFLING GAIT: see cerebellar gait, Korsakoff's syndrome, alcoholism (chronic), ataxia of Bruns, senile gait.

SHUNT: polythene cannula from the lateral ventricle is placed into the cisterna magna; treatment for hydrocephalus; a passage or anastomosis between two natural channels, especially between blood vessels; may be formed physiologically, a structural anomaly, or surgically created.

SIG.: abreviation for signetur; let it be labeled.

SIGN: an objective manifestation of a pathological condition observed by the examiner.

SILLY SENTENCES: (Botwinick & Storandt, 1974) explores the contribution of meaning to retention.

SIMILARITIES AND DIFFERENCES TEST: (Stanford-Binet subtest, age level VIII); test of conceptual functioning.

SIMILARITIES SUBTEST: (WAIS-R) excellent test of general intellectual ability; test of verbal reasoning; least affected by the patient's background and experiences; does not depend upon academic skills; independent of social or educational background and unaffected by the impulsivity and social misjudgments that accompany some kinds of brain injury; brain-damaged patients give more "I don't know" responses and fewer conceptual responses (Spence, 1963);

more sensitive to the effects of brain injury regardless of localization than other verbal subtests (Hirschenfang, 1960); impaired concept formation; left-temporal and frontal-lobe involvement in relatively depressed scores (McFie, 1975; Newcombe, 1969); one of the best predictors of left-hemisphere disease in the WAIS-R battery; left frontal-lobe lesions show significantly lower scores than right frontal-lobe lesions; may be unaffected by right frontal-lobe lesions (Bogen et al., 1972; McFie, 1975); lower scores with bilateral frontal-lobe lesions (Sheer, 1956); demented patients may receive a relatively normal score since overlearned material often survives dementing process for a long time past the patient's ability to care for self; for older people: best test of verbal ability; free of memory component.

SIMULTANAGNOSIA: inability to perceive more than one object or point in space at one time; occipital-lobe disfunction; also called simultaneous agnosia.

SIMPLE SENSORY EPILEPSY: seizure attacks caused by sensory hallucinations which may involve any sensory modality; most often a feeling of numbness or tingling in some part of body which may develop into a motor Jacksonian attack or generalized convulsion; originates in opposite parietal lobe near the postcentral gyrus (Brain, 1985).

SIXTH NERVE: (Abducens); motor nerve; enervates lateral rectus muscle; arises from a paired group of cells in the floor of the fourth ventricle at the level of the lower pons; controls the eye muscles; originates from the front of the brainstem at the ponto-medullary junction, deep in the posterior fossa; ascends on the front of the brainstem and then angles sharply forwards over the tip of the petrous bone to enter the back of the cavernous sinus; lies free in the sinus, enters the orbit through the superior orbital fissure, and passes laterally to reach the lateral rectus muscle.

SIXTH NERVE LESION: paralysis of abduction and a convergent strabismus; diplopia; the sixth nerve may also be affected in the basal area with increased intracranial pressure from hydrocephalus which pushes the brainstem down and the sixth nerve becomes stretched over the petrous tip.

SIXTH NERVE PALSY: weakness of the abducens; causes diplopia because the eye is pulled medially by the unopposed action of the medial rectus muscle; no ptosis; the patient may compensate by turning his head towards the weak muscle.

SKIN WRITING: test used to detect somesthetic defects or tactile-perceptual defects; useful to lateralize the site of brain-damage when there is no obvious signs such as hemiparesis or aphasia.

SLEEP: state of physical and mental inactivity from which the patient may be aroused to normal consciousness; partial inhibition of the

S

ARAS by the pontine nuclei; mediated through the hypothalamus.

SLEEP APNEA: cessation of breathing during sleep; see apnea.

SLEEP AUTOMATISM: see somnambulism, sleep walking.

SLEEP DEPRIVATION: (60-200 hrs.) fatigue, irritability, poor concentration, disorientation, illusions and hallucinations (usually visual and tactile), slowing in motor tasks, lapses in attention, mild nystagmus, slight tremor.

SLEEP DEPRIVATION-PARTIAL: hyperactivity, lability, dysinhibition, excessive appetite, and oversexuality.

SLEEP HYPOCHONDRIAC: see primary insomnia, sleep pedants.

SLEEP PARALYSIS: while falling asleep or awakening, the patient has a helpless feeling of not being able to move or speak; lasts 1-2 minutes.

SLEEP PEDANTS: persons with primary insomnia; suffer the effects of partial sleep deprivation; awaken more often; more rapid pulse; peripheral vasoconstriction; higher body temperature; less REM sleep; more stage II NREM.

SLEEP-REM: occurs after about 70 minutes of sleep; increase in body movements; stage V; eyes roll from side to side; alternates with NREM sleep at about the same intervals four to six times per night.

SLEEP-STAGES: five stages: I through IV-NREM (nonrapid eye movement sleep); V-REM (rapid eye movement sleep), paradoxical sleep (PS) or activated sleep (AS).

SLEEP — UNCONTROLLABLE: narcolepsy.

SLEEP WALKING: see somnambulism, automatic behaviors.

SLOWING: the speed component probably contributes to the association of lowered Object Assembly and Digit Symbol subtest scores with frontal-lobe lesions.

SLOWING/SLOWED COGNITIVE FUNCTIONS: delayed reaction times and longer than average total performance times in the absence of a specific motor disability; common in brain-damage; may be associated with weakness or poor coordination; most often related to frontal-lobe damage.

SLOW VIRUS INFECTIONS: (viral encephalitis) viral infections which continues and produces progressive disability over a period of many months or years; see kuru, Jakob-Creutzfeldt disease, and subacute sclerosing panenchephalitis; there appears to be no treatment for these infections and often progress to death (Reitan & Wolfson, 1985).

SMELL: controlled by the hypothalamus via the medial forebrain bundle.

SNS: Sympathetic Nervous System; controlled by the posterior hypothalamus; for more information, see Nervous System.

SOB: shortness of breath.

SOCIAL ABULIA: social inactivity resulting from inability to select a course of action, although a wish to participate may be present.

SOCIAL ADJUSTMENT RATING SCALES: (Weissman, 1975); 15 scales for examining the social function of psychiatric patients; may also be appropriate for evaluating brain-damaged patients.

SOCIAL BEHAVIOR — FRONTAL-LOBE LESIONS: damage to the orbital regions are associate with more dramatic changes in personality than dorsolateral lesions (Kliest, 1966); two types of personality changes in frontal-lobe patients: (orbital) pseudodepression and (dorsolateral) pseudopsychopathic behavior (Blumer & Benson, 1975); the former may show outward apathy and indifference, loss of initiative, reduced sexual interest, little overt emotion, and little or no verbal output; the latter, immature behavior, lack of tact and restraint, coarse language, promiscuous sexual behavior, increased motor activity, and a general lack of social graces.

SOCIAL DYSFUNCTION: see abulia, social abulia, amygdala, temporal-lobe epilepsy, frontal-lobe dysfunction/lesions, orbital frontal-lobe dysfunction, dorsolateral-frontal, social behavior, frontal-lobe lesions, Korsakoff's syndrome/psychosis, Parkinson's syndrome.

SOCIAL STATUS OUTCOME SCALE: (Cope, 1982) a six category behavioral status questionnaire that specifies functional level and living status of head-injured patients; may be used to track social status over time.

SODIUM AMYTAL MEMORY STUDIES: three principal findings from studies: 1. if the drug is injected ipsilaterally to the lesioned hemisphere, the patient retains 90% to 95% of both the verbal and nonverbal material — implying that both temporal lobes are capable of storing both types of memory; 2. injection of the drug contralateral to the damaged temporal lobe results in substantial memory impairment, retention dropping to around 50%; 3. if injection ipsilateral to a known lesion results in impaired memory, there are strong grounds for predicting that the patient suffers from a bilateral lesion.

SOMA: 1. the body as distinguished from the mind; 2. body tissue as distinguished from the germ cells; 3. cell body; see also neuronal cell body.

SOMASTHENIA: a condition of bodily weakness, poor appetite and sleep, and inability to maintain a normal active life without easy exhaustion.

SOMATESTHETIA: the consciousness of having a body.

SOMATESTHETIA — PRIMARY AREA: see postcentral gyrus.

SOMATIC: pertaining to the body.

SOMATOGNOSIS: see somatosensory agnosias.

SOMATOMOTOR STRIP: precentral gyrus, primary motor cortex.

SOMATOSENSORY AGNOSIAS: astereognosia: the inability to recognize the nature of an object by touch (asymbolia); asomatognosia: the loss of knowledge or sense of one's own body and bodily condition.

S

SOMATOSENSORY FUNCTION TEST: two-point discrimation test (Corkin et al., 1970).

SOMATOSENSORY LESIONS: lesions of the primary somatosensory cortex produce abnormally high sensory thresholds, impaired position sense, and stereognostic deficits; cause difficulty on tests of pressure sensitivity, two-point threshold, and point localization on the skin of the hand contralateral to the lesion (Corkin, Milner, Rasmussen et al., 1970); excisions sparing the postcentral gyrus or in the posterior parietal cortex cause only transient deficits, if any; lesions of the postcentral gyrus may cause afferent paresis (Luria, 1965) in which movements of the fingers are clumsy because the patient has lost the necessary feedback about their exact position; if there is a loss of representation of the face area in the left hemisphere, motor aphasia is also observed; animal studies indicate that lesions of Brodmann's areas 5 and 7 produce defective form discrimination, reduced precision of grasping with the hands, and defective spatial analysis; see Verger-Dejerine syndrome.

SOMATOSENSORY SYSTEM: includes the skin senses of touch, pressure, pain, temperature, itch, vibration, and tickle, as well as the body senses of joint position, muscle tension, and visceral state; somatosenory areas: the primary somatosensory cortex; postcentral gyrus Brodmann's areas 1, 2, & 3 and the secondary, or supplementary, somatosensory cortex located on the superior bank of the Sylvian fissure (Brodmann's area 43); the primary regions produce sensation on the contralateral side while the secondary regions produce sensations simultaneously on both sides of the body; primary regions receive input from the lemniscal system via the ventral basal complex of the thalamus; secondary regions receive input from the extralemniscal or spinothalamic system via the ventral basal complex and posterior thalamus; the ventrobasal complex and posterior thalamus are different from one another in functional organization: the ventrobasal area has a topographical somatosensory map similar to the neocortical maps, whereas the posterior thalamus appears to be arranged haphazardly (Kolb & Whishaw, 1980); hierarchically arranged; receptors in the skin transmit five basic sensations: light touch to the skin, deep pressure to the fascia below the skin, joint movement, pain, and temperature; thalamic cells are highly specific with any given cell being maximally responsive to only one mode of stimulation; cortical cells are just as specific to particular stimuli, but a given cell is responsive to a smaller region of skin; spatial location discrimination increases as one moves up the hierarchy; discrimination of the quality of stimulation does not change.

SOMATOTROPIC HORMONES: secretions of anterior pituitary gland: adrenocorticotropic (ACTH), thyrotropic (TTH), lutenizing (LH), lactogenic (prolactin), gonadotropic, follicle stimulating (FSH) stimulates growth; hyposecretion in the child results in dwarfism; hypersecretion in the child causes giantism; hypersecretion in the adult produces acromegaly.

SOMESTHESIS IN THE COMMISSURED BRAIN: the somatosensory system is completely crossed; if the hemispheres are disconnected by a commissurotomy, the somatosensory functions of the left and right parts of the body become independent.

SOMESTHETIC: somatesthetic.

SOMESTHETIC DEFECTS: tactile recognition and discrimination deficits.

SOMESTHETIC SENSES: information related to touch and pressure is thought to be conveyed to the cord by fast-conducting fibers; once in the cord, the fibers synapse with two ascending tracts: the funiculus gracilis, which collects pressure information from the lower part of the body, and the funiculus cuneatus; from these nuclei a second tract, the medial lemniscus, crosses to the opposite side of the brain and ascends to the ventrobasal complex of the thalamus; on its way to the thalamus the medial lemniscus collects somesthetic information from the head and face via the trigeminal nerve; from the thalamus, the information is projected to the primary and secondary somatosensory areas of the parietal cortex (the posterior part of the postcentral gyrus); the primary area tends to receive somesthetic information that originated from the opposite side of the body, particularly the face.

SOMNAMBULISM: sleep walking; patient arises from bed, walks, gives no outward sign of emotion, eyes open, may awaken at sight of an unfamiliar object; sometimes speaks strange phrases over and over; no memory of episode; hypnotic state.

SOUTHERN CALIFORNIA FIGURE-GROUND PERCEPTION TEST: (Ayres, 1966) basically a children's test, but appropriate for evaluating perceptual disorders in brain-damaged adults; simple to administer.

S/P: status post.

SPASMODIC TORTICOLLIS: rotation of the head brought about by clonic or tonic contraction of the cervical muscles; may occur as the result of organic disease of the nervous system; sometimes a hysterical symptom; characterized by violent clonic movements of rotation of the head to one side and may lead to hypertrophy of the contracting muscles; intractable disorder (Brain, 1985).

SPASTIC: 1. of the nature of or characterized by involuntary spasms; 2. hypertonic; muscles stiff and movements awkward; see also cerebral palsy.

SPASTIC BULBAR PALSY: see supernuclear palsy, pseudobulbar palsy.

S

SPASTIC DIPLEGIA: see Little's disease.

SPASTIC DYSARTHRIA: stuttering.

SPASTIC DYSPHAGIA: see Little's disease.

SPASTIC GAIT: see hemiplegic gait, paraplegic gait, spastic paraparesis.

SPASTIC HEMIPLEGIA: paralysis on one side marked by spasticity of the muscles of the paralyzed part and increased tendon reflexes.

SPASTIC OR RIGID DYSARTHRIA: lesion in the corticobulbar tracts; see also paretic dysarthria.

SPASTIC PARAPARESIS: see cerebral spastic diplegia, multiple sclerosis, syringomyelia, spinal syphilis, spinal cord compression, familial spinal spastic ataxia.

SPASTIC PSEUDOPARALYSIS: see Creutzfeldt-Jakob syndrome.

SPASTICITY: feature of all acute and chronic lesions of the pyramidal system at cerebral, capsular, midbrain, and pontine levels. In cerebral and brainstem lesions spasticity does not usually appear immediately, and in exceptional cases the paralyzed limbs remain flaccid but with reflexes.

SPATIAL AGNOSIAS (visual): deficits of vision caused mainly by right posterior-hemispheric lesions (particularly in the right parietal and occipital cortex); includes defective stereoscopic vision, loss of topographical concepts, and neglect of one side of the environment.

SPATIAL DYSCALCULA: difficulty in carrying numbers, misplacement of numbers relative to one another, confusion of columns or rows of numbers, neglect of one or more numbers; posterior right-hemisphere lesions.

SPATIAL DYSFUNCTION: lesion of Brodmann's areas 7 & 40, right (Benton, 1969b; Semmes et al., 1963).

SPATIAL HEARING DEFECT: impaired ability to locate the source of sounds in space; lesions to the secondary zone of the right auditory cortex.

SPATIAL INATTENTION TESTS: Scene Recall (Bisiach & Luzzatti, 1978); Dotting a Target Circle (Vernea, 1977).

SPATIAL ORIENTATION: ability to relate to the position, direction, or movements of objects or points in space (Lezak, 1983); deficits are associated with damage to different areas of the brain and involve different functions (Benton, 1969b); dysfunction is most often related to posterior right-hemisphere lesions; exceptions: right-left, topographic, and body schema disorientation which are usually due to a lesion of the left-parietal lobe (Weinstein, 1964); spatial disorientation may be due to errors in verbal labeling, specific amnesia, visual scanning, visual agnosia, or a true spatial disorientation; a component of visual perception which may be tested by tests such as Judgment of Line Orientation Test and Bisection of Line Test.

SPATIAL ORIENTATION MEMORY TEST: (Wepman & Turaids,

1975) a test of immediate recall of the orientation of geometric and design figures; Parkinsonian patients have difficulty with this test (Pirozzolo et al., 1982).

SPATIAL ORIENTATION TESTS: Perceptual Functions: Judgment of Line Orientation; Body Orientation; Personal Orientation Test; Body Center Test; Right-Left Orientation; Standardized Road-Map Test of Direction Sense; Distance Estimation tasks; mental transformations in space; (mental rotations, inversions,etc.); Spatial Orientation Memory Test; Spatial Dyscalculias; Topographical Orientation; Geographic Orientation Tests.

SPATIAL RELATIONS TESTS: Semmes locomotor map; right-left differentiation tests.

SPEECH CORTICAL FACE AREA: directs the movements of the face, tongue, etc., necessary for speech.

SPEECH DYSFLUENCY: see stuttering, anarthria, literal dysarthria, dysarthria, aphasia.

SPEECH LATERALIZATION TESTS: handedness questionnaire and Dichotic Digits from the Montreal Neurological Institute Battery, Test of Lateral Dominance (A. J. Harris, 1958), The Handedness Inventory (Annett, 1967; Briggs & Nebes, 1975).

SPEECHLESSNESS: anarthria.

SPEECH MECHANICS: coordinated sequence of contractions of the larynx, pharynx, palate, tongue, lips, and respiratory musculature; innervated by hypoglossal, vagal, facial nerves; controlled through corticobulbar tracts; also extrapyramidal influences from cerebellum and basal ganglia; see also language model (Wernicke-Geschwind).

SPEECH SOUNDS PERCEPTION TEST: (subtest of the Halstead-Reitan battery); sensitive to brain-damage in general; left-hemisphere damage in particular; may be affected by age of patient.

SPELLING APRAXIA: expressive aphasia; disruption of the ability to spell.

SPINA BIFIDA: developmental anomaly characterized by defective closure of the bony encasement of the spinal cord, through which the cord and meninges may or may not protrude.

SPINAL ACCESSORY NERVE (XI, cranial): a parasympathetic and motor nerve formed by cranial roots from the side of the medulla oblongata, and by spinal roots from the side of the upper three or more cervical segments of the spinal cord; the roots unite and the nerve thus formed divides into an internal cranial branch and an external spinal branch; the internal branch supplies the vagus nerve and thereby supplies the palate, pharynx, larynx, and thoracic viscera; the external branch supplies the sternocleido-mastoid and trapezius muscles.

SPINAL CORD: serves as a pathway for communication between the

S

brain and the rest of the body.

SPINAL CORD FUNCTIONING: (all other higher CNS functions removed) reflexes (stretching, withdrawal, support, scratching, paw shaking, etc.) to appropriate sensory stimulation; movements are brief adjustments to the stimulation, are stereotyped, and usually last only for the length of the stimulation.

SPINAL CORD LESION: paralysis on the same side as the lesion.

SPINAL CORD SEGMENTS: 8 cervical (C); 12 thoracic (T); 5 lumbar (L); 5 sacral (S).

SPINAL REFLEXES (basic): Nerve fibers from sensory receptors in or on the body enter the spinal cord through its superior or dorsal roots; project to interneurons or to motor neurons in the same or other segments of the spinal cord; projections go to the muscles or the body through the spinal cord's inferior or ventral roots.

SPINAL SHOCK: a state of profound depression of all reflexes below the level of section/lesion; lasts from one to six weeks and changes to spasticity; some reflexes such as penile erection in males, may not be depressed.

SPINAL STRETCH REFLEX: see stretch reflex-spinal.

SPINOTHALAMIC TRACT: pathways that synapse with sensory neurons from the skin fibers conveying sensations have already crossed in the spinal cord and sympathetic pathways; ascend into the medulla lying in a lateral position with the leg fibers laterally and the arm fibers medially; the tract maintains its position in the dorsolateral brainstem until the medial meniscus merges with it in the midbrain.

SPINOTHALAMIC TRACT LESION: often a Horner's syndrome on one side with pain and temperature loss on the opposite side of the body whenever the dorsolateral brainstem is damaged.

SPLANCHNIC NERVES: nerves of the blood vessels and viscera, especially the visceral branches of the thoracic, lumbar, and pelvic parts of the sympathetic trunks.

SPLENIUM: (of corpus callosum); posterior rounded end of the corpus callosum.

SPLIT BRAIN: see commissurotomy; corpus callosum.

SPONTANEOUS RECOVERY: an inevitable physiological repair process of the brain following injury; may be influenced by age, extent and location of damage, general condition of the patient, and to some degree, the quality of care a patient receives (Goldstein, 1984); edema lessens, blood flow is normalized to undamaged areas, catecholamine levels return to normal, normal function in undamaged brain areas is resumed (Rubens, 1977); may continue up to 6 months or longer; most spontaneous recovery is accomplished in the first 3 months.

SPONTANEITY — REDUCED: orbital frontal-lobe lesion (Jones-

S

Gotman & Milner, 1977; Milner, 1964).

S/T: soft tie restraints.

ST. VITUS' DANCE: see Sydenham's Chorea.

STAGGERING GAIT: characteristic of alcoholic and barbiturate intoxication; the patient totters, reels, tips forward and then backward; steps are irregular and uncertain; balance usually maintained.

STAGNANT ANOXIA: anoxia resulting from inadequate blood flow through the capillaries with resultant abnormal oxygen extraction and low tissue oxygen tension; a generalized or localized lack of oxygen due to deficiency in the volume of blood; may be caused by cardiac failure or arrest, shock, arterial spasm, or thrombosis.

STAMMERING: see stuttering, anarthria literales, speech dysfluency.

STANDARD SCORES: scores that are based on the mean and standard deviation of the same scale.

STANDARDIZATION POPULATION: the group of individuals tested for the purpose of obtaining normative data on the test.

STANDARDIZED ROAD-MAP TEST OF DIRECTION SENSE: (Money, 1976) a quick paper and pencil assessment of right-left orientation.

STANFORD-BINET: provides a wide enough range of item difficulty for testing those neuropsychological patients who are so seriously impaired that they are unable to pass enough WAIS-R items to earn subtest scores much above zero; many of the individual items are excellent test of one or another of the functions and skills that come under investigation in neuropsychological studies (Lezak, 1983); Maze Tracing, Sentence Completion, Differentiation of Abstract Words, Giving of Opposites, Analogies, Speeded Block-manipulation Tasks, and Picture Absurdities are sensitive to brain damage (Hebb, 1942); the age-grades of the subtests serve as points of reference.

Stat.: immediately; at once.

STATIC ENCEPHALOPATHY: below average intellectual functioning with no history of brain trauma.

STATIC TREMOR: see ataxic intention tremor, intention tremor.

STATUS EPILEPTICUS: succession of convulsions without any intervening period of consciousness; may lead to deepened coma, pyrexia or hyperpyrexia, and death if not arrested; may follow abrupt withdrawal of anticonvulsant drugs, especially barbiturates (Brain, 1985).

STEELE-RICHARDSON-OLZEWSKI SYNDROME: dementia associated with specific impairment of conjugate eye movement and pseudo-bulbar palsy.

STEREOANESTHESIA: inability to identify shape and form of an object because of lesions of the cortex, spinal cord, and brainstem due

S

to interruption of tracts transmitting postural and tactile sensation.

STEREOGNOSIS: recognition of objects by touch.

STEREOTYPY: a prolonged, aimless repetition of words, movements, or attitudes.

STERTOROUS RESPIRATIONS: snoring.

STICK TEST: (Benson & Barton, 1970; Butters & Barton, 1970) visuoconstructional task; more sensitive to right-hemisphere lesions; the need for verbal mediation may lower the performance of left-hemisphere lesioned patients.

STIMULANT DRUGS: increase behavioral activity either by producing increases in motor activity or by counteracting fatigue; includes antidepressants such as desipramine, imipramine, amphetamine, cocaine; acts on the ARAS.

STIMULUS BOUND: unable to screen out irrelevant stimuli due to diffuse brain dysfunction or extensive bilateral cortical damage; probably a frontal-lobe dysfunction.

STM: short-term memory.

STOCKTON GERIATRIC RATING SCALE: (Meer & Baker, 1966) a behavior rating scale designed to be used by ward staff to assess social abilities of inpatient geriatric patients such as eating, toileting, self-direction, and sociability.

STORAGE VS RETRIEVAL PROBLEMS: recall depends upon both the amount of information stored and the efficiency of retrieval processes (Lezak, 1983); to evaluate relative performance a comparison can be made between complete recall and a recognition task on a multiple-choice test. A score on the multiple-choice test that is higher than a direct recall test suggests a retrieval problem; recall compared with savings measures storage; if the memory impairment is due to retention problems, then recall will be low and there will be little savings on later learned trials; if the problem is one of retrieval, recall will be down, but relearning at a later time will occur rapidly, indicating that the material had been stored.

STORY TELLING: see Thematic Apperception Test for typical projective organic responses.

STRABISMUS: improper alignment of eyes.

STREET COMPLETION TEST: (Street, 1931); test of perceptual closure capacity; sensitive to right-hemisphere lesions.

STRETCH RECEPTORS: nerve endings that wrap around the nuclear bag; 2 types: the annulospiral endings which wrap around the center of the bag and synapse in the spinal cord with the motor neurons that return to the extrafusal fibers in the stimulated muscle, and the flower-spray endings that wrap around the outer part of the bag and take a different path to the spinal cord, eventually synapsing with motor neurons that travel to the extrafusal fibers of the muscle that is functioning antagonistically to the stimulated muscle; work reciprocally; the annulospiral endings trigger the contraction of extrafusal fibers in the stretched muscle, while the flower-spray endings work to inhibit contractions in the antagonistic muscle.

STRETCH REFLEX-SPINAL: simplest of the spinal reflexes; the contraction of a muscle to stretch a limb. The stretch activates a receptor in the muscle, and its sensory neuron; on stimulation, activates the motor neuron in the spinal cord, which then contracts the stretched muscle. The function of the stretch reflex is to allow the muscle to maintain a limb in position. Stretching a muscle can also influence muscles that work in opposition to it (reciprocal inhibition); the stretch reflex is an automatic leveling function that takes place in the spinal cord; allows the body to adjust quickly to abrupt shifts in weight.

STRIATE CORTEX LESION: disruption of pattern vision but no impairment of orientation to visual stimuli.

STRIATUM: the striate body; one of the components of the basal ganglia; specifically, a subcortical mass of gray and white substance in front of and lateral to the thalamus in each cerebral hemisphere. The gray substance is arranged in two principal masses, the caudate nucleus and lentiform nucleus; the striate appearance on section of the area being produced by connecting bands of gray substance passing from one of these nuclei to the other through the white substance of the internal capsule; see chorea or choreoathetosis, Sydenham's chorea, Huntington's chorea, senile chorea, tardive dyskinesia.

STROKE: (CVA) sudden appearance of neurological symptoms as a result of severe interruption of blood flow; can result from a wide variety of different vascular diseases; not all vascular disorders produce stroke; the onset of dysfunction can be insidious, spanning months or even years; often produces an infarct, an area of dead or dying tissue resulting from an obstruction of the blood vessels normally supplying the area or structure; tend to have one-sided effects; signs of bilateral or diffuse damage during the early stages; symptoms may diminish or disappear over time; focal deficits typically fit into a pattern of dysfunction associated with areas of the brain that share a common artery or network of smaller arterial vessels (Geschwind & Strub, 1975; Hécaen & Albert, 1978).

STROOP COLOR/WORD TEST: (Stroop, 1935) measures the ease with which the patient can shift perceptual set to conform to changing demands; test of the effects of perceptual interference (Talland, 1965a), concentration (Dodrill, 1978c), and ability to to shift sets; particularly sensitive to left frontal-lobe lesions; inability to suppress word naming in favor of color naming (Perret, 1974); probably more a test of impairments in executive functions, particu-

S

larly those relating to mental control and response flexibility; measure of frontal-lobe dysfunction; the Press Test (Baehr & Corsini, 1982) is a paper and pencil form suitable for group administration.

STRUCTURE DEPENDENCY: frontal-lobe pathology; patient needs framework or pattern to follow; can do block designs and perform Raven's Matrices acceptably, but have much more trouble on Object Assembly or the Hooper since these are tests that require the patient to conceptualize, or at least identify, the finished product in order to assemble it mentally or actually.

STUPOR: mental and physical activity is reduced to a minimum; the patient may open eyes; response to spoken commands either absent or slow and monosyllabic; tremulousness, coarse twitching, restlessness, grasping and sucking reflexes present; does not arouse spontaneously.

STUTTERING: anarthria literalis; speech dysfluency; repetitions of parts of/whole words, prolongation of sounds, interjections of sounds or words, unduly prolonged pauses.

STUTTERING HEMIPARESIS: series of cerebral vascular disease attacks with increasing disability; most often a result of progressive thrombosis of the carotid artery.

SUBACUTE SCLEROSING PANENCEPHALITIS: follows a history of measles infection in early childhood; diffuse pathological changes of the brain in both gray and white matter; may progress to death within months or remit for several years (Reitan & Wolfson, 1985).

SUBARACHNOID: between the arachnoid and the pia mater.

SUBARACHNOID HEMORRHAGE: usually due to aneurysms on vessels traversing the sub-arachnoid space; may be transient cardiac arrhythmia or glycosuria; symptoms include headache, acute nausea and vomiting, and neck stiffness.

SUBCLAVIAN "STEAL" SYNDROME: symptoms of vertebrobasilar insufficiency may be due to the diversion of blood from the vertebral artery to the brachial artery; sometimes provoked by arm exercise; may be characterized by symptoms of brainstem dysfunction, reduced blood pressure in one arm, and a bruit at the root of the neck on the same side; flow of blood in the vertebral artery is reversed and the upper extremity "steals" blood from the brainstem (Brain, 1985).

SUBCORTICAL APHASIA: due to lesion interrupting impulses toward the afferent tracts that proceed to the auditory speech center.

SUBCORTICAL DEMENTIAS: symptoms may include decreased initiation, slowing of responses, and specific defects in memory functions; specific behavioral symptoms vary according to the subcortical structures involved and the variations in the production of neurotransmitters (Lishman, 1978; Walton, 1977); see also Parkinson's disease and Huntington's disease.

SUBCORTICAL MOTOR SYSTEM: the red nucleus in the midbrain sends axons that cross in the midbrain and then descend as the rubrospinal tract to synapse with cells in the dorsolateral portion of the intermediate zone; projections from the other subcortical nuclei descend through the ventro-medial system and connect bilaterally with interneurons in the ventromedial intermediate zone.

SUBCORTICAL STROKE, S/P: (thalamus, basal ganglia, and brainstem); also called hypertensive cerebral hemorrhages or intracerebral hemorrhages; symptoms include attention and memory problems, and irritability (Walton, 1977); subtle changes in psychosocial and self-regulatory behavior is typically associated with frontal-lobe lesions.

SUBDURAL: between the dura mater and arachnoid.

SUBDURAL HYGROMA: pool of cerebrospinal fluid which has collected in the subdural space from which it cannot be absorbed; thought to be the result of a tear in the arachnoid.

Subj.: subjective.

SUBLIMATION: unconscious process of transforming the energy of repressed tendencies and directing them to socially useful goals.

SUBSTANTIA NIGRA: important nucleus involved with extrapyramidal motor control; part of the basis pedunculi; contain dark pigment which is depigmented in Parkinson's disease by degeneration of the melatonin-containing neurons of the area; the point of origin of fibers that go to the basal ganglia and also project to the frontal cortex and spinal cord; dopamine is the neurotransmitter at the synapses of the projections; see Parkinson's Disease, Wilson's Disease, Hallervorden-Spatz Disease.

SUBSTANTIVE WORDS: nouns.

SUBTHALAMIC MOVEMENT DISORDER: see choreic, athetotic.

SUBTHALAMIC: see also tegmentum of midbrain; Wilson's Disease; multiple sclerosis, Wilson's disease, arousal.

SUBSTRATE: substance upon which an enzyme acts.

SULCUS OF NEOCORTEX: cleft in the neocortex that is shallower than a fissure and does not indent the ventricles.

SUPERIOR COLLICULI: upper portion of the tectum; one of two structures of the tectum; mediates whole body movements to visual stimuli (visual reflexes); mediates visual, auditory, and tactile tracking behavior.

SUPERIOR COLLICULI LESIONS: interferes with voluntary upward gaze; no convergence or pupillary light reflex; may also involve the tegmentum.

SUPERIOR COLLICULUS (ABLATION): deficits in orientation to visual stimuli with little or no effect on pattern discrimination.

SUPERIOR OBLIQUE MUSCLE: see fourth nerve.

SUPERIOR OLIVARY NUCLEI: dorsal nucleus of trapezoid body; a group of nerve cell bodies dorsolateral in the trapezoid body; receives

S

chochlear fibers and contributes to the formation of the trapezoid body and lateral lemniscus; also called dorsalis corporis trapezoidei; see also auditory system.

SUPPRESSION: a conscious dismissal from consciousness of undesirable thoughts, desires, or experiences.

SUPRAMARGINAL GYRUS: the convolution of the inferior parietal lobe that curves around the upper end of the posterior branch of the lateral fissure and is continuous behind it with the superior temporal gyrus.

SUPRANUCLEAR MOTOR PARALYSIS: always involves a group of muscles, never individual muscles; see also supernuclear palsy.

SUPRANUCLEAR PALSY: spastic weakness of the muscles innervated by the cranial nerves (face muscles, pharynx, and tongue) due to bilateral lesions of the corticospinal tract; often accompanied by uncontrolled weeping or laughing; also called pseudobulbar paralysis and spastic bulbar palsy.

SUPRASPAN NUMBER TEST: sensitive to age, educational level, brain impairment, and anticholinergic medications (Crook et al., 1980; Drachman & Leavitt, 1974).

SWALLOWING MECHANICS: several cranial nerves are involved simultaneously in chewing, bolus formation, and swallowing; the first phase is under voluntary control: the mouth is held shut by the 7th nerve, sensory input via 5th nerve relays position of the food bolus in the mouth, motor input via 5th nerve controls the chewing movements, the 12th nerve pushes the chewed bolus up and back against the soft palate, the 9th nerve senses the arrival of the bolus at the palate; the second phase is the reflex swallowing: the 5th nerve pulls the hyoid up and forward which brings the larynx beneath the back of the tongue, the 9th nerve moves the stylopharyngeus muscle which assists the hyoid elevaton and lifts the larynx forward, the 10th nerve elevates the palate to occlude the nasopharynx and prevents regurgitation up the back of the nose, flips the epiglottis forward over the top of the elevated and tilted larynx which prevents the food from falling into the trachea, dilates the hypopharynx allowing the bolus to fall back into the esophagus, and initiates peristalsis in the esophagus.

SWEARING (COMPULSIVE): see coprolalia, Gilles de la Tourette's disease.

SWEATING: central neck lesions usually affect sweating over the entire head, neck, arm and upper trunk on the same side; lesions in the lower neck affect sweating over the entire face; lesions above the superior cervical ganglion may not affect sweating at all; controlled through the hypothalamus.

SYDENHAM'S CHOREA: continuous irregular choreic movements in standing or walking, affecting the face, neck, hands, and large proximal joints and trunk; movements include jerks of head, grimacing, squirming, twisting, and respiratory noises; an acute, usually self-limited disorder of early life, usually between the ages of five and fifteen, or during pregnancy; closely linked with rheumatic fever; characterized by involuntary movements that gradually become severe, affecting all motor activities including gait, arm movements, and speech; mild psychic component is usually present; may be limited to one side of the body or may take the form of muscular rigidity; usually involves the caudate nucleus, putamen, and striatum; also called St. Vitus' dance.

SYMBOL DIGIT MODALITIES TEST: (SDMT) (Smith, 1973); a test of attentional functions; education level is positively correlated with scores; sensitive to visual perceptual, visual scanning, oculomotor defects, or general mental or motor slowing (Kaufman, 1968), normal aging, and brain dysfunction.

SYMBOLIC APRAXIA: often associate with receptive language disorders (Dee et al., 1970); imitation of symbolic gestures is sensitive to brain damage in general regardless of laterality.

SYMBOLIC GESTURES TESTING: (Christensen, 1979; Luria, 1966; 1973b) Face: stick out tongue, blow kiss; Arms: salute, hitchhike, "OK" sign, "stop" sign; Body: bow, stand like a boxer.

SYMPATHETIC APRAXIA: (in Broca's aphasia) lesion in the subcortical white matter, underlying Broca's area, that destroys the origin of the fibers that connect the left and right motor association cortices; causes an apraxia of command movements of the left hand.

SYMPATHETIC NERVOUS SYSTEM: becomes most active during stress and emergency situations (fight or flight reactions); thoracolumbar portion of the autonomic nervous system.

SYMPATHETIC NERVOUS SYSTEM PATHWAY: (EYE) starts in the hypothalamus; travels to and synapses with a neuron in the lateral grey in the thoracic spinal cord; travels to the superior cervical ganglion where it synapses with a nerve that travels to the pupil and blood vessels of the eye entering the cranial cavity on the surface of the carotid artery; damage to the sympathetic pathway causes Horner's syndrome; sympathetic pathways in the brainstem lie adjacent to the spinothalamic tract throughout its course; Horner's syndrome due to a brainstem lesion is often associated with pain and temperature loss on the opposite side of the body.

SYMPATHOMIMETIC: mimicking the effects of impulses conveyed by adrenergic postganglionic fibers of the sympathetic nervous system; an agent that produces effects similar to those of impulses as above; called also antiadrenergic.

SYMPTOM: a manifestation of a pathological condition.

SYMPTOM VALIDITY TEST: (Lezak, 1983, pp. 621-622; Pankratz, 1979; Pankratz at al., 1975) a test to expose malingering.

S

SYNAPSE: point of functional connection between neurons; usually between axon and dendrite (axodendritic); communication between neurons are chemically mediated.

SYNAPTIC VESICLES: structures on teledendria that contain chemical transmitters.

SYNCOPE: generalized weakness of muscles, with inability to stand upright, and a loss of consciousness.

SYNDROME: a group of symptoms that occur together and constitute a recognizable condition.

SYNERGY: correlated action or cooperation on the part of two or more structures or drugs; in neurology, the faculty by which movements are properly grouped for the performance of acts requiring special adjustments.

SYNKINESIS: an associated movement; an unintentional movement accompanying a volitional movement; imitative synkinesis: an involuntary movement on the healthy side accompanying an attempt at movement on the paralyzed side; spasmodic synkinesis: a movement on the paralyzed side attending a voluntary movement on the healthy side.

SYNTACTICAL APHASIA: jargon a.

SYPHILIS: nervous system disease caused by Treponema pallidum (a spirochete); three stages: primary, secondary and syphilitic meningitis, and tertiary (neurosyphilis); also called general paresis.

SYPHILITIC POSTERIOR SPINAL SCLEROSIS: late syphilis, tabes dorsalis.

SYRINGOMYELIC SYNDROME: dissociated sensory loss occurring in a segmental distribution (normal above and below the affected segment), varying degrees of segmental amyotrophy and reflex loss; caused by lesions of central gray matter at the anterior commissure and sometimes lesions of the corticospinal, spinothalamic tracts, and posterior columns; due to a developmental abnormality in the formation of the central canal of the spinal cord, although trauma to the neck can play a part in precipitating the emergence of symptoms; may also follow complete or incomplete transection in fracture dislocation of the spinal cord; the spinal cord is enlarged with a zone of translucent gelatinous material containing clear or yellow fluid that occupies the central grey matter near the central canal, the posterolateral part of the tegmentum in the medulla; degeneration of the anterior horns of the grey matter; symptoms appear between ages 25 and 40; symptoms include either slow wasting and weakness of one hand or the loss of sensation of pain over one hand and forearm, slight signs of a corticospinal tract lesion unaccompanied by much weakness found in the lower limb on the same side, progression of symptoms to opposite limb, ocular sympathetic paralysis, dorsal kyphoscoliosis (Brain, 1985).

SYSTEMATIC REVERSAL: the patient shows the opposite side to the one requested; often associated with language skill deficiencies (Benton, 1959).

SYSTOLE: the contraction or the period of contraction, of the heart, especially that of the ventricles.

T

T: Thoracic.

TAB./tab.: tablet.

TABES: any wasting of the body; degeneration of the dorsal columns of the spinal cord and of the sensory nerve trunks, with wasting, due to infection of the central nervous system with Treponema pallidum; marked by paroxysms or crises of intense pain, incoordination, disturbances of sensation, loss of reflexes, paroxysms of functional disturbance of various organs; incontinence or retention of urine, failure of sexual power; course of disease is usually slow but progressive; complete cure is very rare; occurs mostly after middle life; more frequent in men; see tabes dorsalis, syphilis (tertiary or late), Duchenne's disease, locomotor ataxia, syphilitic posterior spinal sclerosis, Friedreich's ataxia.

TABES DORSALIS: (locomotor ataxia) 25% of persons with neurosyphilis develop these symptoms that is most often thought to be a spinal cord disease primarily. Reitan & Wolfson (1985) have found that there are also neuropsychological changes; the disease is characterized by thickening of the meninges, particularly the dorsal regions, and atrophy of the dorsal nerve roots and posterior columns.

TACHISTOSCOPE: a special instrument used in testing subjects on right- and left-brain processing of visual information; subjects are asked to fixate on a center point marked by a dot or cross. An image is flashed in one visual field for about 50 milliseconds or images are presented simultaneously in each visual field and then the accurate identification of the images is compared for each right- or left-visual field.

TACHYCARDIA: excessive rapidity in the action of the heart; the term is usually applied to a heartrate above 100 per minute and may be qualified as atrial, junctional, ventricular, or paroxysmal; atrial is usually between 160 and 190 heartbeats per minute, originating from an atrial locus.

TACTILE AGNOSIA: inability to recognize an object by touch or handling in one or both hands (not to be confused with stereoanesthesia, or astereognosis); caused by a lesion lying posterior to the

T

postcentral gyrus of the dominant parietal lobe; Brodmann's areas 5, 7, &, 37 (Brown, 1972; Hécaen & Albert, 1978).

TACTILE APHASIA: inability to name objects which are felt.

TACTILE DYSFUNCTION: Brodmann's areas 1, 2, & 3 (Semmes et al., 1960; Corkin et al., 1970).

TACTILE EXTINCTION: see tactile inattention.

TACTILE FINGER RECOGNITION TEST: (Reitan & Davison, 1974) test for finger agnosia.

TACTILE FORM RECOGNITION: Seguin-Goddard formboard test (Teuber & Weinstein, 1954).

TACTILE INATTENTION: also called tactile extinction, tactile suppression; may occur by itself or accompany visual or auditory inattention; most often occurs with right-hemisphere (particularly right parietal-lobe) damage.

TACTILE INATTENTION TESTS: points on some part of the body on each side are touched first singly and then simultaneously (double simultaneous stimulation); if the patient is experiencing left-hemisphere inattention, he will report a right-sided touch on simultaneous stimulation, although when only one side is touched, he may have no difficulty reporting it correctly; Face-Hand Test; Halstead-Reitan battery, Luria-Nebraska battery; Face-Hand Sensory Test; Quality Extinction Test.

TACTILE RECOGNITION TESTS: skin writing; fingertip Number-Writing Perception.

TACTILE SUPPRESSION: see tactile inattention; finger agnosia, object recognition by touch (stereognosis); somesthetic defects.

TALKING — ABNORMAL: right-hemisphere lesions appear to release talking; left-hemisphere lesions appear to reduce talking — especially with frontal-lobe lesions; right frontal-lobe lesioned patients make poor jokes and puns and also tell pointless stories, often liberally embellished with profanity; usually intensely amused by the stories he or she is telling and will persist even if others are ambivalent to them; lesions of the right-temporal lobe and/or parietal lobe produce talking characterized by excessive concern for their own personal lives; they often go to great lengths to rationalize their personal shortcomings, and are generally unaware that others may be bored with their talking; may show symptoms of paranoia, often being convinced that friends or family either are not supportive or are against them; excessively suspicious of neuropsychological assessments, insisting either that the assessments are unnecessary or that they would rather do them when they are "feeling better" (Lezak, 1983).

TARDIVE DYSKINESIA: impairment of the power of voluntary movement, resulting in fragmentary or incomplete movements induced by long-term administration of neuroleptics and persisting after withdrawal; lesion of putamen, striatum, caudate nucleus.

TASTE-LOSS OF (posterior third of tongue): ageusia; see also glossopharyngeal nerve (IX).

TECTOPULVINAR SYSTEM: involved primarily in locating (detection of) and tracking of visual stimuli in space; combines with the geniculostriate system in Brodmann's areas 20 and 21 where the form and content of the visual stimuli are analyzed by the geniculostriate system; projections are received along the optic nerve from the retina of the eye and go to the superior nucleus of the thalamus, and finally to areas 20 and 21 of the neocortex.

TECTOSPINAL TRACT: a group of nerve fibers, chiefly crossed, which arise mostly in the superior colliculus and descend to the cervical cord, where they lie in the anterior funiculus.

TECTUM: consists of two sets of bilaterally symmetrical nuclei — the superior colliculi (anterior) and inferior colliculi (posterior); one of two main structures in the midbrain; lies above the aqueduct; controls whole body movements to visual and auditory stimuli.

TEGMENTUM: middle part of midbrain; contains four types of structures: 1. next to the aqueduct are nuclei for some of the cranial nerves; 2. beneath these are sensory fibers coming from the body senses; 3. below these are motor fibers coming down from the forebrain; 4. intermingled among these three structures are a number of motor nuclei such as the red nucleus and substantia nigra and some of the nuclei of the reticular system; grayish upper conversion of the pedunculus (crus) cerebri; the upper and larger of the two principal parts of either crus cerebri; most important area of brainstem with respect to motivational and emotional functions: positive (pleasure); negative (fear & anger); paramount importance in determining levels of consciousness (wakefulness, arousal, attention); contains central gray (periaqueductal gray) and reticular formation.

TEGMENTUM LESIONS: interfere with voluntary upward gaze; no convergence or pupillary light reflex; tremors in multiplesclerosis; see also Wilson's disease.

TELEGRAPHIC SPEECH: omission of small words; see Broca's aphasia.

TELENCEPHALON: front or end brain; neocortex; includes the basal ganglia, limbic system, olfactory bulb, lateral ventricles.

TELODENDRIA: terminal processes of axon.

TEMPERATURE REGULATION: see anterior hypothalamus.

TEMPORAL HEMIANOPIA: hemianopia in the lateral vertical half of the visual field (nearest the temple).

TEMPORAL LOBES: all the tissue below the Sylvian fissure anterior to an imaginary line running roughly from the end of that fissure to the boundary of Brodmann's area 37 with area 19, and the boundary

T

of areas 22 and 37 with the parietal association areas 39 and 40; includes the neocortex on the lateral surface as well as the phylogenetically older cortex (archicortex and paleocortex) on the medial surface; neocortical regions include Brodmann's areas 20, 21, 22, 37, 38, 41, & 42; these areas may also be described by the three gyri that form them: Heschl's gyrus (Brodmann's areas 41 and 42), the superior-temporal gyrus (approximately Brodmann's area 22), the middle-temporal gyrus (approximately Brodmann's areas 21, 37, & 38), and the inferior-temporal gyrus (approximately Brodmann's areas 20 & 38). The older cortex includes both the cortex on the medial surface of the temporal lobe, which forms the fusiform gyrus, parahippocampal gyrus, and uncus as well as the hippocampus and amygdala, which are subcortical. The temporal lobe includes the auditory cortex, association cortex, and limbic cortex. The left and right temporal lobes are connected via the corpus callosum and anterior commissure, the neocortex through the former, and archicortex through the latter. Efferent projections go to the parietal and frontal association regions, limbic system, and basal ganglia; afferent projections received from the sensory systems; included are the primary and secondary auditory cortex, tertiary sensory cortex, as well as limbic cortex; bounded dorsally by the lateral fissure; functions include: 1. central representation of auditory and vestibular information; 2. memory function in the hippocampal gyrus; 3. visual association area; 4. central representation of taste and smell; 5. upper homonymous visual field pathways; 6. entire visual radiation at the parieto-occipital-temporal junction; 7. supplementary motor areas concerned with facial expression, eating, and emotional responses to pain and pleasure; 8. control of many aspects of behavior via frontal-lobe connections; 9. central control of visceral motility, sexual and respiratory functions.

TEMPORAL LOBE - AMYGDALA: (together with the medial cortex) influences association of affective properties with particular stimuli; (along with the hippocampus) memory.

TEMPORAL LOBE - ANTERIOR & MEDIAL: feelings of fear (Penfield, 1954).

TEMPORAL LOBE - ANTERIOR LIMBIC CORTEX LESION: approximately Brodmann's area 38; lesions of the anterior zone, including the amygdala, produce deficits in the process of associating visual stimuli with their reinforcement properties.

TEMPORAL LOBE - AUDITORY CORTEX: the primary and secondary auditory cortex are concerned with auditory sensations and auditory and visual perception, one specialized for long-term storage of sensory input, and one functioning to add affective tone to sensory input.

TEMPORAL-LOBE AUTOMATISM: psychomotor epileptic attacks;

transient global amnesia due to migraine headaches.

TEMPORAL-LOBE BOUNDARIES: The sylvian fissure separates the superior surface of each temporal lobe from the frontal and anterior parts of the parietal lobes; no definite anatomical boundary between the temporal and occipital lobes or between posterior temporal and parietal lobes; temporal lobe includes the superior, middle, and inferior temporal, fusiform, and hippocampal convolutions and the transverse convolutions of Heschl, which are the auditory receptive area present on the superior surface within the sylvian fissure; lower fibers of the geniculocalcarine pathway (from the inferior retina) swing in a wide arc over the temporal horn of the ventricle into the white matter of the temporal lobe enroute to the occipital lobes, and lesions that interrupt them characteristically produce a contralateral homonymous upper quadrant defect of visual fields. Hearing, also localized in the temporal lobes, is bilaterally represented, which accounts for the fact that unless both temporal lobes are affected, there is little or no demonstrable loss of hearing.

TEMPORAL-LOBE EPILEPSY (TLE): personality characteristics in which there is an overemphasis on trivia and the petty details of life; pedantic speech, egocentricity, perseveration on discussion of personal problems, paranoia, preoccupation with religion, and proneness to aggressive outbursts; sometimes called temporal-lobe personality with the following symptoms: altered sexual behavior, intensification of emotional reactions, an intense concern about moral and religious issues, tendency to write excessively, and sometimes aggressiveness (Pincus & Tucker, 1978); right denial of depression; display greater affect than left TLE (Bear & Fedio, 1977); left depressed; preoccupation with religious and moral ideation (Bear & Fedio, 1977).

TEMPORAL LOBE - MEDIAL CORTEX: (together with the amygdala) association of affective properties with particular stimuli; long-term memory.

TEMPORAL LOBE - TERTIARY REGION: Brodmann's areas 20, 21, 37, & 38.

TEMPORAL-LOBE LESIONS: Brodmann's areas 41, 42, & 22: disturbance of auditory sensation and perception; Brodmann's areas 20, 21, 22, 37, & 38: disturbance of selective attention of auditory and visual input; disturbance of language; Brodmann's area 21, hippocampus and possibly amygdala: impaired long-term memory; areas 21, & 38 and amygdala: altered personality and affective behavior; altered sexual behavior.

TEMPORAL-LOBE LESIONS (either side): emotional illusions such as feelings of fear, loneliness, or sorrow.

TEMPORAL-LOBE LESION, SUPERIOR GYRUS (BRODMANN'S

T

area 22): (either hemisphere); auditory illusions: sounds seem louder, fainter, more distant, or nearer.

TEMPORAL LOBE, BILATERAL EXCISION: placidity, loss of visual recognition, tendency to examine objects by touch and mouthing, and hypersexuality that is indiscriminantly directed heterosexually and homosexually and toward inanimate objects (Klüver-Bucy syndrome).

TEMPORAL-LOBE PERSONALITY: (Pincus & Tucker, 1978) pedantic speech, egocentricity, perseveration on discussion of personal problems, paranoia, preoccupation with religion, and proneness to aggressive outbursts; sometimes called temporal-lobe personality; right temporal-lobe lesioned patients are more likely to show paranoia, pedantic behavior, egocentricity, talkativeness, and perseveration on discussion of personal problems; altered sexual behavior.

TEMPORAL LOBE - POSTERIOR LESION: (approximately Brodmann's area 20) inability to discriminate and select the essential cues from a visual stimulus and maintain attention to them; (approximately Brodmann's area 21); difficulty distinguishing complex visual stimuli from one another; difficulty in forming visual memories; able to discriminate among complex visual stimuli, but unable to remember the visual image for more than a few minutes; impaired visual memory.

TEMPORAL-LOBE LESION, LEFT: deficits in verbal memory (Milner, 1967); overall drop in the number of words heard (Schulhoff & Goodglass, 1969); impaired recall of content of the right visual field (Dorff et al., 1965); usually produces impaired recall of right visual and aural input; lesion of Brodmann's area 22 (Wernicke's area): disturbance of verbal word recognition — if extreme, produces word deafness; protracted latencies in producing word associations (Jaccarino-Hiatt, 1978); does not interfere with recall of strings of digits (parietal-lobe function); (Brodmann's area 39) lesions of the superior and middle convolutions result in Wernicke's aphasia (jargon aphasia and inability to write, read, or understand the meaning of spoken words); inability to learn auditorially presented material; (Brodmann's area 22, left): disorder of language comprehension; damage to the posterior part of area 22 near Wernicke's area causes deficits in phonemic hearing so that patient confuses oppositional phonemes such as da-la, ba-pa, sa-za.

TEMPORAL-LOBE LESIONS, RIGHT: deficits in nonverbal memory (Milner, 1967); overall drop in the number of tonal sequences recognized (Schulhoff & Goodglass, 1969); impaired recall of content of both visual fields (Dorff et al., 1965); usually impaired recall of bilateral visual and aural input of stimulus; excessive talkativeness; impaired recall of nonverbal material such as geometric drawings, faces, tunes; impairment on any recall figure drawing tests such as

248

Rey Complex figure test, Bender-Gestalt, Wechsler Memory Scale; right temporal-lobe lesioned patients are more likely to show paranoia, pedantic behavior, egocentricity, talkativeness, and perseveration on discussion of personal problems; visual illusions; objects seem nearer, farther, larger, or smaller; illusions of recognition in which present experience seems either familiar (déjà vu) or strange, unreal, and dreamlike; visual hallucinations; inability to learn visually presented material.

TEMPORAL-LOBE LESIONS AND MEMORY: produce significant and often severe deficits in long-term memory; deficits are not modality-specific, as they occur to both visual and auditory material no matter how the material is initially presented or memory is assessed. The deficits are material-specific: left temporal lesions specifically impair memory for verbal material; right-temporal lesions impair memory of nonverbal material.

TEMPORAL-LOBE SEIZURES: foci in medial temporal lobe, amygdaloid nuclei, and hippocampus.

TEMPORAL ORIENTATION TEST: (Benton et al., 1964; 1983) discriminates between bilateral and unilateral frontal-lobe lesioned patients (Benton, 1968).

TEMPORAL RADIATION LESION: produces an upper congruous quadrantic homonymous hemianopia.

TEMPOROPARIETAL APHASIA: see Wernicke's aphasia.

TEMPOROPARIETAL TERTIARY ZONE: location of cognition, thought, reasoning functions.

TENSION HEADACHE TREATMENT: muscle-relaxant drugs, minor tranquilizers, application of heat to the affected muscles, and improvement of posture; avoidance of tension producing situations.

TENSOR TYMPANI: tensor muscle of the tympanic membrane; originates in the cartilaginous portion of auditory tube; enervated by the mandibular division of the trigeminal; functions to tense the tympanic membrane.

TENTH CRANIAL NERVE: vagus nerve; parasympathetic, motor, and general sensory nerve; see vagus nerve for complete description.

TENTH CRANIAL NERVE LESION: weakness of the palate may cause nasal regurgitation of food and nasal speech; paralysis of one vocal cord will allow that cord to lie permanently and limply in the midline causing hoarseness, loss of volume of voice and an inability to cough explosively (bovine cough).

TERTIARY CORTICAL ZONE - FRONTAL: prefrontal, or granular frontal, cortex; Brodmann's areas 9, 10, 45, 46, & 47; formation of intentions; most highly integrated area of function (the superstructure above all other parts of the cerebral cortex) (Luria (1973b).

TERTIARY VISUAL AREA LESION: deficit in ability to abstract function or significance of object seen.

T

TERTIARY ZONES - SENSORY (LURIA): lie on the boundary of the occipital, temporal, and parietal cortex; Brodmann's areas 5, 7, 21, 22, 37, 39, & 40; function of the tertiary zones is to integrate the excitation arriving from the different sensory systems and this sensory input is translated into symbolic processes; concrete perception translated into abstract thinking.

TESTS USED FOR NEUROPSYCHOLOGICAL EVALUATION: see neuropsychological evaluation tests/batteries.

TETRAPARESIS: muscular weakness affecting all four extremities; also see quadriparesis.

TETRAPLEGIA: paralysis affecting all four extremities; also see quadriplegia.

THALAMIC LESIONS: see Dejerine-Roussy syndrome; deep sensory loss to pinprick and touch in face, arm, and leg; may give rise to intellectual impairment associated with altered activation and arousal; may cause memory defects, atrophy of language mechanisms leading to mutism, apathy, disorientation, and confusion.

THALAMIC PAIN: see paresthesia, causalgia.

THALAMIC SYNDROME: a combination of 1. superficial persistent hemianesthesia, 2. mild hemiplegia, 3. mild hemiataxia, and more or less complete asterognosis, 4. severe and persistent pains in the hemiplegic side, 5. choreoathetoid movements in the members of the paralyzed side; also called Dejerine-Roussy s. and thalamic hyperesthetic anesthesia.

THALAMOPARIETAL PROJECTION LESION (ASSOC. AREA): astereognosis; either hemisphere.

THALAMOSTRIATE SYSTEM LESION: speech disorders, stoppage or paraphasia.

THALAMUS: two areas: ventral and dorsal thalami; principal component of the diencephalon; right and left lobes; located immediately dorsal to the hypothalamus; receives fiber projections from, and projects to, the hypothalamus, basal ganglia, midbrain, limbic system, and neocortex relays; primary sensory information projected to appropriate receiving areas of neocortex; all the special senses with the exception of olfaction (smell) have thalamic relay nuclei; relays extrapyramidal motor information between brainstem and basal ganglia and the motor and premotor areas; mediates the focal orienting reflex or arousal reaction; controls focusing of attention; mediates defensive-aggressive behavior; links areas of hypothalamus and limbic system that are involved with emotional behavior; "felt" emotion most primitively represented at thalamic level; participates in higher cognitive processes (learning, memory, etc.) through an interplay with the associational areas of the neocortex; serves both a relay function of somatosensry pathways and a modulator of ascending sensory information; three major divisions:

1. lateral geniculate nuclei which relays visual information; 2. the medial geniculate nuclei which relays auditory information; 3. the ventrobasal complex which relays sensory information traveling through the thalamus.

THALAMUS, ANTERIOR LESION: see athetosis, dystonia, cerebral palsy, Wilson's Disease, Huntington's Chorea (rigid form), postanoxic sequela, posthemiplegic states.

THALAMUS, DORSAL: see dorsal thalamus.

THALAMUS, VENTRAL: provides a general, nonspecific input into the neocortex that may modulate the activity of the neocortex.

THEMATIC APPERCEPTION TEST: a story telling task; demonstrates ability to handle sequential verbal ideas (organization, complexity, and abstractions); sensitive to frontal-lobe lesions; the organically impaired patient is more likely to give short interpretations, longer response times and pauses, concrete descriptions rather than stories or brief stories with few characters and little action, few of the most common themes, perseverative themes; may show inflexibility, expressions of self-doubt, catastrophic reactions, and difficulties in dealing with the whole picture; may show confusion, simplification or vagueness.

THERMOREGULATION: heat regulation.

THIAMINE DEFICIENCY: thought to cause damage to the dorsomedial thalamus which results in memory loss; see also Korsakoff-Wernicke disease.

THINKING: selective ordering of symbols for problem solving and capacity to reason and form sound judgments; any mental operation that relates two or more bits of information explicitly or implicitly; comparing, compounding, abstracting, ordering, reasoning (Lezak, 1983).

THINKING DISORDERS: see incoherence, flight of ideas, loose associations, blocking, poverty of ideas, and delusions.

THIRD CRANIAL NERVE: oculomotor nerve; controls levator palpebrae (eye muscles); two nerves emerge together between the cerebral peduncles; splay out as they pass anteriorly; lie between the posterior cerebral arteries and the superior cerebellar arteries, and then run parallel to the posterior communicating arteries until they enter the cavernous sinus, and then lie between the two layers of dura that form the lateral wall of the sinus; enters the orbit through the superior orbital fissure and divides into two main branches; the upper branch supplies the eyelid and superior rectus muscle; the lower branch supplies all the other eye muscles and the pupil.

THIRD NERVE LESIONS: aneurysmal dilation of the upper basilar artery may cause multiple nerve palsies and in particular bilateral third nerve lesions.

THIRD NERVE PALSY: paralysis of the eyelid; ptosis; a complete

T

third nerve lesion causes total paralysis of the eyelid and diplopia when the lid is held up; severe diplopia occurs in all directions except on lateral gaze to the side of the third nerve lesion (lateral rectus muscle intact); pupil may be normal or dilated and fixed to light.

THIRD VENTRICAL LESION: lowered cortical tone, disturbance of consciousness, possible oneiroid state, disorientation in surroundings, confabulation; may also involve the hypothalamic region, the hippocampus; to test for deficiencies produced by a third ventrical lesion: ask the patient to repeat a story with two semantic themes or give an interference test.

THIRST: controlled by the hypothalamus which mediates the medial forebrain bundle.

THIRST, LOSS OF: adipsia.

THIRST (MORBID): dipsosis.

THOUGHT: located in the left tertiary zones of the parietal lobes (Brodmann's areas 39 & 40).

THOUGHT DISORDERS: mental confusion; loose or tangential associations between ideas; impaired rate of thought production; blocking; confabulation; circumstantiality; rationalizations; flight of ideas; sometimes called derailment.

THREE-DIMENSIONAL CONSTRUCTIONAL PRAXIS TEST: (Benton, 1967); simplification and neglect of half the model are not uncommon; sensitive to right-hemisphere lesions including right frontal lobe lesions; also differentiates well between moderate left- and right-hemisphere patients where two-dimensional tasks do not.

THREE THINGS TEST: Similarities subtest; Stanford-Binet, age level XI; test of conceptual functioning.

THRESHOLD OF DEPOLARIZATION OF AXON: level of depolarization at which a nerve impulse is generated.

THROMBOCYTIN: serotonin.

THROMBOSIS: the formation of a thrombus; in the brain, usually due to a complication of infection of the scalp, skull, face, middle ear, mastoid air cells, paranasal sinuses, or nasopharynx, heart disease or failure, severe dehydration, post-traumatic states following closed-head injuries, cerebral arterial thrombosis or hemorrhage, and blood dyscrasias such as leukemia; symptoms of the superior longitudinal sinus include severe headache, seizures, hemiparesis or hemiplegia, homonymous hemianopia, dysphasia, confusion, and loss of orientation; symptoms of the cavernous sinus include fever, headache, nausea and vomiting, signs of third, fourth, sixth nerve involvement and the ophthalmic divisions of the fifth cranial nerves (Reitan & Wolfson, 1985).

THROMBUS: aggregation of blood factors, primarily platelets and fibrin; may cause vascular obstruction; see also thrombosis.

THURSTONE PRIMARY MENTAL ABILITIES TEST: average 18

year old can produce 65 written words that begin with the letter S in 5 minutes and the letter C in 4 minutes. Milner, (1964) uses a cutting score of 45 to identify fluency problems; left-frontal lobectomy patients may be significantly impaired.

THURSTONE WORD FLUENCY TEST: say or write as many words as possible begining with a given letter in five minutes, and then as many four-letter words beginning with a given letter in four minutes; patients with lesions of the prefrontal cortex will probably do poorly on this test, but patients with face-area lesions perform the worst with orbital lesioned patients performing only slightly better; left-hemisphere lesions cause the poorest performance.

THURSTONES' REASONING TESTS: Primary Mental Abilities battery (Thurstone, 1962); a deductive reasoning task as well as a conceptual sequencing test.

THYROID GLAND: controlled by the anterior pituitary; secretes thyroxin which regulates the ATP production; plays a critical role in the formation of the nervous system of the developing fetus; regulates general metabolism.

THYROID DISEASE: hyposecretion of Thyroxin in childhood results in cretinism; hyposecretion in adults leads to myxedema; hypersecretion causes symptoms that resemble mania.

THYROID DYSFUNCTION: causes cretinism; myxedema; mania-like symptoms; idiocy.

THYROTROPIC HORMONE: stimulates secretion of thyroid, secretion of the anterior pituitary gland.

THYROXIN: metabolic regulation hormone; produced by thyroid gland; hypersecretion may cause mania, hyperthyroidism, goiter; hyposecretion causes cretinism; also see hypothyroidism, myxedema.

TIA: see transient ischemic attacks.

t.i.d.: three times a day.

t.i.w.: three times a week.

TIME ESTIMATION TASK: (Benton et al., 1964) sensitive to brain-damage; manic patients often will underestimate the passage of time during a mental status exam.

TIME AGNOSIA: loss of comprehension of the succession and duration of events.

TIME ORIENTATION TESTS: date and time of day, appreciation of temporal continuity; Temporal Orientation Test; Temporal Disorientation Questionnaire; Time Estimation Test; Discrimination of Recency task.

TINNITUS: a noise in the ears, as ringing, buzzing, roaring, clicking, etc.; see also cerebello-pontine angle lesions, auditory-vestibular nerve (VIII), cochlea.

TNS: Transcutaneous neuronal stimulation.

TODD'S PARALYSIS: see motor epilepsy.

T

TOKEN TEST: (Boller & Vignolo, 1966; De Renzi & Vignolo, 1962) assesses language comprehension (aphasia test); simple to administer; sensitive to the disrupted linguistic processes that are central to the aphasic disability; also involves immediate memory span for verbal sequences and capacity to use syntax (Lesser, 1976); can identify those brain-damaged patients whose other disabilities may be masking a concomitant aphasic disorder or whose symbolic processing problems are relatively subtle and not readily recognizable; not useful for severe aphasic conditions (Wertz, 1979); a few nonaphasic patients may perseverate on the Token Test as a result of conceptual inflexibility or an impaired capacity to execute a series of commands (Lezak, 1982b).

TONGUE: see glossopharyngeal nerve (IX), hypoglossal nerve (XII).

TONGUE WEAKNESS: see twelfth cranial nerve (hypoglossal).

TONGUE, DEVIATION TO SIDE OF LESION ON PROTRUSION: see hypoglossal nerve (XII).

TONGUE, WASTING OF: see hypoglossal nerve (XII).

TONE DEAFNESS: amusia.

TONIC INNERVATION: inability to relax a voluntary movement.

TONIC STAGE: (major motor seizures) stiffening of body muscles/ rigidity.

TONIC-CLONIC EPILEPSY: see Grand Mal epilepsy.

TOPOGRAPHICAL LOCALIZATION TEST: (Lezak, 1983) sensitive to diffuse brain-damage and right-sided lesions.

TOPOGRAPHICAL ORIENTATION: memory for familiar routes or locations in space; impairment of ability to retrieve established visuospatial knowledge (Benton, 1969a); inability to perform tasks; may involve visuographic disabilities, unilateral spatial inattention, a global memory disorder, or a confusional state (Lezak, 1983); Brodmann's areas 18 & 19.

TORSION: also see dystonia; related to athetosis, differing only in that the larger axial muscles (trunk and limb girdles) are involved; results in bizarre, grotesque movements and position of body.

TORTICOLLIS: see spasmodic torticollis.

TOUCH DYSFUNCTION: see astereognosis.

TOURETTE'S DISEASE: see Gilles de la Tourette's Disease.

TOXIC CONFUSIONAL STATES: may be due to drug overdose or idiosyncratic reactions to drugs; pneumonia may cause confusion as a result of hypoxia, fever, or general toxicity; other causes include congestive cardiac failure, uremia, liver failure, meningitis, subarachnoid hemorrhage, or hypoglycemia; see also alcohol withdrawal (delirium tremens); alcohol hallucinosis.

TPR: temperature, pulse, respiration.

TRACHEOSTOMY: the surgical creation of an opening into the trachea through the neck, with the tracheal mucosa being brought into continuity with the skin; also, the opening so created; the term is also used by some to refer to a tracheotomy done for insertion of a tube.

TRACHEOTOMY: the incision of the trachea through the skin and muscles of the neck.

TRACING, TAPPING, AND DOTTING: (MacQuarrie Test for Mechanical Ability Subtests) sensitive to impairments in fine motor regulation; may show motor slowing; test of frontal-lobe functioning.

TRACKING (OCULAR): occipital lobe.

TRACT: large collection of axons grouped together; also called fiber pathway or commissure.

TRACTS (cerebral): see inferior occipital frontal tract, uncinate tract, superior occipital frontal tract, superior longitudinal tract, inferior longitudinal tract, cingulum, corpus callosum, arcuate fibers, inferior longitudinal tract, anterior commissure.

TRACKING (mental): sustained attention to a stimulus or concentration on a direct train of thought.

TRAIL MAKING TEST: a paper and pencil test of visual conceptual and visuomotor tracking; highly sensitive to brain-damage (Armitage, 1946; Reitan, 1958; Spreen & Benton, 1965); sensitive to aging (Davies, 1968; Harley et al., 1980; Lindsey & Coppinger, 1969); scores on Part A which are much less than Part B scores suggest difficulties in complex simultaneous conceptual tracking; slow scores on one or both Parts A & B are highly suggestive of brain-damage; brain-damaged patients may show problems in motor slowing, incoordination, visual scanning, poor motivation, or conceptual confusion; visual scanning and tacking problems suggested by this test may demonstrate how the patient responds to sequential stimuli, double tracking (Eson et al., 1978), or flexibility in shifting sets (Pontius & Yudowitz, 1980).

TRAIL MAKING TEST-PART B: low scores may suggest an inability to shift sets; or faulty double simultaneous tracking; particularly sensitive to frontal-lobe dysfunction.

TRANSCORTICAL ALEXIA: reading without comprehension; usually associated with transcortical sensory aphasia or recovering Wernicke's aphasia.

TRANSCORTICAL APHASIA: caused by a lesion of a pathway between the speech center and other cortical centers; may be either motor aphasia or sensory aphasia or a combination of both; may be caused by extensive crescent shaped infarcts within borderzones between major cerebral vessels or within the frontal-lobe between the anterior and cerebral arteries; *transcortical sensory aphasia*: lesion is located in the posterior borderzone; some causes include anoxia, decreased cerebral circulation from cardiac arrest, occlusion or significant stenosis of the carotid artery, anoxia due to carbon monoxide poisoning; spontaneous speech is restricted, may be fluent,

T

but paraphasic speech (Wernicke's a.); comprehension impaired, repetition intact, naming intact; may be able to repeat words but unable to comprehend what is heard or repeated; presumed to be caused by loss of the secondary sensory cortex (association cortex). Comprehension could be poor because words fail to arouse associations. Production of meaningful speech could be poor because even though the the production of words is normal, words are not associated to other cognitive activity in the brain (Kolb & Whishaw, 1980); also called isolation syndrome; *transcortical motor aphasia*: intact repetition of spoken language, but disruption of other language functions; able to repeat, and read well; restricted spontaneous speech — like Broca's aphasia;

TRANSCUTANEOUS NEURONAL STIMULATION: a method of treating intractable pain with electrical stimulation.

TRANSFERENCE: unconscious transfer to someone in present day life of feelings and attitudes that were originally attached to important persons in one's early life.

TRANSIENT BRAINSTEM ISCHEMIC ATTACKS: most likely to affect the medulla; symptoms include vertigo, dysarthria, and tingling around the mouth suggesting central medullary dysfunction; *at pontine level*: vertigo, hearing abnormalities, tingling, numbness or weakness of the limbs and diplopia; *mesencephalic level*: diplopia, sudden loss of consciousness, weakness of limbs and subsequently transient hemianopia if the calcarine cortex becomes involved.

TRANSIENT ISCHEMIC ATTACKS: (TIA) repeated identical brief episodes of hemiparesis with full recovery; may be a sign of an impending stroke; episodic encephalomalacia; cerebral vascular insufficiency; onset often abrupt, frequently occuring as fleeting sensations of giddiness or impaired consciousness; last between a few minutes and 24 hours; if neurological deficits persist for more than 24 hours, they are customarily called vascular infarcts; of the carotid system recurring attacks of symptoms involving only one eye, such as dimness of vision or complete blindness due to diminution of blood flow in the ophthalmic artery on the same side as the involved eye; may have various degrees of homonymous hemianopia, hemiparesis, and hemihypesthesia on the side opposite the diseased carotid artery; transient dysphasia or losses in ability to deal with spatial configurations (Reitan & Wolfson, 1985); vertebral-basilar system: most often in the elderly; occurrence varies from several times a day to several months; occipital headaches, dimness of vision or transient blindness, the experience of "flashing lights" and sometimes homonymous visual field defects; brainstem symptoms, including diplopia, ptosis, facial weakness, tinnitus, vertigo, nausea and vomiting, dysphagia, slurring of speech, and feelings of numbness, especially around the mouth; cerebellar dysfunction, including ataxia; when vertebral arteries are involved, patient may suddenly collapse without loss of consciousness; frequently precede cerebral infarction or myocardial infarcts (Reitan & Wolfson, 1985).

TANSIENT ISCHEMIC ATTACKS - COGNITIVE DEFICITS: slowing and tracking suggestive of bilateral or diffuse brain-damage and focal deficits indicating that lateralized damage had occurred in those areas in which blood flow is most commonly disrupted by stroke (Delaney et al., 1980).

TRANSIENT GLOBAL AMNESIA: (Fisher & Adams, 1958) sudden and transient loss of memory; onset sudden and includes both retrograde and anterograde amnesia, without apparent precipitating cause; most probable explanation: vascular interruption in the territory of the posterior cerebral artery, by either a transient ischemic attack or an embolism.

TRANSVERSE TEMPORAL GYRI: see gyri temporalis transversi.

TRAUMATIC AMNESIA: (posttraumatic amnesia) head injuries commonly produce a form of amnesia; severity of injury determines the characteristics of the amnesia; retrograde amnesia generally shrinks over time, frequently leaving a residual retrograde amnesia of only a few seconds to a minute for events immediately preceding the injury; usually an additional period of posttraumatic amnesia (PTA) (i. e., anterograde amnesia) as well; duration of PTA varies and may end quite sharply, often after a period of natural sleep (Whitty & Zangwill, 1966).

TRAUMATIC BRAIN INJURIES: the brain may be injured by any blow to the head (with or without skull fracture), penetrating head wounds, compound fractures; may result in direct damage to the brain, such as a gunshot wound in which neurons and support cells are damaged directly, disruption of blood supply resulting in ischemia, necrosis, and/or infarction, or infection as a result of penetrating head injuries or compound fractures. Head trauma can produce scarring of brain tissue which becomes a focus for later epileptic seizures; see also penetrating head trauma, acceleration/deceleration head trauma, concussion, cerebral contusion, cerebral laceration, cerebral compression.

TREMOR: more or less regular rhythmic oscillations of a part of the body around a fixed point; usually involves the distal part of the limbs, the head, tongue, or jaw; see Parkinson's disease, alcohol withdrawal, extrapyramidal reaction, akasthisia; afferent disorder.

TREMOR-AT-REST: alternating movements of one or both of the distal limbs when at rest, but which stop during voluntary movements or during sleep; seen in Parkinson's disease and extrapyramidal reaction to neuroleptic drugs.

TRIGEMINAL NERVE (V): conveys sensation from the face and provides the motor supply to the muscles of mastication; splits into three

T

divisions: ophthalmic, maxillary, mandibular (a large area over the angle of the jaw is supplied by nerve roots C2 and C3).

TRIGEMINAL NERVE LESION: see brainstem lesions.

TRIGEMINAL SENSORY SYSTEM: information from the right side of the face enters the brainstem in the fifth nerve at mid-pontine level. Fibers subserving the corneal reflex and simple tactile sensation enter the nucleus of the fifth nerve in the pons, and decussate at mid-pontine level to the opposite side of the pons. Fibers subserving pain and temperature sensation descend parallel to the descending nucleus of cranial nerve V and enter it to relay to the opposite side in the lower medulla and upper cervical cord; the crossed fibers become the secondary ascending tract of cranial nerve V (the quinto-thalamic tract), lying adjacent to the medial lemniscus throughout the brainstem.

TRIGEMINAL SENSORY SYSTEM LESION: a lesion in the dorso-lateral medulla on the left will cause numbness of the left side of the face and numbness of the right side of the body. The crossed sensory loss is typical of a dorsolateral brainstem lesion, between mid-pontine level and C2.

TRISOMY 21: see Down's Syndrome.

TROCHLEAR NERVE: (IV) controls eye movement, upward & downward; originates just inferior to those of the oculomotor nerves, along with the abducens nerves; fibers from each side decussate across the median plane and emerge from the back of the brainstem below the corresponding inferior colliculus; runs forward in lateral wall of cavernous sinus, traverses the superior orbital fissure; enervates superior oblique and the external rectus muscles.

TROPIC HORMONES: effect targeted at other endocrine glands.

TRUE HEMIANOPIA: hemianopia in one vertical half of each eye; usually due to a single lesion of the optic tract, at or above the level of the chiasm.

TRUNCAL ATAXIA OF BRUNS: inability to stand because of decomposition of gait and upright stance; wide base, flexed posture, and small shuffling steps.

TRYPANOSOMIASIS: see hypersomnia.

T-SCORES: derived scores; mean of 50; standard deviation of 10.

TSH: thyrotropin; thyroid stimulating hormone secreted by the adenohypophysis.

TTH: thyrotropic hormone, secreted by the anterior pituitary gland.

TUMOR: a new growth of tissue in which the multiplication of cells is uncontrolled and progressive; see also neoplasm, glioma, meningioma, metatastic, medulloblastoma, glioblastoma, astrocytoma.

TUMOR-BRAIN: symptoms may include heachache, vomiting, swelling of the optic disc (papilledema), slowing of the heart rate (bradycardia), mental dullness, double vision (diplopia), and convulsions;

other symptoms will be location related; treatment is usually surgical; chemotherapy may not be successful because of the difficulty in getting drugs passed the blood-brain barrier; see also under specific types of tumor.

TUMOR (ASTROCYTOMA): a glioma tumor resulting from the growth of astrocytes and is usually slow growing; accounts for about 40% of the gliomas; most common in adults over age 30; not very malignant; prognosis usually good; sometimes over a 20 year survival.

TUMOR (GLIOBLASTOMA): highly malignant, rapidly growing tumor; most common in adults, especially males, over 35; accounts for roughly 30% of gliomas; results from the sudden growth of spongioblasts, cells that are ordinarily formed only during development of the brain; life expectancy beyond surgery is seldom beyond one year.

TUMOR (GLIOMA): general term for those brain tumors that arise from glial cells and infiltrate the brain substance; roughly 45% of all brain tumors are gliomas; range from relatively benign to highly malignant; frequently occurring types: astrocytomas, glioblastomas, and medulloblastomas.

TUMOR (MEDULLOBLASTOMA): highly malignant tumors that are found almost exclusively in cerebellum of children; account for about 11% of gliomas; results from the growth of germinal cells that infiltrate the crebellum or underlying brainstem; prognosis is poor; postoperative survival 1 1/2 to 2 years.

TUMOR (MENINGIOMA): a hard, slow growing, usually vascular tumor which occurs mainly along the meningeal vessels and superior longitudinal sinus, invading the dura and skull and leading to erosion and thinning of the skull.

TUMOR (METASTATIC): a tumor that has become established by a transfer of tumor cells from some other region of the body, most commonly lung and breast; usually multiple; treatment is complicated and prognosis poor.

TUMOR (NEOPLASM): a mass of new tissue that persists and grows independently of its surrounding structures and that has no physiologic use; tumors grow from either glia or other support cells; tumors account for a relatively high proportion of neurological disease; no region of the brain is immune to tumor formation; may be benign or malignant, encapsulated or infiltrating; may destroy normal cells and occupy their space or surround existing cells and interfere with their normal functioning; account for high proportion of neurological disease; may be encapsulated (distinct entity in the brain) and produce pressure on the rest of the brain; often cystic (fluid-filled cavity in the brain, lined with tumor cells).

TURNER'S SYNDROME: a genetic syndrome characterized by short stature, undifferentiated (streak) gonads, and variable abnormalities that may include webbing of neck, low posterior hair line, increased carrying angle of elbow, cubitus valgus, and cardiac defects; associate with a defect or absence of the second sex chromosome (X0 instead of XY); phenotype is female; intellectual deficits include lower spatial abilities and average verbal abilities.

TWELFTH CRANIAL NERVE: (hypoglossal nerve) motor nerve to the tongue; originates from several rootlets in the anterolateral sulcus between the olive and the pyramid of the medulla oblongata; passes through the hypoglossal canal to the tongue; unilateral damage to the nerve supply leads to wasting, weakness, and fasciculation of that side of the tongue; if the tongue is protruded the muscle on the weak side cannot balance the forward push of the muscle on the intact side, and as a result the tongue deviates towards the weak side.

TWINKLING OR PUSATING LIGHTS: a symptom of a lesion or seizure of lateral surface of occipital lobes (Brodmann's areas 18 & 19).

TWO THINGS TEST: Similarities subtests; Stanford-Binet, Age level VII; test of conceptual functioning.

TWO-POINT DISCRIMINATION TEST: tests the somatosensory function; parietal-lobe dysfunction; lesion is most often in the postcentral gyrus which controls the contralateral side of the body.

Tx: abreviation for treatment.

U

U: units.

UA: urinalysis.

UE: upper extremities.

UNCAL SEIZURES (or amygdala seizures): typically cause brief olfactory or gustatory hallucinations; usually unpleasant like rotting cabbage or burning rubber; may involve lip smacking, chewing movements; involuntary defecation; also known as uncinate attacks.

UNCINATE FASCICULUS: long cerebral association fiber bundle; a collection of association fibers which interconnect the cortex of the orbital surface of the frontal lobe with the parahippocampal gyrus and perhaps with the amygdala; other temporofrontal connections probably also exist.

UNCINATE EPILEPSY/SEIZURE: dreamy state, olfactory or gustatory hallucinations, and masticatory movements.

UNCUS: the medial curved anterior end of the parahippocampal gyrus; see also uncinate fasciculus.

UNDERSHOOTING GOAL: see hypometria, dysmetria, cerebellar disease.

UNILATERAL: one sided.

UNILATERAL ANESTHESIA: see hemianesthesia.

UNILATERAL DISEASE - PARIETAL LOBE: (right or left) cortical sensory syndrome and sensory extinction (or total hemianesthesia with large acute lesions of white matter); mild unilateral hemiparesis; muscular atrophy in children; homonymous hemianopia or visual inattention, and sometimes anosognosia, neglect of one-half of the body and of extrapersonal space; abolition of opticokinetic nystagmus to one side.

UNILATERAL DISEASE - PARIETAL LOBE (DOMINANT SIDE): disorders of language (especially alexia); Gerstmann's syndrome; bimanual astereognosis (tactile agnosia); bilateral apraxia of the ideomotor type.

UNILATERAL DISEASE - PARIETAL LOBE (NONDOMINANT): dressing apraxia; constructional apraxia; misidentification of opposite arm and leg; bland mood; indifference to illness.

UNILATERAL DISEASE - TEMPORAL LOBE (DOMINANT): homonymous quadrantanopia; Wernicke's aphasia; impairment in verbal tests of material presented through auditory sense; dysnomia or amnesic aphasia.

UNILATERAL DISEASE - TEMPORAL LOBE (NONDOMINANT): homonymous quadrantanopia; impairment of mental function with inability to judge spatial relationships in some cases; impairment in nonverbal tests of visually presented material.

UNILATERAL HEMIANOPIA: hemianopia in half of the visual field of one eye only.

UNILATERAL PREFRONTAL LESIONS: less debilitating than bifrontal lesions with little or no effect on certain tasks.

UNILATERAL SPATIAL NEGLECT: right parietal-lobe plus occipital-lobe damage; also see visual inattention.

UPPER HEMIANOPIA: hemianopia in the upper half of the visual field.

UPPER NEURON LESION (7TH NERVE): see seventh nerve lesion; causes paralysis of the lower face.

UPWARD GAZE IMPAIRMENT: under-activity of the basal ganglia; early sign of parkinsonism and Huntington's chorea; attempted upward gaze may cause jerky vertical nystagmus due to weakness of the movement; also see oculargyral crisis.

UREMIC POISONING: result of kidney failure; progressive development of lethargy, apathy, and cognitive dysfunction with accompanying loss of sense of well-being as the uremic conditon develops (Lishman, 1978; Yager, 1973); attentional deficits that interfere with performance on memory tasks and impaired performance on several different visual perceptual tasks (Beniak, 1977) which do not

V

always improve following dialysis.

URI: upper respiratory infection.

URINARY INCONTINENCE: the cortical center for micturition is in the second frontal gyrus located on the medial surface of the frontal lobe; if urinary incontinence occurs along with intellectual decline, a frontal lesion might be in progress.

URINATION: micturition.

USE OF OBJECTS TESTS: (Christensen, 1979; Luria, 1966, 1973a); *face*: blow out match, suck on a straw; *arms*: brush teeth, hammer nail, cut paper, flip coin; *legs*: kick ball, put out cigarette with foot; body: swing baseball bat, sweep with broom; distinguishes convergent thinking from divergent thinking; Test for Mental Inflexibility (Zangwill, 1966); a frontal-lobe lesioned patient tends to elaborate on the main or conventional use of an object, often failing to think up other, less probable uses (Getzels & Jackson, 1962).

UTRICLE/UTRICULUS: the larger of the two divisions of the membranous labyrinth, located in the posterosuperior region of the vestibule; major organ of the vestibular system which gives information about the position and movements of the head.

V

VA: visual acuity; Veteran's Administration.

VAGINISMUS: painful spasm of the vagina due to local hyperesthesia; may be mental as a result of extreme aversion to coitus by the female, attended with contraction of the muscles when the act is attempted.

VAGUS NERVE (cranial nerve X): a parasympathetic, visceral afferent, motor, and general sensory nerve which supplies sensory fibers to the ear, tongue, pharynx, and larynx; supplies motor fibers to the pharynx, larynx, and esophagus, and parasympathetic and visceral afferent fibers to the thoracic and abdominal viscera; controls the heart, blood vessels, viscera, and movement of larynx and pharynx; originates by numerous rootlets from the lateral side of the medulla oblongata in the groove between the olive and the inferior cerebellar peduncle which descend through the jugular foramen; superior and an inferior ganglion; continues through the neck and thorax into the abdomen.

VALIDITY: the degree to which a test measures what it is intended to measure.

VASCULITIS: inflammation of blood vessels.

VASOCONSTRICTION: the diminution of the caliber of vessels, especially constriction of arterioles leading to decreased blood flow to a part.

V

VASOCONSTRICTION: the diminution of the caliber of vessels, especially constriction of arterioles leading to decreased blood flow to a part.

VASOPRESSIN: a hormone manufactured by the supraoptic nucleus in the hypothalamus and stored in the posterior pituitary gland; suppresses urination and increases blood pressure; also prepared synthetically or obtained from the posterior lobe of the pituitary of domestic animals, and is used, in solution, for injection as an antidiuretic; also called antidiuretic hormone (ADH).

V. D.: venereal disease.

V. D. G.: venereal disease — gonorrhea.

VDRL: sometimes used to indicate a blood test for syphilis; actually stands for Venereal Disease Research Laboratories.

V. D. S.: venereal disease — syphilis.

VEGETATIVE NERVOUS SYSTEM: autonomic nervous system.

VEGETATIVE STATE: see locked-in syndrome.

VENTRAL: toward the base of the brain or the belly side of an animal; opposite of dorsal; pertaining to the front (anterior) portion of the body.

VENTRAL ROOT: the area of the spinal cord from which motor neurons leave enroute to a muscle.

VENTRAL THALAMUS: provides a general, nonspecific input into the neocortex that may modulate the activity of the neocortex.

VENTRICULAR NUCLEI: the nuclear group in the thalamus containing several of the ventral nuclei of the nuclei laterales thalami; see also athetosis, dystonia, cerebral palsy, Wilson's Disease, Huntington's chorea (rigid form), postanoxic state, posthemiplegic states.

VENTRICLES: see cerebral ventricles.

VENTRICULO-VENUS SHUNT: see shunt.

VENTRICULOATRIOSTOMY: surgical creation of a passage by means of subcutaneously placed catheters with a one-way valve, permitting drainage of cerebrospinal fluid from a cerebral ventricle to the right atrium by way of the jugular vein; performed for relief of hydrocephalus.

VENTRICULOGRAPHY: x-ray after air or opaque medium is introduced into the ventricle through a cannula inserted through the skull; chiefly used when there is an increase in intracranial pressure and when other procedures have not proven enlightening.

VENTRICULOSTOMY: a surgical procedure to establish a free communication between the floor of the third ventricle and the underlying cisterna interpeduncularis; for the treatment of hydrocephalus.

VENTROBASAL COMPLEX: an area in the thalamus believed to transmit pressure information to primary and secondary somatosensory areas of the parietal lobe.

V

VENTROMEDIAL CORTICOSPINAL TRACT: pyramidal tract; arises chiefly in the sensorimotor regions of the cerebral cortex and descends in the internal capsule, cerebral peduncle, and pons to the medulla oblongata; most of the fibers cross in the decussation of the pyramids and descend in the spinal cord as the lateral pyramidal (lateral corticospinal) tract; most of the uncrossed fibers form the anterior pyramidal (anterior corticospinal) tract; synapse with internuncial and motor neurons.

VENTROMEDIAL MOTOR SYSTEM: controls movements of the body and the proximal portion of the limbs bilaterally.

VENTROMEDIAL NUCLEI: a pair of nuclei in the hypothalamus believed to play a role in the regulation of eating behavior; see also satiety center.

VENTROMEDIAL SYSTEM LESION: patients walk with a narrow-based gait, veering off target, bump into things; distal parts of the limbs and hands are less impaired; flexion of the head, limbs, and trunk; impaired ability to achieve upright posture, difficulty in moving the body or in moving the limbs at the proximal joints.

VERBAL ABSURDITIES SUBTEST: (Stanford-Binet) may be used to assess impairments in the ability to evaluate and integrate all elements of a problem; test of reasoning and judgment.

VERBAL AND WRITTEN MATH TEST - EXAMPLES: (Strub & Black, 1977, mental status examination) inability to respond correctly to the simplest and automatic levels such as addition, division, and multiplication suggests an impairment in symbol formulation characteristic of aphasic disorders or a severe breakdown in conceptual functions; more complex math operations, such as carrying, test the immediate memory span, attention, and mental tracking functions.

VERBAL APHASIA: Broca's aphasia, ataxic a, frontocortical a.

VERBAL COMPREHENSION TESTS: Token test; Peabody Picture Test; Quick Test.

VERBAL DEFICITS S/P DIFFUSE HEAD INJURY: following a period of recovery, verbal tests that measure overlearned material or behaviors such as culturally common information and reading, writing, and speech may appear close to premorbid levels (Lezak, 1983) impairment in word retrieval (dysnomia) may continue (Levin et al., 1981).

VERBAL FLUENCY: impairments in speed and ease of verbal production may change the ability to produce words in uninterrupted strings following brain injury; reduced verbal productivity accompanies most aphasic disabilities, but it does not necessarily signify the presence of aphasia (Lezak, 1983); impaired verbal fluency is also associated with frontal-lobe damage, particularly the left frontal-lobe anterior to Broca's area (Milner, 1967; Ramier & Hécaen, 1970;

Tow, 1955); fluency problems may show up in speech, reading, and writing (Perret, 1974; Taylor, 1979).

VERBAL FLUENCY DISORDER: low verbal fluency may be associated with word-finding difficulty, or may occur in the absence of any other language disturbances; dominant frontal-lobe lesions may reduce word output even though no other deficits in language use or production are known.

VERBAL MEMORY TEST: Wechsler Memory Scale (Logical Stories & Paired Associates subtests).

VERBAL PARAPHASIA: faulty word selection.

VERBAL REASONING: a category of thinking that may involve the ordering, comparing, analyzing, and synthesizing words (Lezak, 1983).

VERMIS: (cerebelli) the median part of the cerebellum between the two hemispheres.

VERNET'S SYNDROME: paralysis of the 9th, 10th, and 11th cranial nerves due to a lesion in the region of the jugular foramen; paralysis of the superior constriction of the pharynx and difficulty in swallowing solids; paralysis of the soft palate and fauces with anesthesia of these parts and of the pharynx; loss of taste in the posterior third of the tongue; paralysis of the vocal cords and anesthesia of the larynx; paralysis of the sternocleidomastoid and trapezius muscles; also called jugular foremen syndrome.

VERTEBRA: any of the thirty-three bones of the spinal column, comprising the seven cervical, twelve thoracic, five lumbar, five sacral, and four coccygeal vertebrae.

VERTEBROBASILAR ARTERIAL SYSTEM: supplies all the structures in the posterior fossa, and through the posterior cerebral arteries, the visual cortex on both sides (Brain, 1985).

VERTEBROBASILAR ARTERY NARROWING: transitory attacks of hemianopia or complete cortical blindness; ophthalmoplegia may lead to diplopia, vertigo, nystagmus, symptoms and signs of involvement of one or both corticospinal tracts, and of the long ascending sensory pathways on one or both sides; cerebellar symptoms may occur; paroxysmal symptoms of vertigo, drop attacks, and syncope may be precipitated by head movement; coma may result from large lesions (Brain, 1985); see also subclavian "steal" syndrome.

VERTICAL GAZE IMPAIRMENT: under-activity of the basal ganglia; often found in elderly persons.

VERTICAL HEMIANOPIA: defective vision or blindness in a lateral half of the visual field.

VERTIGIOUS SENSATIONS: a sensation of revolving caused by a lesion in the superior posterior temporal region or at the junction between the parietal and temporal lobes; may be accompanied by auditory sensations.

V

VERTIGO: feeling of whirling or rotation, as well as nonrotatory swaying, weakness, faintness, and light headedness; patient may have an illusion of movement as if the external world were revolving around the patient or as if the patient were revolving in space; sometimes erroneously used as a synonym for dizziness; may be caused by a lesion in the superior posterior temporal region or at the junction between the parietal and temporal lobes, from diseases of the inner ear, or disturbances of the vestibular centers or pathways in the CNS; common symptom of brainstem vascular disease (ischemic attacks); major causes: benign positional vertigo; vestibular neuronitis; Meniere's disease; migraine; multiple sclerosis; temporal-lobe epilepsy; may also be caused by drugs and alcohol as a side effect; see also Meniere's disease, eighth nerve lesion.

VESICLES: tiny structures in the axonal endings which contain the chemical transmitter released during synaptic transmission.

VESTIBULAR NERVE: carries nerve impulses from the sensory receptors of the vestibular system to the brainstem; part of the eighth cranial nerve which is concerned with equilibrium, consisting of fibers that arise from bipolar cells in the vestibular ganglion and divide peripherally into a superior and inferior part, with receptors in the semicircular canals, utricle, and saccule.

VESTIBULAR NERVE TUMOR: see Cerebello-Pontine angle lesions; decerebrate functioning.

VESTIBULAR SYSTEM: cranial nerve VIII; vestibular receptors in the middle ear: 1. saccule signals when the head is oriented in the normal position; and, 2. utricle signals changes in orientation; upright posture of the head and body is probably maintained by the saccule or its motor nuclei in the hindbrain; part of this system's function is to maintain and adjust posture; probably mediated by the macula and its motor nuclei; branch of the auditory nerve which is solely concerned with sensing movement and maintaining posture.

VIGILANCE: wakefulness; watchfulness; arousal; normal vigilance requires sustained attention to tasks; hypervigilance may be present in paranoid disorders (including schizophrenia), RAS dysfunction and frontal-lobe dysfunctions; testing of vigilance may be performed by presentation of sequential stimuli verbally or paper and pencil test over an extended period of time with instructions for the patient to identify a target stimulus (Diller et al., 1974; Franz, 1970; Strub & Black, 1977); see Cancellations Tests; sensitive to general response slowing, inattentiveness of diffuse brain-damage, acute brain syndromes, or specific defects of response shifting, motor smoothness, or unilateral spatial neglect; sensitive to right-hemisphere spatial neglect, and left-hemisphere temporal processing of information.

VILLARET'S SYNDROME: unilateral paralysis of the 9th, 10th, 11th,

& 12th cranial nerves and sometimes the 7th due to a lesion in the retroparotid space, and characterized by paralysis of the superior constriction of the pharynx and difficulty in swallowing solids; paralysis of soft palate and fauces with anesthesia of these parts and of the pharynx; loss of taste in the posterior third of the tongue; paralysis of the vocal cords and anesthesia of the larynx; paralysis of the sternocleidomastoid and trapezius muscles; and paralysis of the cervical sympathetic nerves (Horner's Syndrome).

VINELAND SOCIAL MATURITY SCALE: (Doll, 1953; 1965) a check list that assesses social-adaptive behavior of normal adults, children, and infants; measures general self-help, self-help in eating, self-help in dressing, self-direction, occupation, communication, locomotion, and socialization; yields a Social Age Score.

VIOLENCE /RAGE: see amygdala, TLE, sham rage.

VIRAL ENCEPHALITIDES: a group of diseases in which there is direct invasion of the CNS and the meninges by any of a large number of viruses; two distinct syndromes: aseptic meningitis and encephalitis (Gilroy & Meyer, 1979); see also slow virus infections; most common viruses are Coxsackie B, mumps, ECHO, and lymphocytic choriomeningitis, mosquito-borne viruses, tick-borne viruses, rabies, poliomyelitis, Coxsackie A, herpes simplex, herpes zoster, measles, encephalomyocarditis, infectious mononucleosis, influenza, infectious hepatitis (see Reitan & Wolfson, 1985 for descriptions).

VIRAL INFECTIONS (CEREBRAL): may be caused by either neurotropic or pantropic viruses; diseases such as rabies and poliomyelitis usually produce nonspecific lesions affecting widespread regions of the brain.

VIRUS: an encapsulated aggregate of nucleic acid that may be made up of either DNA or RNA; may be either neurotropic or pantropic.

VISCERA: plural of viscus.

VISCERAL DISTURBANCE - INDEFINITE: see Vagus nerve (X).

VISCERAL SENSATIONS - PRESEIZURE OF THORAX, EPIGASTRIUM, AND ABDOMEN: seizure discharge located in upper bank of Sylvian fissure or upper intermediate or medial frontal areas near cingulate gyrus.

VISCUS: any large interior organ in any one of the three great cavities of the body, especially the abdomen; plural: viscera.

VISION: Brodmann's area 17 (primary); areas 18 & 19 (secondary); areas 5, 7, 21, 22, 37, 39 & 40 (tertiary).

VISUAL AGNOSIAS: see apperceptive visual agnosia; associative visual agnosia; simultaneous agnosia; simultanagnosia; color agnosia, visual object agnosia, visual agnosia for drawing, prosopagnosia (agnosia for faces), color agnosia (achromatopsia), color anomia, color agnosia, visual spatial agnosias.

VISUAL AGNOSIA: patient is able to see but cannot recognize objects

V

unless they hear, smell, taste, or palpatate them; inability to combine individual visual impressions into complete patterns, thus, the inability to recognize objects or their pictorial representations; unable to draw or copy objects; defect in perception resulting from damage to a gnostic area; random eye movements; may be caused by lesions to Brodmann's areas 5, 7, & 37 (Brown, 1972; Hécaen & Albert, 1978), left calcarine cortex combined with interruption of secondary and tertiary visual cortical areas (Brodmann's areas 18 & 19), angular gyrus of dominant hemisphere, left calcarine cortex combined with interruption of fibers crossing from the right occipital lobe; see also visual object agnosia, visual agnosia for drawing, prosopagnosia (agnosia for faces), color agnosia (achromatopsia), color anomia, color agnosia, visual spatial agnosias.

VISUAL AGNOSIA (associative): can recognize objects and demonstrate their use, but cannot name them or describe them; visual perception demonstrated by simple visual matching tests: ask patient to verbally identify common objects presented visually. If the patient fails to identify visually, allow manual manipulation; if identification is made manually, the visual system is involved; if the patient cannot describe or name the object, the lesion causing the agnosia is usually an infarct that destroys the left occipital lobe and the posterior corpus callosum; alexia without agraphia may also be present.

VISUAL AGNOSIA FOR DRAWING: impaired ability to recognize drawn stimuli, including realistic representations of simple objects, complex scenes, schematic reproductions of objects, geometric figures, meaningless forms, incomplete figures, and abstract drawings; lesion is most likely located in the secondary and tertiary visual cortex (Brodmann's areas 18 through 21 in either hemisphere, although lesions in the right hemisphere may be more damaging.

VISUAL ALLESTHESIA: illusory displacement of images from one side of the visual field to the other.

VISUAL AND AUDITORY INPUT SELECTION - DISORDERS: Brodmann's areas 20, 21, 22, 37, & 38; temporal lobe.

VISUAL ANESTHESIA: blindness.

VISUAL ASSOCIATION CORTEX: Brodmann's areas 20, & 21.

VISUAL CLOSURE TEST: subtest of the ITPA; involves visual search and recognition of parts of objects or of objects at unusual angles; test of visual agnosia.

VISUAL COMPREHENSION DISORDER: deficits in reading (alexia) accompany deficits in auditory comprehension. A disturbance of reading is commonly associated with impaired comprehension of auditory material, but these two symptoms may occur independently of one another; defects in visual comprehension may involve a deficit in recognizing individual letters or words as being letters or words, or a deficit in attaching meaning to the symbols written on a page.

VISUAL COMPREHENSION TESTS: Raven's progressive matrices tests; Fostig Test.

VISUAL COORDINATION CENTER: superior colliculus.

VISUAL DISCONNECTION SYNDROME: the visual neuronal system is crossed; in the commissurotomy patient (sectioned corpus callosum), visual stimuli of a verbal nature (e.g., words) presented to the left visual field will be disconnected from verbal associations because the input goes to the right, nonlingustic hemisphere; the patient will be aphasic, agnosic, and alexic; complex visual material presented to the right visual field would be inadequately processed, because it would not have access to the visuospatial abilities of the right hemisphere; the patient will be acopic.

VISUAL DISCRIMINATION TEST: Raven's Progressive matrices tests; Fostig Test.

VISUAL DISPLACEMENT: visual allesthesia.

VISUAL DISTORTION: may be caused by lesions of the visual association areas of the occipital lobe.

VISUAL DISTURBANCES: see agnosia, alexia, amaurosis, amblyopia, nyctalopia, strabismus, nystagmus, oscilliopsia, opsoclonus, ocular dysmetria, mydriasis, miosis, constriction, dilatation, diplopia, blindness, visual anesthesia, prosopagnosia.

VISUAL HALLUCINATIONS: (complex) may be caused by lesion(s) anterior to occipital lobe in the association area (junction of occipital, parietal and posterior part of temporal lobe); may be associated with auditory hallucinations; often distorted or seem too small (micropsia); damage to the visual pathways may cause irritative phenomena, appreciated by the patient as flashes of light or color; more complicated visual images are usually the result of abnormal activity in visual association areas, particularly the temporal lobes; seeing "stars" may be the result of damage or ischemia of the retina due to a blow or migraine headache onset; unformed blobs of color or zig-zag lines or circular lines may be caused by ischemia of the occipital poles occurring during or preceding a migraine attack; formed visual images like a tableaux (déjà vu), or micropsia or macropsia are often a symptom of temporal-lobe epilepsy or migrainous vascular spasm; more complicated and persisting visual hallucinations may occur as part of a temporal-lobe attack, but occurs more frequently in toxic confusional states or schizophrenia.

VISUAL HALLUCINATIONS-LIGHT/DARK/COLOR: lesion of striate cortex of occipital lobe.

VISUAL HALLUCINATIONS-TWINKLING LIGHTS: lesion of the lateral surface of occipital lobes (Brodmann's areas 18 & 19).

VISUAL ILLUSIONS: lesion of the right temporal lobe; objects seem

V

nearer, farther larger, smaller.

VISUAL INATTENTION: also referred to as visual neglect, visual extinction; involves absence of awareness of visual stimuli in the left field of vision, reflecting its common association with right-hemisphere lesions; more likely to occur with posterior (usually parietal lobe) than anterior lesions (Frederiks, 1969), but may result from frontal-lobe lesions as well (Heilman & Valenstein, 1972); homonymous hemianopia increases the likelihood of visual inattention, but is not necessarily linked (De Renzi, 1978; Diller & Weinberg, 1977); usually more apparent during acute stages of brain-injury; may be inattentive to people on neglected side or eat only food on one side of a plate; also called unilateral spatial neglect; most often a result of right parietal-lobe and occipital-lobe damage.

VISUAL INATTENTION TESTS: Test of Visual Neglect (M. L. Albert, 1973); Line Bisection tests (Diller et al., 1974; Kinsbourne, 1974; Schenkenberg et al., 1980); Meaningful Pictures (Battersby et al., 1956); Picture Matrix Memory Task (Deutsch et al., 1980).

VISUAL INCOMPREHENSION/ IMPERCEPTION: see visual agnosia.

VISUAL INTERFERENCE TASKS: visual recognition tasks complicated by distracting embellishments/masking; visual interference tasks differ from tests of visual organization in that the latter call on synthesizing activities whereas visual interference tests require the subject to analyze the figure-ground relationship in order to distinguish the figure from the interfering elements (Lezak, 1983); perceptual flexibility, perceptual focusing, and the ability to hold a closure against distraction (Thurstone, 1944); Cross-hatching or shading over simple drawings, letters, or words may destroy the underlying percept for patients whose lesions involved the occipital lobe (Luria, 1965, 1966).

VISUAL INTERFERENCE TESTS: Hidden Figures Test, Overlapping Figures Test, Southern California Figure-Ground, Visual Perception Test, Visual Closure Test, Optical Illusions.

VISUAL FORM AGNOSIA: receptive aphasia; unable to attach the correct verbal label to forms (objects) although physical vision is intact.

VISUAL LETTER AGNOSIA: (receptive aphasia); cannot correctly label all the letters of the alphabet; may substitute letters; may be unable to read letters or may give correct response after a delay.

VISUAL MASKING /CROSS-HATCHING/ SHADING: cause simple drawings, letters or words to be unidentifiable by occipital-lobe lesioned patients (Luria, 1965, 1966); left-hemisphere lesioned patients have difficulty with letters and right-hemisphere lesioned patients have difficulty with simple drawings for well-known objects.

VISUAL MEMORY DEFECTS: lesion of Brodmann's area 21.

VISUAL NEGLECT TEST: (M. L. Albert, 1973); a line crossing-out test.

VISUAL OBJECT AGNOSIA: the patient can see an object but is unable to name it, demonstrate its use, or remember having seen it before; probably a result of a lesion of the left occipital lobe extending into subcortical white matter; may be bilateral, often including the corpus callosum and the inferior longitudinal fasiculus in the right hemisphere.

VISUAL PERCEPTION: ability to distinguish verbal/symbolic stimuli and configural stimuli; perception of angular relationships tends to be a predominantly right-hemisphere function (Benton et al., 1975) except when the angles readily lend themselves to verbal mediation (Berlucchi, 1974; Kimura & Durnford, 1974); visual field defects do not necessarily affect facial recognition scores, but facial recognition deficits tend to occur with spatial agnosias and dyslexias, and with dysgraphias that involve spatial disturbances (Tzavaras et al., 1970).

VISUAL PERCEPTION TESTS: Gollin Incomplete Figures Test; Mooney Closure Test.

VISUAL PERCEPTUAL ORGANIZATION TESTS: tests requiring the patient to make sense out of ambiguous, incomplete, fragmented, or otherwise distorted visual stimuli call for perceptual organizing activity beyond that of simple perceptual recognition; tests with incomplete visual stimuli: WAIS Picture Completion; Mutilated Pictures; Recognition of Incomplete Stimuli: Mooney's Closure Test (Closure Faces Test); Street Completion Test (Gestalt Completion Test); Gollin Figures; Fragmented Visual Stimuli: Hooper Visual Organization Test; Minnesota Paper Form Board Test; Rorschach.

VISUAL PERCEPTUAL TESTS WITH INTERFERENCE: (figure-ground tests): Hidden Figures Test; Closure Flexibility (Concealed Figures); Overlapping Figures Test; Southern California Figure-Ground Visual Perception Test; Visual Closure; Optical Illusions; Muller-Lyer Illusion.

VISUAL PROCESSING: McGill Picture Anomalies.

VISUAL RECOGNITION/PERCEPTION TESTS: Judgment of Line Orientation (Benton et al., 1975, 1978, 1983); Recognition of Pictured Objects (Warrington & Taylor, 1973); Face Recognition of Well-known Persons (Milner, 1968;Warrington & James, 1967b); Facial Recognition without Memory Component (Benton & Van Allen, 1968; Benton et al., 1983); Recognition of the Facial Expression of Emotion (DeKosky et al., 1980).

VISUAL REPRODUCTION SUBTEST: (Wechsler Memory Scale) tests immediate visual memory drawing.

V

VISUAL SCANNING DEFECTS: visual scanning defects that often accompany brain lesions can seriously compromise such important activities as reading, writing, performing paper and pencil calculations, and telling time (Diller et al., 1974); may be associated with accident-prone behavior (Diller & Weinberg, 1970); most common and most severe in patients with right-hemisphere lesions (Weinberg et al., 1976); high incidence in brain-damaged populations; tests of visual scanning can be used to screen for brain damage; tests for inattention and cancellation tasks will often disclose scanning problems; deficits also show up on purely perceptual tests involving scanning behavior.

VISUAL SEARCH TEST: a timed test which is sensitive to brain-damage; requires patient to match a specific stimulus figure; frontal-lobe patients are severely handicapped in focusing in on the specific stimulus figures and will randomly scan the page without locating the identical stimulus pattern (Goldstein et al., 1973).

VISUAL SEARCH TESTS: Perceptual Maze Test; Visual Search; Counting Dots.

VISUAL SPATIAL AGNOSIAS: see spatial agnosias, visual.

VISUAL SYSTEM: optic nerve; geniculostriate system; tectopulvinar system; Brodmann's areas 17, 18, 19, 20, & 21; the successively higher levels of the visual system are more involved than lower levels in processing complex aspects of stimulation.

VISUAL TRACKING TESTS: Line Tracing Task; Pursuit.

VISUOGRAPHIC TESTS: Bicycle Drawing Test; Bender-gestalt Test; Visual Reproduction Test (WMS); Benton Visual Retention Test; Complex Figure Test (Rey); Memory for Designs Test.

VISUOSPATIAL CONCEPTUAL DEFICITS ON VISUOMOTOR ACT: right parietal-lobe damage; patients with these deficits perform both Block Design and Object Assembly by using trial and error to manipulate their way to acceptable solutions without having to rely solely on discrete features or verbal guidance; performance much worse on purely perceptual tasks such as the Hooper; unable to form visuospatial concepts before seeing the actual objects, but their perceptions are sufficiently accurate and their self-correcting abilities sufficiently intact that as they manipulate the pieces, they can identify correct relationships and thus use their evolving visual concepts to guide them; unable to visualize or conceptualize what the Object Assembly constructions should be, but can put them together in piecemeal fashion by matching lines and edges in a methodical manner; may not recognize what they are making until the puzzle is almost completed; capable of accepting grossly inaccurate constructions as correct solutions; fail Block Design items that do not lend themselves to a verbalized solution; do not benefit from visuomotor stimulation, although their visuomotor coordination and control

272

may be excellent.

VOCABULARY SUBTEST: (WAIS-R) single best measure of both verbal and general mental ability; more likely to reflect the patient's socioeconomic and cultural origins and less likely to have been affected by academic motivation or achievement than Information or Arithmetic subtests (Lezak, 1983); least affected subtest with diffuse or bilateral brain injury (Gonen & Brown, 1968); relatively sensitive to lesions in the left hemisphere (Parsons et al., 1969), but not greatly depressed by left-hemisphere damage; may be a relatively normal score in dementia (Lezak, 1983); psychosurgery patients tend to give illustrations, poor explanations, repetitions with slight modifications, demonstrations, and loose associations; may be useful to differentiate between a functional thought disorder and brain disease because patients with thought disorders occasionally let down their guard to reveal a thinking problem in "clangy" expressions, ideosyncratic association, or personalized or confabulatory responses (Lezak, 1983).

VOCABULARY TESTS: Wide Range Vocabulary Test (Atwell & Wells, 1937); Mill Hill Vocabulary Scale (Raven, 1965); sensitive to dominant hemisphere disease (Brooks & Aughten, 1979a, b); Peabody Picture Vocabulary Test (PPVT).

VOLUNTARY GAZE MECHANISM: lateral gaze: located in the frontal lobe (Brodmann's area 8); connected with the parietal control area (Brodmann's area 19) which the frontal lobe can override to change the direction of gaze; the descending pathways pass in the corona radiata through the internal capsule; after rotating they lie medially and dorsally in the cerebral peduncle; main pathway passes to the pons and decussates to the opposite side and is assumed to end in the para-abducen nucleus or the vestibular nucleus; 6th nerve is activated as well as the opposite paired medial rectus muscle; crosses back over the midline and up to the opposite third nerve nucleus; the pathway controlling the vertical gaze is presumed to be mediated via the basal ganglia and the area underlying the superior colliculus; whenever there is weakness of conjugate movement, nystagmoid movements in the direction of weak gaze are a common feature.

VOLUNTARY LOCOMOTIVE MOVEMENTS: units of motivated behavior that take an animal to a specific place such as turning, walking, climbing, swimming; present at the level of the midbrain and below; present in the high decerebrate animal.

VOLUNTARY MOVEMENTS: also called appetitive, instrumental, purposive, or operant.

VOYEURISM: a form of paraphilia in which sexual gratification is derived from watching or looking at others, particularly the genitals, or from observing sexual objects or acts.

W

VOYT'S SYNDROME: usually due to birth trauma; characterized by bilateral athetosis, walking difficulties, spasmodic outbursts of laughing or crying, speech disorders, excessive myelination of the nerve fibers of the corpus striatum and sometimes mental deficiency.

W

WADDLING GAIT: uncertain but regular steps; exaggerated elevation of one hip and depression of the other; body inclines to side weight is on; seen in progressive muscular dystrophy; see also lordosis.

WAIS: Wechsler Adult Intelligence Scale.

WAIS-R: Wechsler Adult Intelligence Scale — Revised; consists of 6 verbal scale subtests and 5 performance scale subtests; a difference of 10 or more points between the verbal and performance scores is usually considered abnormal; a relatively lower score on the verbal subtests should alert the examiner to the possibility of a well-defined left-hemisphere lesion; a relatively lower score on the performance subtest should alert the examiner to the possibility of a well-defined right-hemisphere lesion; diffuse brain damage may produce a relatively low performance scale score with a near normal verbal scale score.

WAIS/WAIS-R ARITHMETIC SUBTEST: see Arithmetic Subtest; not an adequate test for testing basic arithmetic, symbol recognition, or spatial dyscalculia (Lezak, 1983); assesses knowledge of and ability to apply arithmetic operations only.

WAIS/WAIS-R BLOCK DESIGN SUBTEST: see Block Design Subtest.

WAIS/WAIS-R COMPREHENSION SUBTEST: see Comprehension subtest.

WAIS/WAIS-R DIGIT SPAN SUBTEST: see Digit Span subtest.

WAIS/WAIS-R DIGIT SYMBOL SUBTEST: see Digit Symbol Subtest.

WAIS/WAIS-R INFORMATION SUBTEST: see Information Subtest.

WAIS/WAIS-R OBJECT ASSEMBLY SUBTEST: see Object Assembly subtest.

WAIS/WAIS-R PICTURE ARRANGEMENT SUBTEST: see Picture Arrangement subtest.

WAIS/WAIS-R PICTURE COMPLETION SUBTEST: see Picture Completion Subtest.

WAIS/WAIS-R SIMILARITIES SUBTEST: see Similarities subtest.

WAIS/WAIS-R SUBTEST SCORES: (IN ALZHEIMER'S DISEASE)

the highest scores are obtained on tests of overlearned behaviors presented in a familiar format and of immediate memory recall (Coolidge et al., 1982); Information, Vocabulary, many Comprehension and Similarities subtest items, and Digits Forward will be performed relatively well, even long after the patient is not capable of caring for himself; the more the task is unfamiliar, abstract, speed-dependent, and taxes the patient's capacity for attention and learning, the more likely it is that there will be poor performance; Block Design, Digit Symbol, and Digits Backward often rank among the bottom test scores; Object Assembly generally runs a little higher than Block Design and Digit Symbol; a Vocabulary subtest score that is at least twice as large as the Block Design subtest score is a highly likely indicator of dementia and rarely, if ever, occurs among depressed patients (Coolidge et al., 1982); immediate and short-term memory tend to be relatively spared (Tweedy et al., 1982).

WAIS/WAIS-R VOCABULARY SUBTEST: see Vocabulary Subtest.

WAIS-R SUBTEST DISCREPANCIES: four scaled score points between the subtests is approaching a significant difference and five or more scaled score points are nonchance (Field, 1960); immediate memory, attention, and concentration problems show up in depressed performances on Digit Span and Arithmetic; attention and response speed primarily affect Digit Symbol scores (Russell, 1972).

WAKEFULNESS: see midbrain; ascending reticular formation; insomnia.

WALKING: mediated through the medial cerebellum.

WALLENBERG'S SYNDROME: caused by occlusion of the posterior inferior cerebral artery; marked by ipsilateral loss of temperature and pain sensations of the face and contralateral loss of these sensations of the extremities and trunk; ipsilateral ataxia, dysphagia, dysarthria, and nystagmus; see also medullary vascular lesions, brainstem lesions.

WASHINGTON PSYCHOSOCIAL SEIZURE INVENTORY: (Dodrill, 1978a) a 132-item inventory designed to assess social maladaptations associated with chronic epilepsy.

W.B.C./WBC: white blood cell; white blood-cell count.

WC; w/c: wheel chair.

w/d: well-developed.

WEAKNESS OF FACE: lesion of the trigeminal nerve (V).

WEBER'S SYNDROME: paralysis of the oculomotor nerve on the same side as the lesion, producing ptosis, strabismus, and loss of light reflex and accommodation; also produces spastic hemiplegia on the side opposite the lesion with increased reflexes and loss of superfical reflexes; paralysis of contralateral face, arm, and leg; due to damage to the corticospinal and cortico-brainstem tracts in the upper portion of the brainstem.

W

WECHSLER ADULT INTELLIGENCE SCALE: see WAIS.

WECHSLER ADULT INTELLIGENCE SCALE — REVISED: see WAIS-R.

WECHSLER MEMORY SCALE (WMS): (Stone et al., 1946; Wechsler, 1945) a battery consisting of seven subtests: Personal and Current Information, Orientation, Mental Control, Logical Memory, Digit Span, Visual Reproduction, Associate Learning; right temporal-lobe lesioned patients are impaired in recall of geometric figures; left temporal-lobe lesioned patients are impaired on verbal memory (paired associates and logical stories).

WECHSLER INTELLIGENCE SCALE FOR CHILDREN: see WISC.

WECHSLER INTELLIGENCE SCALE FOR CHILDREN — REVISED: see WISC-R.

WECHSLER PRESCHOOL AND PRIMARY SCALE OF INTELLIGENCE: see WPPSI.

WEIGL'S TEST: (modified version) (DeRenzi et al., 1966); modification of the Color Form Sorting Test; conceptual functioning test; sensitive to left-hemisphere lesions.

WERNICKE's APHASIA: receptive aphasia; spontaneous speech is fluent with normal rhythm but often pressured; comprehension of written or verbal speech, repetition, and naming are impaired; object naming poor; in its most severe form the patient speaks with incomprehensible syllables, can only make illegible marks on a page in attempts at writing, cannot be made to repeat aloud or copy at sight correctly; echoes words with faulty pronunciation; faulty comprehension; errors in word structure with improper tenses, prefixes, suffixes, etc.; because of confusion of phonematic characteristics (paraphasic speech), speaks nonsense with inappropriate words thrown in (word salad); cannot comprehend written or verbal speech; writing form may be correct, but content is nonsense; unaware of deficits; visual field defects may be present; inability to isolate significant phonematic characteristics and classification of sounds into known phonematic systems; writing impairment because the patient does not know the graphemes that combine to form a word; sound substitution errors (literal); neologisms; overuse of contentless nouns and verbs; hemiparesis mild or absent; hemianopia or quadrantopia may be present; not depressed and often euphoric; linguistically opposite to Broca's a.; paranoid attitude and combative behavior may be present; the more severe the deficit in auditory comprehension the more likely the lesion is of the posterior portion of the superior temporal gyrus; if single word comprehension is good more likely to involve the parietal lobe; may be caused by embolic occlusion of the lower posterior division of the left middle cerebral artery, slit hemorrhage in the subcortex of the temporoparietal region or temporal isthmus, extension of small putaminal or thalamic tumor, or in the posterior sylvian region, comprised of the left posterior superior temporal, opercular suypramarginal, and posterior insular gyri; called also impression a, sensory a, temporoparietal a, and receptive a.

WERNICKE'S AREA: (Brodmnnn's area 22) transforms auditory input into meaningful units (words); if this area is lesioned, comprehension of both spoken and written language is impaired; lies next to the primary auditory cortex and involves the understanding of auditory input as language and monitors speech output.

WERNICKE'S ENCEPHALOPATHY: serious complication of alcoholism; gross confusion with memory loss; potentially fatal disturbance of the brainstem function; extra-ocular nerve palsies, usually 6th nerve; conjugate gaze palsies; nystagmus and ataxia; may be reversable with Vitamin B1 therapy.

WERNICKE-MANN HEMIPLEGIA: partial hemiplegia of the extremities.

WESTERN APHASIA BATTERY: (Kertesz, 1979) many items taken from the Boston Diagnostic Aphasia Exam; a profile of performance and the "Aphasia Quotient" (AQ) determine the patient's diagnostic subtype according to pattern descriptions for eight aphasia subtypes.

W/F: white female.

WHIPLASH INJURIES: injury to the cervical spine as a result of sudden hyperextension and flexion of the neck; may also cause brain damage (Ommaya, Faas, & Yarnell, 1968) by involving the vertebral arteries, causing possible occlusion of these vessels and ischemia of the brainstem and occipital areas; the linear acceleration produced by the extreme movement of the head may also result in concussion and contusion of the brainstem and brain; patient most often remains conscious, but after a short period of time, has a feeling of weakness and unsteadiness and sometimes ataxia, vertigo, and vomiting; may be due to ischemia of the brainstem; occipital headache which may spread to the temporal areas within a relatively short period of time after the injury; pain and tenderness in the neck area may disappear after a few days, but headache often persists for weeks or even months (Reitan & Wolfson, 1985).

WHITE MATTER: area of the nervous system rich in axons covered with glial cells; the conducting portion of the brain and spinal cord; composed mostly of myelinated nerve fibers, association fibers, commissural fibers, and projection fibers.

WICKENS RELEASE FROM PROACTIVE (PI) INHIBITION TEST: (Wickens, 1970) test of short-term retention; anterior left-hemisphere damaged patients have normal recall with no release from PI, left temporal lobe lesions do poorly on the recall task but show release from PI; right-hemisphere patients show release from PI regardless of the site of lesion; uses the phenomenon of proactive inhibition to determine the level at which material to be learned is encoded; normal persons who encode in terms of semantic categories show a release from PI in that recall of the new category of material returns to the level of recall on the first list, although level of recall gradually lowers on the subsequent trials using lists of items in the same category as the first list.

WIDE BASE/SHORT STEP GAIT: see alcoholism; cerebellar gait; Korsakoff's syndrome; ataxia of Bruns.

WIDE RANGE ACHIEVEMENT TEST (WRAT): the arithmetic subtest is useful to the neuropsychologist so that when a patient's math performance is defective, the examiner can determine by inspection of the worksheet whether the difficulties are due to a dyscalculia of the spatial type, a figure or number alexia, or an anarithmetria in which number concepts or basic operations have been lost; may be used with patients who are so impaired that they have difficulty with the WAIS-R.

WIDE RANGE VOCABULARY TEST: sensitive to dominant hemisphere disease (Brooks & Aughton, 1979a,b).

WILSON'S DISEASE: Parkinson-like picture of tremor, rigidity, slowness of movement, and flexion dystonia of trunk, sometimes athetosis, tonic innervation, phasic dystonia, and intention tremor; lesion of substantia nigra; anterior thalamus, or ventricular nuclei; hepatolenticular degeneration; progressive disorder of early life which is frequently familial; degeneration of the corpus striatum; cirrhosis of the liver; caused by a disturbance of copper metabolism and also aminoaciduria; low serum copper level which is deposited in the tissues and excreted in the urine; inherited as an autosomal recessive gene; degeneration of ganglion cells with neuroglial overgrowth, most marked in the putamen of the lenticular nucleus (Brain, 1985).

WISC/WISC-R: Wechsler Intelligence Scale for Children ages five to fifteen years; comprised of 12 subtests although only 10 are most often used: 1. Information subtest: 30 questions are arranged in level of difficulty which explore general knowledge; considered to be related to school achievement; learning problems may be exposed; 2. Similarities subtest: 17 paired concepts arranged in level of difficulty; best measure of general intelligence; 3. Arithmetic subtest; 18 problems which are solved mentally; 4. Vocabulary subtest: 38 words listed in increasingly difficult order; requires some abstract responses; one of the best measures of intellectual functioning; 5. Comprehension subtest: 17 questions; explores familiarity with social mores and values; 6. Digit Span: groups of numbers to be repeated after oral presentation, both forward and backwards; this subtest is an alternative test and is not always used; 7. Picture Completion subtest: 26 sketches of objects with missing parts; test of visual acuity; 8. Picture Arrangement subtest: 12 sets of comic strip-type illustrations of social situations; 9. Block Design subtest: 11 designs of increasing difficulty constructed from colored blocks; visual motor task which is correlated with general intelligence; 10. Object Assembly subtest: 4 cut-up puzzles which are to be assembled within a time limit; a visual motor task; 11. Coding subtest: a substitution test that requires sustained attention; 12. Mazes subtest: an optional test of 9 mazes which test planning ability.

WISCONSIN CARD SORT TEST: (Berg, 1948; Grant & Berg, 1948); devised to study abstracting abilities and shift of set; particularly sensitive to left frontal-lobe lesions; some impairment with right frontal-lobe lesions; best available test of dorsolateral frontal-cortex function; demonstrates perseveration, inability to change sets/strategies; no effect post-surgically in inferior frontal-lobe and orbital excisions; right frontal-lobe damaged patients perform worse than left frontal-lobe damaged patients; left medial frontal-lobe lesioned patients have difficulty sorting according to category; dorsolateral frontal-lobe lesioned patients have difficulty shifting set.

WISCONSIN NEUROPSYCHOLOGICAL TEST BATTERY: (Harley at al., 1980) a modified Halstead-Reitan test battery used to evaluate motor disturbances associated with brain dysfunction (Haaland et al., 1977; Matthews & Harley, 1975); includes the Wisconsin Motor Battery which contains five measures of motor proficiency.

W/M: white male.

w/n: well-nourished.

WNL: within normal limits.

WORD BLINDNESS: see Wernicke's aphasia, alexia, aphasia.

WORD DEAFNESS: auditory aphasia due to disease of the hearing center of the brain.

WORD FINDING DISORDER: words are formed by combining sounds; to do so correctly, it is necessary to choose the appropriate words from the large available repertoire; all aphasics suffer from some restriction in the repertoire of words available, even when words are produced it takes longer than normal to do so. If this difficulty in finding words occurs in the absence of other aphasic symptoms, the disorder is called anomia. Difficulty in word finding often results in the person deliberately choosing a word that approximates the intended idea when the intended word cannot be found; test by asking for names of common objects presented to patient; listen to spontaneous speech; ask patient to describe a picture containing objects and actions; lesion of the left temporal lobe.

WORD FLUENCY DEFICITS: severely impaired patients with lesions of the left-frontal lobe anterior to Broca's (orbital-frontal) area; loss of spontaneity of speech (Zangwill, 1966), difficulty in evoking appropriate words or phrases; lesions in the right orbital-frontal

W

region may also produce a large reduction in verbal fluency.

WORD LEARNING TESTS: word span, Auditory-Verbal Learning Test, Associate Learning subtest of the Wechsler Memory Scale, New Word Learning and Retention Test, Modified Word Learning Test, Wicken's Release from PI Test, Serial Word-Learning Test, Pictorial Verbal Learning Test.

WORD RECOGNITION: a recognition trial can be used with any of the word recall tests; may clarify the nature of the patient's recall problem; if the the recognition list contains words from previously administered tests and the patient shows intrusions this may suggest impaired frontal-lobe functions where the patient can learn readily but cannot keep track or make order out of what they have learned or the context within which they learned it (Lezak, 1983, pp. 620-621; Rey, 1941); a method of exposing malingering.

WORD RECOGNITION DEFICIT: see word blindness, alexia, dyslexia, Wernicke's aphasia.

WORD SALAD: incoherent sentences of otherwise normal words; often seen in Wernicke's aphasia; speech defect in which phonematic characteristics are confused .

WORD SPAN: influenced by familiar-unfamiliar, concrete-abstract, low-high imagery, low-high association levels, ease of categorization, low-high emotional charge, and structural dimensions such as rhyming, or phonetically similar qualities (Baddeley, 1976; Mandler, 1967; Poon et al., 1980) and ease of retention (Schonen, 1968).

WORD SUBSTITUTION: see amnestic dysnomic aphasia, circumlocution, paraphasia.

WORD-NAMING TESTS: tests of verbal fluency which also involve short-term memory in keeping track of words already said (Estes, 1974); age, sex, and education have been found to influence performance (Benton & Hamsher, 1976; Verhoff et al., 1979; Wertz, 1979); women's performances hold up better than men's after age 55; Stanford-Binet; Controlled Oral Word Association Test (Benton, 1968; Benton & Hamsher, 1976; 1978) — first used F, A, & S (FAS); 1976 version included in the Multilingual Aphasia Exam (Benton & Hamsher, 1978) and uses C, F, & L or P, R, & W.

WPPSI: Wechsler Preschool and Primary Scale of Intelligence; suitable for children ages 4 though 6 1/2; not usually any more appropriate to use with adult neuropsychologically impaired patients than the WISC-R (Lezak, 1983); 11 subtests: Information, Vocabulary, Arithmetic, Similarities, Comprehension, Sentences (in place of Digit Span), Animal Houses (in place of Digit Symbol), Picture Completion, Mazes, Geometric Designs (in place of Object Assembly), and Block Design.

WRAT ARITHMETIC SUBTEST: a test of basic arithmetic including recognition of symbols, ability to calculate spatially, and calculation of adult level mathematical concepts such as fractions, decimals, squares, and algebraic functions; a test for spatial dyscalculia.

WRITING DISORDERS: may be disturbed in a wide variety of ways: may result from disturbance in movements of the limb to produce letters and words (not a language disorder); may be unable to write (agraphia) because of inability to recall the form of letters or the correct movements necessary to produce them; paragraphia (writing of an incorrect word) and perseveration (writing the same word repeatedly).

WRITING FLUENCY TEST: Thurstone Primary Mental Abilities Test; the average 18 year old can produce 65 written words that begin with the letter S in 5 minutes and the letter C in 4 minutes; Milner (1964) uses a cutting score of 45 to identify fluency problems; left-frontal lobectomy patients may be significantly impaired; right-hemisphere lesioned patients may produce lengthy responses (Lezak & Newman, 1979); aphasia and agraphia are often combined; *tests*: write numbers and letters to dictation; write names of common objects or body parts; write short sentences describing weather, job, or picture from magazine.

WRITING/SPELLING IMPAIRMENTS: right hemisphere lesioned patients tend to repeat elements of letters and words and to leave a wider than normal margin on the left hand side of the paper; left visuospatial inattention may be elicited by copying tasks; small perseverative errors may show up in the writing of patients with right-brain lesions, such as extra bumps on n's and m's; left hemisphere lesioned patients are more likely to have a wide right-sided margin and tend to leave separations between letters or syllables that disrupt the continuity of the writing line; aphasic patients tend to print when asked to write; demented/confused patients often show dysgraphia in the form of motor impairments (scribbling), and spatial disorders (alignment, overlapping, cramping), agrammatisms, spelling, and other linguistic errors (Chédru & Geschwind, 1972).

WRITING/SPELLING TESTS: Sentence Building (Terman & Merrill, 1973); tests verbal and sequential organizing abilities, use of syntax, spelling, punctuation, and graphomotor behavior.

WRONGLY COLORED PICTURES TEST: test to discriminate between color agnosia and color anomia.

wt.: weight.

XYZ

X: times; for.

X-RAY: computerized transaxial tomography (CT-scan); radioisotope scanning (brain scan) used to view the skull for evidence of fractures, calcification, or erosion of bone; see also angiography, ventriculography.

ZUNG SELF-RATING DEPRESSION SCALE: (Zung, 1965, 1967); a 20-item scale; can be scored in symptom categories: affect, physiological disturbances, psychomotor disturbance, and psychological disturbances.

References

Adams, R. D. Altered cerebrospinal fluid dynamics in relation to dementia and aging. In L. Amaducci, A. N. Davison, & P. Antuono (Eds.), *Aging of the brain and dementia*. New York: Raven Press, 1980.

Aita, J. A. Armitage, S. G., Reitan, R. M., & Rabinowitz, A. The use of certain psychological tests in the evaluation of brain injury. *Journal of General Psychology*, 1947, *47*, 25-44.

Albert, M. L., A simple test of visual neglect. *Neuropsychology*, 1973, *23*, 658-664.

Albert, M. L. Subcortical dementia. In R. Katzman, R. D. Terry, & K. L. Bick (Eds.), *Alzheimer's disease: senile dementia and related disorders*. New York: Raven Press, 1978.

Albert, M. S., Butters, N., & Brandt, J. Memory for remote events in chronic alcoholics and alcoholic Korsakoff's disease. *Journal of Studies on Alcohol*, 1980, *41*, 1071-1081.

Albert, M. S., Butters, N., & Levin, J. Temporal gradients in the retrograde amnesia of patients with alcoholic Korsakoff's disease. *Archives of Neurology*, 1979, *36*, 211-216.

Allison, J., Blatt, S. J., & Zimet, C. N. *The interpretation of psychological tests*. New York: Harper & Row, 1968.

Aminoff, M. J., Marshall, J., Smith, E. M., & Wyke, M. A. Pattern of intellectual impairment in Huntinton's chorea. *Psychological Medicine*, 1975, *5*, 169-172.

Annnett, M. The binomial distribution of right, mixed, and left handedness. *Quarterly Journal of Experimental Psychology*, 1967, *19*, 327-333.

Archibald, Y. M. *Simplification in the drawings of left hemisphere patients — a function of motor control?* Unpublished manuscript, no date.

Archibald, Y. M., Wepman, J. M., & Jones, L. V. Performance on nonverbal cognitive tests following unilateral cortical injury to the right and left hemispheres. *Journal of Nervous and Mental Disease*, 1967, *145*, 25-36.

Arenberg, D. Equivalence of information in concept identification. *Psychological Bulletin*, 1970, *74*, 355-361.

Armitage, S. G. An analysis of certain psychological tests used for the evaluation of brain injury. *Psychological Monographs*, 1946, *60*, (Whole No. 277).

Atwell, C. R., & Wells, F. L. Wide range multiple-choice vocabulary tests. *Journal of Applied Psychology*, 1937, *21*, 550-555.

Arthur, G. A. *Point Scale of Performance Tests*. Revised Form II. New

York: Psychological Corp., 1947.

Artiola i Fortuny, L., Briggs, M., Newcome, F., Ratcliff, G., & Thomas, C. Measuring the duration of post traumatic amnesia. *Journal of Neurology, Neurosurgery,* and *Psychiatry,* 1980, *43,* 377-379.

Ayres, A. J. *Southern California Figure-Ground Visual Perception Test Manual.* Los Angeles: Western Psychological Services, 1966.

Babcock, H. An experiment in the measurement of mental deterioration. *Archives of Psychology,* 1930, *117,* 105.

Babcock, H., & Levy, L. *The measurement of efficiency of mental functioning (revised examination). Test and manual of directions.* Chicago: C. H. Stoelting, 1940.

Baddeley, A. D. *The psychology of memory.* New York: Basic Books, 1976.

Baehr, M. E., & Corsini, R. J. *The Press Test.* Chicago: Human Resources Center, University of Chicago, 1980; Park Ridge, Ill.: London House Press, 1982.

Baker, G. Diagnosis of organic brain damage in the adult. In B. Klopfer (Ed.), *Developments* in the *Rorschach Technique.* New York: World Book, 1956.

Balint, R. Die seelenlähmung des "Schauens." Cited in T. Incagnoli, G. Goldstein, & C. J. Golden (Eds.), *Clinical application of neuropsychological test batteries.* New York: Plenum, 1986.

Balthazar, E. E. *Balthazar Scales of Adaptive Behavior for the profoundly and severely mentally retarded.* Champaign, Ill.: Research Press, 1956.

Bannister, R. *Brain's clinicial neurology* (5th ed.). London: Oxford University Press, 1977.

Barbizet, J., & Cany, E. Clinical and psychometrical study of a patient with memory disturbances. *International Journal of Neurology,* 1968, *7,* 44-54.

Barr, M. L., & Kiernan, J. A. *The human nervous system. An anatomical viewpoint,* (4th ed.). Philadelphia: Harper & Row, 1983.

Barrett, R., Merritt, H. H., & Wolf, A. Depression of consciousness as a result of cerebral lesions. *Research publications of the Association for research in nervous and mental disease,* 1967, *45,* 241-276.

Barton, M. Perception of the Mueller-Lyer illusion in normal and aphasic adults. *Perceptual and Motor Skills,* 1969, *28,* 403-406.

Battersby, W. S., Bender, M. B., Pollack, M., & Kahn, R. L. Unilateral "spatial agnosia" (inattention) in patients with cortical leasions. *Brain,* 1956, *79,* 68-93.

Bauer, J. H., & Copper, R. M. Effects of posterior cortical lesions on performance on a brightness discrimination task. *Journal of Comparative and Physiological Psychology,* 1964, *58,* 84-92.

Bear, D., & Fedio, P. Quantitative analysis of interictal behavior in temporoal lobe epilepsy. *Archives of Neurology*, 1977, *34*, 454-467.

Beard, R. M. The structure of perception: a factorial study. *British Journal of Educational Psychology*, 1965, 210-221.

Beatty, P. A., & Gange, J. J. Neuropsychological aspects of multiple sclerosis. *Journal of Nervous and Mental Disease*, 1977, *164*, 42-50.

Beck A. T., Ward, C. H., Mendelson, M., Mock, J., & Erbaugh, J. K. An inventory for measuring depression. *Archives of General Psychiatry*, 1961, *4*, 561-571.

Belleza, T., Rappaport, M., Hopkins, H. K., & Hall, K. Visual scanning and matching dysfunction in brain-damaged patients with drawing impairment. *Cortex*, 1979, *15*, 19-36.

Bender, L. A visual motor gestalt test and its clinical use. *American Orthopsychiatric Association Research Monographs*, 1938, *66*, 167-193.

Bender, M. B., Fink, M., & Green, M. Patterns in perception on simultaneous tests of face and hand. *A. M. A Archives of Neurology and Psychiatry*, 1951, *66*, 355-362.

Beniak, T. E. *The assessment of cognitive deficits in uremia.* Paper presented at European meeting of the International Neuropsychological Society, Oxford, England, 1977.

Benson, D. F. The hydrocephalic dementias. In D. F. Benson & D. Blumer (Eds.), *Psychiatric aspects of neurologic disease.* New York: Grune & Stratton, 1975.

Benson, D. F., & Barton, M. I. Distrubances in constructional ability. *Cortex*, 1970, *6*, 19-46.

Benton, A. L. *Right-left discrimination and finger localization: development and pathology.* New York: Hoeber-Harper, 1959.

Benton, A. L. Constructional apraxia and the minor hemisphere. *Confinia Neurologica*, 1967, *29*, 1-16.

Benton, A. L. Differential behavioral effects in frontal lobe disease. *Neuropsychologia*, 1968, *6*, 53-60.

Benton, A. L. Constructional apraxia: some unanswered questions. In A. L. Benton, *Contributions to clinical neuropsychology.* New York: Aldine, 1969a.

Benton, A. L. Disorders of spatial orientation. In P. J. Vinken & G. W. Bruyn (Eds.), Handbook of clinical neurology (Vol. 3), *Disorders of higher nervous activity.* New York: Wiley, 1969b.

Benton, A. L. *The Revised Visual Retention Test* (4th ed.). New York: Psychological Corporation, 1974.

Benton, A. L. Interactive effects of age and brain disease on reaction time. *Archives of Neurology*, 1977, *34*, 369-370.

Benton, A. L. Visuoperceptive, visuospatial, and visuoconstructive disorders. In K. M. Heilman & E. Valenstein (Eds.), *Clinical neuropsychology.* New York: Oxford University Press, 1979.

Benton, A. L., & Hamsher, K. deS. *Multilingual Aphasia Examination.*

Iowa City: University of Iowa, 1976; (*Manual*, revised), 1978.

Benton, A. L., Hamsher, K. deS., Varney, N. R., & Spreen, O. *Contributions to neuropsychological assessment*. New York: Oxford University Press, 1983.

Benton, A. L., Hannay, H. J., & Varney, N. R. Visual perception of line direction in patients with unilateral brain disease. *Neurology*, 1975, *25*, 907-910.

Benton, A. L., & Van Allen, M. W. Impairment in facial recognition in patients with cerebral disease. *Cortex*, 1968, *4*, 344-358.

Benton, A. L., Van Allen, M. W., & Fogel, M. L. Temporal orientation in cerebral disease. *Journal of Nervous and Mental Disease*, 1964, *139*, 110-119.

Benton, A. L., Varney, N. R., & Hamsher, K. deS. Visuospatial judgment. A clinical test. *Archives of Neurology*, 1978, *35*, 364-367.

Berg, E. A. A simple objective test for measuring flexibility in thinking. *Journal of General Psychology*, 1948, *39*, 15-22.

Berglund, M., Gustafson, L., & Hagberg, B. Amnestic-confabulatory syndrome in hydrocephalic dementia and Korsakoff's psychosis in alcoholism. *Acta Psychiatrica Scandinavica*, 1979, *60*, 323-333.

Berlucchi, G. Cerebral dominance and interhemispheric communication in normal men. In F. O. Schmitt & F. G. Worden (Eds.), *The Neurosciences. Third Study Program*. Cambridge, Mass: Massachusetts Institute of Technology Press, 1974.

Berry, R. G. Pathology of dementia. In J. G. Howells (Ed.), *Modern perspectives in the the psychiatry of old age*, Edinburgh/London: Churchill Livingstone, 1975.

Billingslea, F. Y. The Bender-Gestalt. A review and a perspective. *Psychological Bulletin*, 1963, *60*, 233-251.

Binder, L. M. Constructional strategies on complex figure drawings after unilateral brain damage. *Journal of Clinical Neuropsychology*, 1982, *4*, 51-58.

Bisiach, E., & Luzzatti, C. Unilateral neglect of representational space. *Cortex*, 1978, *14*, 129-133.

Black, F. W., & Strub, R. L. Constructional apraxia in patients with discrete missile wounds of the brain. *Cortex*, 1976, *12*, 212-220.

Blessed, G., Tomlinson, B. C., & Roth, M. The association between quantitative measures of dementia and senile change in the cerebral gray matter of elderly subjects. *British Journal of Psychiatry*, 1968, *114*, 797-811.

Blumer, D., & Benson, D. F. Personality changes with frontal and temporal lobe lesions. In D. F. Benson and D. Blumer, (Eds.), *Psychiatric aspects of neurologic disease*. New York: Grune and Stratton, 1975.

Blumstein, S. Neurolinguistic disorders: Language — brain relationships. In S. B. Filskov & T. J. Boll (Eds.), *Handbook of Clinical*

Neuropsychology. New York: Wiley — Interscience, 1981.

Boder, E. Developmental dyslexia: a diagnostic approach based on three atypical reading-spelling patterns. *Developmental Medicine and Child Neurology*, 1973, *15*. 663-687.

Bogen, J. E., DeZure, R., Tenhouten, W. D., & March, J. F. The other side of the brain IV: the A/P ratio. *Bulletin of the Los Angeles Neurological Societies*, 1972, *37*, 49-61.

Boll, T. J., Heaton, R., & Reitan, R. M. Neuropsychological and emotional correlates of Huntington's chorea. *Journal of Nervous and Mental Disease*, 1974, *158*, 61-69.

Boller, F., & Vignolo, L. A. Latent sensory aphasia in hemisphere-damaged patients: an experimental study with the Token Test. *Brain*, 1966, *89*, 815-831.

Bolter, J. F., & Hannon, R. Cerebral damage associated with alcoholism: a reexamination. *The Psychological Record*, 1980, *30*, 165-179.

Bond, M. R. Assessment of the psychosocial outcome after severe head injury. In Ciba Fondation Symposium, No. 34 (New Series). *Symposium on the outcome of severe damage to the central nervous system*. Amsterdam: Elsevier. Excerpta Medica, 1975.

Bond, M. R. The stages of recovery from severe head injury with special reference to late outcome. *International Rehabilitation Medicine*, 1979, *1*, 155-159.

Bondareff, W., Baldy, R., & Levy, R. Quantitative computed tomography in senile dementia. *Archives of General Psychiatry*, 1981, *38*, 1365-1368.

Borod, J. C., Goodglass, H., & Kaplan, E. Normative data on the Boston Diagnostic Aphasia Examination, Parietal Lobe Battery, and the Boston Naming Test. *Journal of Clinical Neuropsychology*, 1980, *2*, 209-216.

Botez, M. I., & Barbeau, A. Neuropsychological findings in Parkinson's disease: a comparison between various tests during long-term Levodopa therapy. *International Journal of Neurology*, 1975, *10*, 222-232.

Botez, M. I., Botez, T., Leveille, J. Bielmann, P., & Caddotte, M. Neuropsychological correlates of folic acid deficiency: facts and hypotheses. In M. I. Botez & E. H. Reynolds (Eds)., *Folic acid in neurology, psychiatry, and internal medicine*. New York: Raven Press, 1979.

Botez, M. I., Leveille, J., Berube, L., & Botez-Marquard, T. Occult disorders of the cerebrospinal fluid dynamics. *European Neurology*, 1975, *13*, 203-223.

Botwinick, J. Intellectual abilities. In J. E. Birren & K. W. Schaie (Eds.), *Handbook of the psychology of aging*. New York: Van Nostrand, 1977.

Botwinick, J. *Aging and behavior* (2nd ed.). New York: Springer, 1978.

Botwinick, J., & Storandt, M. *Memory, related functions, and age.* Springfield, Ill.: C. C. Thomas, 1974.

Bowen, F. P. Behavioral alterations in patients with basal ganglia lesions. In M. D. Yahr (Ed.), *The basal ganglia.* New York: Raven Press, 1976.

Boyd, R. D. *The Boyd Developmental Progress Scale.* San Bernardino, Calif.: Inland Counties Regional Center, 1974.

Bradley, C. Benzedrine and dexedrine in the treatment of children's behavior disorders. *Pediatrics,* 1950, *5,* 24-37.

Brain, Walter R. *Brain's Clinical Neurology,* 6th ed, Revised by Sir Roger Bannister. New York: Oxford University Press, 1985.

Briggs, G. G., & Nebes, R. D. Patterns of hand preference in a student population. *Cortex,* 1975, *11,* 230-238.

Broadbent, D. E. *Perception and communication.* London: Pergamon Press, 1958.

Broadbent, D. E. Recent analyses of short-term memory. In K. H. Pribram & D. E. Broadbent (Eds.), *Biology of memory.* New York: Academic Press, 1979.

Brodal, A. Self-observations and neuro-anatomical considerations after a stroke. *Brain,* 1973, *96,* 675-694.

Brooks, D. N. Memory and head injury. *Journal of Nervous and Mental Disease,* 1972, *155,* 350-355.

Brooks, D. N. Psychological deficits after severe blunt head injury: their significance and rehabilitation. In D. J. Osborne, M. M. Gruneberg, & J. R. Eiser (Eds.), *Research in psychology and medicine* (Vol. 2). London: Academic Press, 1979.

Brooks, D. N. & Aughton, M. E. Cognitive recovery during the first year after severe blunt head injury. *International Rehabilitation Medicine,* 1979a, *1,* 166-172.

Brooks, D. N. & Aughton, M. E. Psychological consequences of blunt head injury. *International Rehabilitation Medicine,* 1979b, *1,* 160-165.

Brooks, D. N., McKinlay, W., & Bond, M. R. *The burden on the relatives of head injured adults.* Paper presented to the second European Conference of the International Neuropsychological Society, Noordvijkerhout, The Netherlands, June, 1979.

Brown, J. *Aphasia, apraxia and agnosia.* Springfield, Ill.: C. C.Thomas, 1972.

Buchsbaum, M. *Positron emission tomography.* Paper presented at the Laterality Conference, Banff, 1982.

Buchsbaum, M. S., & Ingvar, D. H. New version of the schizophrenics brain: regional differences in electrophysiology, blood flow, and cerebral glucose use. In F. A. Henn and H. A. Nasrallah (Eds.), *Schizophrenia as a brain disease.* New York: Oxford University Press, 1982.

Buck, N. W. *Dysphasia*. Englewood Cliffs, N. J.: Prentice-Hall, 1968.

Burch, P. R. J. Huntington's Disease: Types, frequency, and progression. In T. N. Chase, N. S. Wexler, & A Barbeau (Eds.), *Advances in neurology* (Vol. 23). New York: Raven Press, 1979.

Burton, C. Unilateral spatial neglect after cerebrovascular accident. In G. V. Stanley & K. W. Walsh (Eds.), *Brain impairment. Proceedings of the 1977 Brain Impairment Workshop*, Parkville, Victoria, Australia: Neuropsychology Group, Dept. of Psychology, University of Melbourne, 1978.

Buschke, H., & Fuld, P. A. Evaluating storage, retention, and retrieval in disordered memory and learning. *Neurology*, 1974, *11*, 1019-1025.

Butters, N. *Position paper on neuropsychology and Huntington's disease: a current assessment.* (Commission for the control of Huntington's disease and its consequences. Vol. 3, Part 1.) Washington, D. C.: U. S. Department of Health, Education, and Welfare, 1977.

Butters, N., & Barton, M. Effect of parietal lobe damage on the performance of reversible operations in space. *Neuropsychologia*, 1970, *8*, 205-214.

Butters, N., & Brody, B. A. The role of the left parietal lobe in the mediation of intra- and cross-modal associations. *Cortex*, 1968, *4*, 328-343.

Butters, N., & Cermak, L. S. The role of cognitive factors in the memory disorders of alcoholic patients with the Korsakoff syndrome. *Annals of the New York Academy of Sciences*, 1974, *233*, 61-75.

Butters, N., & Cermak, L. S. Some analyses of amnesic syndromes in brain-damaged patients. In R. L. Isaacson & K. H. Pribram, *The Hippocampus*, Vol. 2. New York: Plenum Press, 1975.

Butters, N., & Cermak, L. S. Neuropsychological studies of alcoholic Korsakoff patients. In G. Goldstein & C. Neuringer (Eds.), *Empirical studies of alcoholism*. Cambridge, Mass.: Ballinger, 1976.

Butters, N., & Cermak, L. S. *Alcoholic Korsakoff's syndrome*. New York: Academic Press, 1980

Butters, N., Cermak, L. S., Montgomery, K., & Adinolfi, A. Some comparisons of the memory and visuoperceptive deficits of chronic alcoholics and patients with Korsakoff's disease. *Alcoholism: Clinical and Experimental Research*, 1977, *1*, 73-80.

Butters, N., Sax, D., Montgomery, K., & Tarlow, S. Comparison of the neuropsychological deficits associated with early and advanced Huntington's disease. *Archives of Neurology*, 1978, *35*, 585-589.

Caine, E. D., Ebert, M. H., & Weingartner, H. An outline for the analysis of dementia. *Neurology*, 1977, *23*, 1087-1092.

Caine, E. D., Hunt, R. D., Weingartner, H., & Ebert, M. H. Huntington's dementia. *Archives of General Psychiatry*, 1978, *35*, 377-384.

Campbell D. C., & Oxbury, J. M. Recovery from unilateral visuo-spatial neglect. *Cortex*, 1976, *12*, 303-312.

Canter, A. A background interference procedure to increase sensitivity of the Bender-Gestalt test to organic brain disorder. *Journal of Consulting Psychology*, 1966, *30*, 91-97.

Canter, A. A BIP Bender test for the detection of organic brain disorder modified scoring method and replication. *Journal of Consulting and Clinical Psychology*, 1968, *32*, 522-526.

Canter, A. *The Canter Background Interference Procedure for the Bender Gestalt Test: Manual for administration, scoring, and interpretation.* Los Angeles: Western Psychological Services, 1976.

Caramazza, A., Zurif, E. B., & Gardner, H. Sentence memory in aphasia. *Neuropsychologia*, 1978, *16*, 661-669.

Casey, V. A., & Fennell, E. B. *Emotional consequences of brain injury: effect of litigation, sex, and laterality of lesion.* Paper presented at the ninth annual meeting of the International Neuropsychological Society, Atlanta, February, 1981.

Chédru, F., & Geschwind, N. Writing disturbances in acute confusional states. *Neuropsychologia*, 1972, *10*, 343-353.

Christensen, A. -L. *Luria's neuropsychological investigation.* Text (2nd ed.). Copenhagen: Munksgaard, 1979.

Cohen, L. Perception of reversible figures after brain injury. *A. M. A. Archives of Neurology and Psychiatry*, 1959, *81*, 765-775.

Cohn, R. Role of "body image concept" in pattern of ipsilateral clinical extinction. *A. M. A. Archives of Neurology and Psychiatry*, 1953, *70*, 503-509.

Collier, H. L., & Levy, N. *A preliminary study employing the Sequential Matching Memory task in an attempt to differentially diagnose brain damage.* Unpublished manuscript, undated.

Colombo, A., De Renzi, E., & Faglioni, P. The occurrence of visual neglect in patients with unilateral cerebral disease. *Cortex*, 1976, *12*, 221-231.

Colonna, A., & Faglioni, P. The performance of hemisphere-damaged patients on spatial intelligence tests. *Cortex*, 1966, *2*, 293-307.

Coolidge, F. L., Brown, R. E., & Harsch, T. L. Differential diagnosis of dementia or depression with the WAIS. *Journal of Clinical Neuropsychology*, 1983.

Cooper, I. S., Amin, I., Chandra, R., & Waltz, J. H. A surgical investigation of the clinical physiology of the LP-pulvinar complex in man. *Journal of Neurological Science*, 1973, *18*, 89-110.

Cope, D. N. *Psychosocial recovery trends: Findings of the head injury project.* Paper presented at the 5th annual Head Trauma Rehabilitation Conference: Coma to Community. San Jose, Calif., February, 1982.

Corkin, S., Milner, B., & Rasmussen, T. Somatosensory thresholds.

Archives of Neurology, 1970, *23*, 41-58.

Corsi, P. M. *Human memory and the medial temporal region of the brain*. Unpublished Ph. D. thesis, McGill University, 1972.

Costa, L. D. The relation of visuospatial dysfunction to digit span performance in patients with cerebral lesions. *Cortex*, 1975, *11*, 31-36.

Costa, L. D. Interest variability on the Raven Coloured Progressive Matrices as an indicator of specific ability deficiency in brain-leasioned patients. *Cortex*, 1976, *12*, 31-40.

Costa, L. D., Vaughn, H. G., Jr., Howitz, M., & Ritter, W. Patterns of behavioral deficits associated with visual spatial neglect. *Cortex*, 1969, *5*, 242-263.

Craik, F. I. M., & Birtwistle, J. Proactive inhibition in free recall. *Journal of Experimental Psychology*, 1971, *91*, 120-123.

Crook, T., Ferris, S., McCarthy, M., & Rae, D. Utility of digit recall tasks for assessing memory in the age. *Journal of Consulting and Clinical Psychology*, 1980, *48*, 228-233.

Cronbach, L. J. *Essentials of psychological testing*. New York: Harper & Row, 1970.

Dahlstrom, W. G., & Welsh, G. S. *An MMPI handbook*. Minneapolis: University of Minnesota Press, 1960.

Dahlstrom, W. G., Welsh, G. S., Dahlstrom, L. E. *An MMPI handbook* (Vol. 1. *Clinical interpretation*, Rev. ed.). Minneapolis University of Minnesota Press, 1975.

Dailey, C. A. Psychological findings five years after head injury. *Journal of Clinical Psychology*, 1956, *12*, 440-443.

Damasio, A. R. The frontal lobes. In K. M. Heilman & E. Valenstein (Eds.), *Clinical neuropsychology*. New York: Oxford University Press, 1979.Damasio, A. R., & Benton, A. L. Impairment of hand movements under visual guidance, *Neurology*, 1979, *32*, 170-178.

Damasio, A. R., McKee, J., & Damasio, H. Determinants of performance in color anomia. *Brain and Language*, 1979, *7*, 74-85.

Darley, F. L. The efficacy of language rehabilitation. *Journal of Speech and Hearing Disorders*, 1972, *37*, 3-21.

Davies, A. The influence of age on Trail Making test performance. *Journal of Clinical Psychology*, 1968, *24*, 96-98.

Davis, M. E., Binder, L. M., & Lezak, M. D. *Hemisphere side of damage and encoding capacity*. Paper presented at the eleventh annual meeting of the International Neuropsychological Society, Mexico City, February, 1983.

Dee, H. L., Benton, A. L., & Van Allen, M. W. Apraxia in relation to hemisphere locus of lesion and aphasia. *Transactions of the American Neurological Association*, 1970, *95*, 147-148.

Deelman,B. *Memory deficits after closed head injury*. Paper presented at the first European Conference of the International Neuropsychological Society, Oxford, England, 1977.

DeKosky, S. T., Heilman, K. M., Bowers, D., & Valenstein, E. Recognition and discrimination of emotional faces and pictures. *Brain and Language*, 1980, *9*, 206-214.

Delaney, R. C., Wallace, J. D., & Egelko, S. Transient cerebral ischemic attacks and neuropsychological deficit. *Journal of Clinical Neuropsychology*, 1980, *2*, 107-114.

Denney, N. W. Evidence for developmental changes in categorization criteria for children and adults. *Human Development*, 1974, *17*, 41-53.

De Renzi, E. Hemispheric asymmetry as evidenced by spatial disorders. In M. Kinsbourne (Ed.), *Asymmetrical function of the brain*. Cambridge, England: Cambridge University Press, 1978.

De Renzi, E., & Faglioni, P. The comparative efficiency of intelligence and vigilance tests in detecting hemispheric cerebral damage. *Cortex*, 1965, *1*, 410-433.

De Renzi, E., & Scotti, C. Autotopagnosia: fiction or reality? *A. M. A Archives of Neurology*, 1970, *23*, 221-227.

De Renzi, E., & Spinnler, H. Visual recognition in patients with unilateral cerebral disease. *Journal of Nervous and Mental Disease*, 1966, *142*, 515-525.

De Renzi, E., & Spinnler, H. Impaired performance on color tasks in patients with hemispheric damage, *Cortex*, 1967, *3*, 194-217.

De Renzi, E., & Vignolo, L. A. The Token Test: a sensitive test to detect disturbance in aphasias. *Brain*, 1962, *85*, 665-678.

De Renzi, E., Faglioni, P., Savoiardo, M., & Vignolo, L. A. The influence of aphasia and of the hemisphere side of the cerebral lesion on astract thinking. *Cortex*, 1966, *2*, 399-420.

Deutsch, G., Tweedy, J. R., & Lorinstein, I. B. *Some temporal and spatial factors affecting visual neglect*, Paper presented at the eighth annual meeting of the International Neuropsychological Society, San Francisco, February, 1980.

Dikmen, S., & Reitan, R. M. Minnesota Multiphasic Personality Inventory correlates of dysphasic language disturbance. *Journal of Abnormal Psychology*, 1974a, *83*, 675-679.

Diller, L. Brain damage, spatial orientation, and rehabilitation. In S. J. Freedman (Ed.), *The neuropsychology of spatially oriented behavior*. Homerwood, Ill.: Dorsey, 1968.

Diller, L., & Weinberg, J. Bender Gestalt Test distortions in hemiplegia. *Perceptual and Motor Skills*, 1965, *20*, 1313-1323.

Diller, L., & Weinberg, J. Evidence for accident-prone behavior in hemiplegic patients. *Archives of Physical Medicine and Rehabilitation*, 1970, *51*, 358-363.

Diller, L., & Weinberg, J. Differential aspects of attention in brain-damaged persons. *Perceptual and Motor Skills*, 1972, *35*, 71-81.

Diller, L., & Weinberg, J. Hemi-inattention in rehabilitation: the evolution of a rational remediation program. In E. A. Weinstein & R. P Friedland (Eds.), *Advances in neurology* (Vol. 18). New York: Raven Press, 1977.

Diller, L., Ben-Yishay, Y., Gerstman, L. J., Goodkin, R., Gordon, W., & Weinberg, J. *Studies in cognition and rehabilitation in hemiplegia* (Rehabilitation Monograph No. 50). New York: New York University Medical Center Institute of Rehabilitation Medicine, 1974.

Dodrill, C. B. Diphenylhydantoin serum levels, toxicity, and neuropsychological performance in patients with epilepsy. *Epilepsia*, 1975, *16*, 593-600.

Dodrill, C. B. The hand dynamometer as a neuropsychological measure. *Journal of Consulting and Clinical Psychology*, 1978a, *46*, 1432-1435.

Dodrill, C. B. *Neuropsychological assessment in epilepsy rehabilitation*. Paper presented at the 86th annual convention of the American Psychological Association, Toronto, 1978b.

Dodrill, C. B. A neuropsychological battery for epilepsy. *Epilepsia*, 1978c, *19*, 611-623.

Dodrill, C. B., & Wilkus, R. J. Relationships between intelligence and electroencephalographic epileptiform activity in adult epileptics. *Neurology*, 1976, 525-531.

Doll, E. A. *Measurement of social competence*. Minneapolis: Educational Publishers, 1953.

Doll, E. A. *Vineland Social Maturity Scale: Manual of directions* (Revised ed.). Minneapolis: American Guidance Service, 1965.

Dorff, J. E., Mirsky, A. F., & Mishkin, M. Effects of unilateral temporal lobe removals on tachistoscopic recognition in the left and right visual fields. *Neuropsychologia*, 1965, *3*, 39-51.

Drachman, D. A., & Leavitt, J. Human memory and the cholinergic system. *Archives of Neurology*, 1974, *30*, 113-121.

Elithorn, A., Jones, D., Kerr, M., & Lee, D. The effects of the variation of two physical parameters on empirical difficulty in a perceptual maze test. *British Journal of Psychology*, 1964, *55*, 31-37.

Erber, J. T., Botwinick, J., & Storandt, M. The impact of memory on age differences in Digit Symbol performance. *Journal of Gerontology*, 1981, *36*, 586-590.

Eson, M. E., & Bourke, R. S. *Assessment of information processing deficits after serious head injury*. Paper presented at the eighth annual meeting of the International Neuropsychological Society, San Francisco, February, 1980a.

Eson, M. E., & Bourke, R. S. *Assessment of long-term information processing deficits after serious head injury*. Paper presented at the

NATO Advanced Study Institute of Neuropsychology and Cognition, Augusta, Georgia, September 1980b.

Eson, M. E., Yen, J. K., & Bourke, R. S. Assessment of recovery from serious head injury. *Journal of Neurology, Neurosurgery, and Psychiatry*, 1978, *41*, 1036-1042.

Estes, W. K. Learning theory ad intelligence. *American Psychologist*, 1974, *29*, 740-749.

Evans, M. Cerebral disorders due to drugs of dependence and hallucinogens. In J. G. Rankin (Ed.), *Alcohol, drugs and brain damage*. Proceedings of Symposium. Toronto: Addiction Research Foundation, 1975.

Exner, J. E., Jr. *The Rorschach: a comprehensive system.* Vol. 1, 2nd ed. New York: Wiley-Interscience, 1986.

Farnsworth, D. Farnsworth-Munsel 100 hue and dichotomous test for color vision. *Journal of the Optical Society of America*, 1943, *33*, 568-578.

Fedio, P., Cox, C. S., Neophytides, A. Neuropsychological profile of Huntington's disease: patients and those at risk. In T. N. Chase, N. S. Wexler, & A. Barbeau (Eds.), *Advances in Neurology* (Vol. 23). New York: Raven Press, 1979.

Ferro, J. M., Santos, M. E., Caldas, A. C., & Mariano, G. Gesture recognition in aphasia. *Journal of Clinical Neuropsychology*, 1980, *2*, 277-292.

Field, J. G. Two types of tables for use with Wechsler's Intelligence Scales. *Journal of Clinical Psychology*, 1960, *16*, 3-7.

Filskov, S. B., & Boll, T. J. *Handbook of clinical neuropsychology.* New York: Wiley Interscience, 1981.

Filskov, S. B., & Leli, D. A. Assessment of the individual in neuropsychological practice. In S. B. Filskov & T. J. Boll (Eds.), *Handbook of clinical neuropsychology*. New York: Wiley Interscience, 1981.

Finlayson, M. A. J., & Reitan, R. M. Effect of lateralized lesions on ipsilateral and contralateral motor functioning. *Journal of Clinical Neuropsychology*, 1980, *2*, 237-243.

Finlayson, M. A. J., & Johnson, K. A., & Reitan, R. M. Relationship of level of education to neuropsychological measures in brain-damaged and non-brain-damaged adults. *Journal of Consulting and Clinical Psychology*, 1977, *45*, 536-542.

Fisher, C. M., & Adams, R. O. Transient global amnesia. *Transactions of the American Neurological Association*, 1958, *83*, 143.

Flor-Henry, P. Lateralized temporal-limbic dysfunction and psychopathology. *Annals of the New York Academy of Sciences*, 1976, *280*, 777-797.

Flor-Henry, P., & Yeudall, L. T. Neuropsychological investigation of schizophrenia and manic depressive psychosis. In J. Gruzelier & P.

Flor-Henry (Eds.), *Hemisphere asymmetries of function in psychopathology*. Amsterdam: Elsevier/North Holland Biomedical Press, 1979.

Flor-Henry, P., Yeudell, L. T., Stefanyo, W., & Howarth, B. The neuropsychological correlates of the functional psychoses. *International Research Communication Systems: Medical Science*, 1975, *3*, 34.

Folstein, M. F., Folstein, S. E., & McHugh, P. R. Mini-Mental State. *Journal of Psychiatric Research*, 1975, *12*, 189-198.

Fowler, R. S. A simple non-language test of new learning. *Perceptual and Motor Skills*, 1969, *29*, 895-901.

Franz, S. E. *Handbook of mental examination methods.* New York: Journal of Nervous and Mental Disease, 1912; Reprint, New York: Johnson Reprint Co., 1970.

Frederiks, J. A. M. Constructional apraxia and cerebral dominance. *Psychiatria, Neurologia, Neurochirurgia*, 1963, *66*, 522-530.

Frederiks, J. A. M. The agnosias. In P. J. Vinken & G. W. Bruyn (Eds.), *Handbook of clinical neurology* (Vol. 4). Amsterdam: North-Holland, 1969a.

Fuld, P. A. *Fuld Object-Memory Evaluation.* New York: Saul R. Korey Department of Neurology, Albert Einstein College of Medicine, 1977; Chicago: Stoelting, no date.

Fuld, P. A. Psychological testing in the differential diagnosis of the dementias. In R. Katzman, R. D. Terry, & K. L. Bick (Eds.), *Alzheimer's disease: senile dementia and related disorders (Aging, Vol. 7)*. New York: Raven Press, 1978.

Fuld, P. A., Katzman, R., Davies, P., & Terry, R. D. Intrusions as a sign of Alzheimer dementia: chemical and pathological verification. *Annals of Neurology*, 1982, *11*, 155-159.

Fuller, G. B. *Minnesota Percepto-Diagnostic Test* (Revised Ed.). Brandon, Vt.: Clinical Psychology Publishing Co., 1969.

Fuller, G. B., & Laird, J. T. The Minnesota Percepto-Diagnostic Test. *Journal of Psychology, Monograph Supplement*, 1963, No. 16.

Gainotti, G. Emotional behavior and hemispheric side of the lesion. *Cortex*, 1972, *8*, 41-55.

Gainotti, G., Caltagirone, C., Masullo, C., & Miceli, G. Patterns of neuropsychological impairment in various diagnostic groups of dementia. In L. Amaducci, A. N. Davison, & P. Antuono (Eds.), *Aging of the brain and dementia*. New York: Raven Press, 1980.

Gainotti, G., Cianchetti, C., & Tiacci, C. The influence of the hemispheric side of lesion on nonverbal tasks of finger localization. *Cortex*, 1972, *8*, 364-381.

Gainotti, G., & Tiacci, C. Patterns of drawing disability in right and left hemisphere patients. *Neuropsychologia*, 1970, *8*, 379-384.

Gardner, H., Ling, P. K., Flamm, L., & Silverman, J. Comprehension and appreciation of humorous material following brain damage. *Brain*, 1975, *98*, 399-412.

Garron, D. C., & Cheifetz, D. I. Comment on 'Bender Gestalt discernment of organic pathology.' *Psychological Bulletin*, 1965, *63*, 197-200.

Gates, A. I., & MacGinitie, W. H. *Gates-MacGinitie Reading Test*. New York: Teachers College Press, Teachers College, Columbia University, 1965, 1969.

Gazzaniga, M. S. Determinants of cerebral recovery. In D. G. Stein, J. J. Rosen, & N. Butters (Eds.), *Plasticity of function in the central nervous system*. New York: Academic Press, 1974.

Gerstmann, J. Problems of imperception of disease and of impaired body territories with organic lesions. *Archives of Neurology and Psychiatry*, 1942, *48*, 890-913.

Geschwind, M. Language and the brain. *Scientific American*, 1972, *226*, 76-83.

Geschwind, N. The apraxias: neural mechanisms of disorders of learned movement. *American Scientist*, 1975, *63*, 188-195.

Geschwind, N. Specializations of the human brain. *Scientific American*, 1979, *241*, 180-199.

Geschwind, N., & Levitsky, W. Left-right asymmetries in temporal speech region. *Science*, 1968, *161*, 186-187.

Geschwind, N., & Strub, R. Gerstmann syndrome with aphasia: a reply to Poeck and Orgass. *Cortex*, 1975, *11*, 296-298.

Gesell, A. *The first five years of life*. New York: Harper and Row, 1940.

Gesell, A. & Associates. *Gesell Developmental Schedules*. New York: Psychological Corporation, 1949.

Getzels, J. W., & Jackson, P. W. *Creativity and intelligence*. New York: Wiley, 1962.

Ghent, L. Perception of overlapping and embedded figures by children of different ages. *American Journal of Psychology*, 1956, *69*, 575-587.

Gilroy, J., & Meyer, J. S. *Medical neurology*. New York: Macmillan, 1979.

Gloning, K., & Hoff, H. Cerebral localization of disorders of higher activity. In P. J. Vinken & G. W. Bruyn (Eds.), *Handbook of clinical neurology* (Vol. 3): Disorders of higher nervous activity. New York: Wiley, 1969.

Glosser, G., Butters, N., & Kaplan, E. Visuoperceptual processes in brain damaged patients on the digit symbol substitution test. *International Journal of Neuroscience*, 1977, *7*, 59-66.

Goddard, G. V. Component properties of the memory machine: Hebb revisited. In P. W. Jusczyk and R. M. Klein, (Eds.), *The nature of thought: Essays in honour of D. O. Hebb*. Hillsdale, N. J.: Lawrence

Erlbaum Associates, 1980.

Goddard, G. V., & D. McIntyre. Some properties of a lasting epilepto-genic trace kindled by repeated electrical stimulation of the amygdala in mammals. In L. V. Laitinen and K. E. Livingston, (Eds.), *Surgical approaches in Psychiatry.* Baltimore: University Park Press, 1973.

Golden, C. J. *Clinical interpretation of objective psychological test.* New York: Grune & Stratton, 1979.

Golden, C. J. A standardized version of Luria's Neuropsychological tests. In S. Filskov & T. J. Boll (Eds.), *Handbook of clinical neuropsychology.* New York: Wiley-Interscience, 1981.

Golden, C. J. *Cerebral blood flow.* Paper presented at the Laterality Conference, Banff, 1982.

Golden, C. J., Hammeke, F. A., & Purisch, A. D. *Manual for the Luria-Nebraska Neuropsychological Battery.* Los Angeles Western Psychological Services, 1980.

Goldfried, M. R., Stricker, C., & Weiner, I. B. *Rorschach handbook of clinical and research applications.* Englewood Cliffs, N. J.: Prentice-Hall, 1971.

Goldman, H., Kleinman, K. M., Snow, M. W., et al. Correlation of diastolic blood pressure and signs of cognitive dysfunction in essential hypertension. *Diseases of the Nervous System,* 1974, *35,* 571-572.

Goldman, H., Kleinman, K. M., Snow, M. Y., et al. Relationship between essential hypertention and cognitive functioning: Effects of Biofeedback. *Psychophysiology,* 1975, *12,* 569-573.

Goldstein, G. (Ed.) *Advances in clinical neuropsychology,* Vol. 1 New York: Plenum, 1984.

Goldstein, G., & Shelly, C. H. Neuropsychological diagnosis of multiple sclerosis in a neuropsychiatric setting. *Journal of Nervous and Mental Disease,* 1974, *158,* 280-290.

Goldstein G., Welch, R. B., Rennick, P. M., & Shelly, C. H. The validity of a visual searching task as an indication of general brain disease. *Journal of Consulting and Clinical Psychology,* 1973, *41,* 434-437.

Goldstein, K. *The organism: A holistic Approach to Biology, Derived from Pathological Data in Man.* New York: American Book, 1939.

Goldstein K., & Scheerer, M. Abstract and concrete behavior: an experimental study with special tests. *Psychological Monographs,* 1941, *53,* No. 2 (Whole No. 239).

Goldstein K., & Scheerer, M. Tests of abstract and concrete behavior. In A. Weider, *Contributions to medical psychology* (Vol. 2). New York: Ronald Press, 1953.

Goldstein, S. G., Filskov, S. B., Weaver, L. A. & Ives, J. O. Neuropsychological effects of electroconvulsive therapy. *Journal of Clinical Psychology,* 1977, *33,* 798-806.

Gollin, E. S. Developmental studies of visual recognition of incomplete objects. *Perceptual and Motor Skills*, 1960, *11*, 289-298.

Golper, L. C., & Binder, L. M. Communicative behaviors in aging and dementia. In J. Darby (Ed.), *Speech evaluation in medicine and psychiatry (Vol. 2)*. New York: Grune & Stratton, 1981.

Gonen, J. Y., & Brown, I. Role of vocabulary in deterioration and restitution of mental function. *Proceedings of the 76th Annual Convention of the American Psychological Association*, 1968, *3*, 469-470. (Summary)

Goodale, M., & Cooper, R. M. Cues utilized by normal and posterior neodecorticate rats in the Yerkes brightness discrimination task. *Psychonomic Science*, 1965, *3*, 513-514.

Gooddy, W., & Reinhold, M. The sense of direction and the arrow-form. In E. Halpern (Ed.), *Problems of dynamic neurology*. Jerusalem, Israel: Hebrew University Hadassah Medical School, 1963.

Goodglass, H., & Kaplan, E. *The assessment of Aphasia and Related Disorders*. Philadelphia: Lea and Febiger, 1972.

Goodwin, D. M. *Cognitive and physical recovery trends in severe closed-head injury*. Dissertation Abstracts International, 43(9), 3066-B, 1983a.

Goodwin, D. M. *Prediction of psychosocial outcome following diffuse head-injury with a neuropsychological test battery*. Paper presented at the 11th annual conference of the International Neuropsychological Society, February, 1983b.

Gordon, H. W. Auditory specialization of the right and left hemispheres. In M. Kinsbourne & W. L. Smith (Eds.), *Hemispheric disconnection and cerebral function*. Springfield, Ill.: C. C. Thomas, 1974.

Gorham, D. R. A Proverbs Test for clinical and experimental use. *Psychological Reports*, 1956, *1*, 1-12.

Gottschaldt, K. Über den Einfluss der Erfahrung aug die Wahrnehmung von Figuren. *Psychologische Forschung*, 1928, *8*, 18-317.

Graham F. K., & Kendall, B. S. Memory-for-Designs-Test: revised general manual. *Perceptual and Motor Skills, Monograph Suppliment* No. 2—VIII, 1960, *11*, 147-188.

Granger, C. V., Albrecht, G. L., & Hamilton, B. B. Outcome of comprehensive medical rehabilitation: measurement by PULSES Profile and the Barthel Index. *Archives of Physical Medicine & Rehabilitation*, 1979, *60*, 145-154.

Grant D.A., & Berg, E. A. A behavioral analysis of degree of reinforcement and ease of shifting to new responses in a Weigl-type card-sorting problem. *Journal of Experimental Psychology*, 1948, *38*, 404-411.

Grant, I., & Adams, K. M. *Neuropsychological assessment of neuropsychiatric disorders*. New York: Oxford University Press, 1986.

Greenberg, F. R. Neurosensory Center Comprehensive Examination for Aphasia (NCCEA) (Review). In F. L. Darley (Ed.), *Evaluation of appraisal techniques in speech and language pathology.* Reading, Mass.: Addison-Wesley, 1979.

Gronwall, D. M. A. *Information processing capacity and memory after closed head injury.* Paper presented at the ninth annual meeting of the International Neuropsychological Society, San Francisco, 1980.

Gronwall, D., & Sampson, H. *The psychological effects of concussion.* Auckland, N. Z.: Auckland University Press/Oxford University Press, 1974.

Gronwall, D., & Wrightson, P. Recovery from minor head injury. *Lancet,* 1974, *2,* 1452.

Gronwall, D., & Wrightson, P. Memory and information processing capacity after closed head injury. *Journal of Neurology, Neurosurgery, and Psychiatry,* 1981, *44,* 889-895.

Grubb, R. L., & Coxe, W. S. Trauma to the central nervous system. In S. G. Eliasson, A. L. Prensky, & W. B. Hardin, Jr. (Eds.), *Neurological pathophysiology.* New York: Oxford University Press, 1978.

Gur, R. E., Levy, J., & Gur, R. C. Clinical studies of brain organization and behavior. In A. Frazer & A. Winokur (Eds.), *Biological bases of psychiatric disorders.* New York: Spectrum Publications, 1977.

Gurdjian, E. S., & Gurdjian, E. S. Acute head injuries. *Surgery, Gynecology, and Obstetrics,* 1978, *146,* 805-820.

Haaland, K. Y., Cleeland, C. S., & Carr, D. Motor performance after unilateral hemisphere damage in patients with tumor. *Archives of Neurology,* 1977, *34,* 556-559.

Haaland, K. Y., & Delaney, H. D. Motor deficits after left or right hemisphere damage due to stroke or tumor. *Neuropsychologia,* 1981, *19,* 17-27.

Hachinsky, V. C., Iliff, L. D., Zilhka, E., DuBoulay, G. M., McAllister, V. L., Marshall, J., Russell, R. W. R., & Symon, L. Cerebral blood flow in dementia. *Archives of Neurology,* 1975, *32,* 632-637.

Hall, M. M., & Hall, G. C. Antithetical ideational modes of left versus right unilateral hemisphere lesions as demonstrated on the Rorschach. *Proceedings of the 76th Annual Convention of the American Psychological Association,* 1968, *3,* 657-658.

Halstead, W. C., & Wepman, J. M. The Halstead-Wepman aphasia screening test. *Journal of speech and hearing disorders,* 1959, *14,* 9-15.

Hamsher, K. deS., Benton, A. L., & Digre, K. Serial digit learning: normative and clinical aspects. *Journal of Clinical Neuropsychology,* 1980, *2,* 39-50.

Hamsher, K. deS., Levin, H. S., & Benton, A. L. Facial recognition in patients with focal brain lesions. *Archives of Neurology,* 1979, *36,* 837-839.

Hanfmann, E. Concept Formation Test. In A. Weider (Ed.), *Contribu-*

tions toward medical psychology. New York: Ronald Press, 1953.

Hardy, C. H., Rand, G., & Rittler, J. M. C. *H-R-R Pseudoisochromatic Plates.* Buffalo, New York: American Optical Co., 1955.

Harley, J. P., Leuthold, C. A., Matthews, C. G., & Bergs, L. E. *Wisconsin Neuropsychological Test Battery T-score norms for older Veterans Administration Medical Center patients.* Madison, Wis: C. G. Matthews, May 1980.

Harris, A. J. *Harris Tests of Lateral Dominance. Manual of directions for administration and interpretation* (3rd ed.). New York: Psychological Corporation, 1958.

Harris, D. B. *Childrens drawings as measures of intellectual maturity.* New York: Harcourt Brace, 1963.

Harrison, M. J. G., Thomas, G. H., DuBoulay, G. H., Marshall, J. Multi-infarct dementia. *Journal of Neurological Sciences,* 1979, *40,* 97-103.

Hathaway, S. R., & McKinley, J. C. *The Minnesota Multiphasic Personality Inventory Manual* (Revised). New York: Psychological Corporation, 1951.

Heaton, R. K., & Crowley, T. J. Effects of psychiatric disorders and other somomatic treatments on neuropsychological test results. In S. B. Filskov and T. J. Boll (Eds.), *Handbook of clinical neuropsychology.* New York: Wiley-Interscience, 1981.

Heaton, R. K., Chelune, G. J., & Lehman, R. A. W. *Relation of neuropsychological and personality test results to patient's complaints of disability.* Unpublished manuscript. University of Colorado Health Sciences Center, 1981.

Heaton, R. K., Smith, H. H., Jr., Lehman, R. A. W., & Vogt, A. T. Prospects for faking believable deficits on neuropsychological testing. *Journal of Consulting and Clinical Psychology,* 1978, *46,* 892-900.

Hebb, D. O. The effect of early and late brain injury upon test scores, and the nature of normal adult intelligence. *Proceedings of the American Philosophical Society,* 1942, *85,* 275-292.

Hebb, D. O. *Organization of behavior.* New York: John Wiley and Sons, 1949.

Hebb, D. O., & Morton, N. W. The McGill Adult Comprehension Examination: 'Verbal Situation' & 'Picture Anomaly' series. *Journal of Educational Psychology,* 1943, *34,* 16-25.

Hécaen, H. Aphasia, apraxic and agnosic syndromes in right and left hemisphere lesions. In P. Vinken and G. Bruyn, (Eds.). *Handbook of Clinical Neurology,* (Vol. 4). Amsterdam: North-Holland Publishing Co., 1969a

Hécaen, H. Cerebral localization of mental functions and their disorders. In P. Vinken and G. Bruyn, (Eds.). *Handbook of Clinical Neurology,* (Vol. 3), *Disorders of higher nervous activity.* New York: Wiley, 1969b.

Hécaen, H., Ajuriaguerra, J. de, & Massonet, J. Les troubles visuocon-structifs par lèsion pariéto-occipitale droite. *L'Encéphale*, 1951, *40*, 122-179.

Hécaen, H., & Albert, M. L. Disorders of mental functioning related to frontal lobe pathology. In D. F. Benson and D. Blumer (Eds.), *Psychiatric Aspects of Neurologic Disease*. New York: Grune and Stratton, 1975.

Hécaen, H., & Albert, M. L. *Human neuropsychology*. New York: John Wiley, 1978.

Hécaen, H., & Assal, G. A comparison of constructive deficits following right and left hemispheric lesions. *Neuropsychologia*, 1970, *8*, 289-303.

Heilman, K. M. Apraxia. In K. M. Heilman & E. Valenstein (Eds.), *Clinical neuropsychology*. New York: Oxford Press, 1979.

Heilman, K. M., & Valenstein, E. Frontal lobe neglect in man. *Neurology*, 1972, *22*, 660-664.

Heilman, K. M., & Watson, R. T. The neglect syndrome — a unilateral defect of the orienting response. In S. Harnad, R. W. Doty, L. Goldstein, J. Jaynes, and G. Krauthamer (Eds.), *Lateralization in the nervous system*. New York: Academic Press, 1977.

Heimburger, R. F., & Reitan, R. M. Easily administered written test for lateralizing brain lesions. *Journal of Neurosurgery*, 1961, *18*, 301-312.

Hicks, L. H., & Birren, J. E. Aging, brain damage, and psychomotor slowing. *Psychological Bulletin*, 1970, *74*, 377-396.

Hierons, R., Janota, I., & Corsellis, J. A. N. The late effects of necrotizing encephalitis of the temporal lobes and limbic areas: a clinico-pathological study of 10 cases. *Psychological Medicine*, 1978, *8*, 21-42.

Hines, T. M., & Posner, M. I. *Slow but sure: a chronometric analysis of the process of aging*. Department of Psychology, University of Oregon, Eugene, Oregon. Unpublished manuscript, undated.

Hirschenfang, S. A comparison of Bender Gestalt reproductions of right and left hemiplegic patients. *Journal of Clinical Psychology*, 1960, *16*, 439.

Hirschenfang, S., Silber, M., & Benton, J. G. Psychosocial factors influencing the rehabilitation of the hemiplegic patient. *Disorders of the Nervous System*, 1968, *29*, 373-379.

Holland, A. L. *Communicative Abilities in Daily Living: A test of functional communication for aphasic adults*. Baltimore: University Park Press, 1980).

Hooper, H. E. *The Hooper Visual Organization Test: Manual*. Los Angeles: Western Psychological Services, 1958.

Horan. M., Ashton, R., & Minto, J. Using ECT to study hemispheric specialization for sequential processes. *British Journal of Psychiatry*, 1980, *137*, 119-125.

Horowitz, M. J., Cohen, F. M., Skolnikoff, A. Z., & Saunders, F. A. Psychomotor epilepsy: rehabilitation after surgical treatment. *Journal of Nervous and Mental Disease*, 1970, *150*, 273-290.

Horvath, R. B. Clinical spectrum and epidemiological features of alcoholic dementia. In J. G. Rankin (Ed.), *Alcohol, drugs, and brain damage*, Proceedings of Symposium. Toronto Addiction Research Foundation, 1975.

Houlard, N., Fraisse, P., & Hécaen, H. Effects of unilateral hemispheric lesions on two types of optico-geometric illusions. *Cortex*, 1976, *12*, 232-239.

Howieson, D. B. *Confabulation*. Paper presented at the meeting of the North Pacific Society of Neurology and Psychiatry, Bend, Oregon, March 1980.

Hulicka, I. M. Age differences in Wechsler memory Scale scores. *Journal of Genetic Psychology*, 1966, *109*, 135-145.

Hutt, M. L. *The Hutt adaptation of the Bender-Gestalt test* (3rd ed.). New York: Grune & Stratton, 1977.

Inglis, J. An experimental study of learning and "memory function" in elderly psychiatric elders. *Journal of Mental Science*, 1957, *103*, 796-803.

Ingham, J. G. Memory and intelligence. *British Journal of Psychiatry*, 1952, *43*, 20-32.

Ishihara, S. *Tests for color-blindness* (11th ed.). Tokyo: Kanehara Shuppan, 1954.

Ivnick, R. J. Neuropsychological stability in multiple sclerosis. *Journal of Consulting and Clinical Psychology*, 1978, *46*, 913-923.

Jaccarino-Hiatt, G. *Impairment of cognitive organization in patients with temporal-lobe lesions*. Unpublished Ph. D. thesis, McGill University, 1978.

James, W. *The principles of psychology*. New York: Henry Holt, 1890.

Jennett, B., & Bond, M. Assessment of outcome after severe brain damage. A practical scale. *Lancet*, 1975, *i*, 480-484.

Jennett, B., Teasdale, G., & Knill-Jones, R. Prognosis after severe head injury. Ciba Foundation Symposium, No 34 (New Series). *Symposium on the outcome of severe damage to the CNS*. Amsterdam: Elsevier, Excerpta Medica, 1975.

Jones-Gotman, M., & Milner, B. Design fluency: the invention of nonsense drawings after focal cortical lesions. *Neuropsychologia*, 1977, *15*, 653-674.

Josiassen, R. C., Curry, L., Roemer, R. A. Patterns of intellectual deficit in Huntington's disease. *Journal of Clinical Neuropsychology*, 1982, *4*, 173-183.

Joynt, R. J., & Goldtein, M. N. Minor cerebral hemisphere. In W. J.

Friedlander (Ed.), *Advances in neurology* (Vol. 7). New York: Raven Press, 1975.

Joynt, R. J., Benton, A. L., & Fogel, M. L. Behavioral and pathological correlates of motor impersistence. *Neurology*, 1962, *12*, 876-881.

Kaplan, E., Goodglass, H., & Weintraub, S. *The Boston Naming Test*. Philadelphia: Lea & Febiger, 1983.

Kaplan, R., & Tsaros, L. *Is psychological deficit in multiple sclerosis related to neurological and functional disability?* Paper presented at the seventh annual meeting of the International Neuropsychological Society, New York City, 1979.

Kapur, N., & Butters, N. Visuoperceptive deficits in long-term alcoholics and alcoholics with Korsakoff's psychosis. *Journal of Studies on Alcohol*, 1977, *38*, 2025-2035.

Kaszniak, A. W., Garron, D. C., & Fox, J. Differential effects of age and cerebral atrophy upon span of immediate recall and paired-associate learning in older patients suspected of dementia. *Cortex*, 1979, *15*, 285-295.

Katz, M. M., & Lyerly, S. B. Methods for measuring adjustment and social behavior in the community: I. Rational, description, discriminative validity and scale development. *Psychological Reports*, 1963, *13*, 503-535.

Kaufman, A. The substitution test: a survey of studies on organic mental impairment and the role of learning and motor factors in test performance. *Cortex*, 1968, *4*, 47-63.

Kear-Colwell, J. J. The structure of the Wechsler memory Scale and its relationship to brain damage. *Journal of Social and Clinical Psychology*, 1973, *12*, 384-392.

Kempinsky, W. H. Experimental study of distant effects of acute focal brain injury. *A. M. A. Archives of Neurology and Psychiatry*, 1958, *79*, 376-389.

Kertesz, A. *Aphasia and associated disorders*, New York: Grune & Stratton, 1979.

Kessler, I. I. Parkinson's disease in epidemiologic perspective. In B. S. Schoenberg (Ed.), *Advances in neurology* (Vol. 19). New York: Raven Press, 1978.

Kimura, D. Cerebral dominance in the perception of verbal stimuli. *Canadian Journal of Psychology*, 1961, *16*.

Kimura, D. Right temporal lobe damage. *Archives of Neurology* (Chicago), 1963, *8*, 264-271.

Kimura, D. Functional asymmetry of the brain in dichotic listening. *Cortex*, 1967, *3*, 163-178.

Kimura, D. The asymmetry of the human brain. *Scientific American*, 1973, *228*, 70-78.

Kimura, D. Acquisition of a motor skill after left hemisphere damage. *Brain*, 1977, *100*, 527-542.

Kimura, D. Neuromotor mechanisms in the evolution of human communication. In H. D. Steklis and M. J. Raleigh (Eds.), *Neurobiology of social communication in primates: An evolutionary perspective*. New York: Academic Press, 1979.

Kimura, D., & Durnford, M. Normal studies on the function of the right hemisphere in vision. In S. J. Dimond & J. G. Beaumont (Eds.), *Hemisphere function in the human brain*. New York: Halsted Press, 1974.

Kinsbourne, M. Lateral interactions in the brain. In M. Kinsbourne & W. L. Smith (Eds.), *Hemispheric disconnection and cerebral function*. Springfield, Ill.: C. C. Thomas, 1974.

Kinsbourne, M., & Warrington, E. K. A study of finger agnosia. *Brain*, 1962, *85*, 47-66.

Klebanoff, S. G., Singer, J. L., & Wilensky, H. Psychological consequences of brain lesions and ablations. *Psychological Bulletin*, 1954, *51*, 1-141.

Kliest, K. Cited in O. L. Zangwill, Psychological deficits associated with frontal lobe lesions. *International Journal of Neurology*, 1966, *5*, 395-402.

Kløve, H. Clinical neuropsychology. In F. M. Forster (Ed.), *The Medical clinics of North America*. New York: Saunders, 1963.

Kløve, H., & Doehring, D. G. MMPI in epileptic groups with differential etiology. *Journal of Clinical Psychology*, 1962, *18*, 149-153.

Klüver, H. *Behavior Mechanisms in Monkeys*. Chicago: University of Chicago Press, 1957.

Kolansky, H., & Moore, W. T. Toxic effects of chronic marijuana use. *Journal of the American Medical Association*, 1972, *222*, 35-41.

Kolb, B. *Neural mechanisms in facial expression in man and higher primates*. Paper presented at The Canadian Psychological Association, Vancouver, 1977.

Kolb, B., & Milner, B. *Performance of complex arm and facial movements after focal brain lesions*. Unpublished manuscript, 1980.

Kolb, B., Taylor, L., & Milner, B. *Affective behavior in patients with localized cortical excisions: an analysis of lesion site and side*. Unpublished manuscript, 1980.

Kolb, B., & Whishaw, I. *The behavior of the neonatally decorticated rat*. In preparation.

Kolb, B., & Whishaw, I. *Fundamentals of human neuropsychology*. San Francisco: W. H. Freeman, 1980.

Kramer, N. A., & Jarvik, L. Assessment of intellectual changes in the elderly. In A. Raskin & L Jarvis (Eds.), *Psychiatric symptoms and cognitive loss in the elderly*. Washington, D. C.: Hemisphere, 1979.

Krashen, S. D. Lateralization, language learning and the critical period: some new evidence. *Language Learning*, 1973, *23*, 63-74.

Krauss, I. K. Epidemiologic features of head and spinal cord injury. In

B. S. Schoenberg (Ed.), *Advances in neurology,* (Vol. 19). New York: Raven Press, 1978.

Kronfol, Z., Hamsher, K., Digre, K., & Waziri, R. Depression and hemispheric function: changes associated with unilateral ECT. *British Journal of Psychiatry,* 1978, *132,* 560-567.

Ladurner, G., Iliff, L. D., & Lechner, H. Clinical factors associated with dementia in ischaemic stroke. *Journal of Neurology, Neurosurgery, and Psychiatry,* 1982, *45,* 97-101.

Lansdell, H., & Donnelly, E. F. Factor analysis of the Wechsler Adult Intelligence Scale sub-tests and the Halstead-Reitan Category and Tapping tests. *Journal of Clinical Psychology,* 1977, *45,* 412-416.

Larrabee, G. J., Kane, R. L., Morrow, L., & Goldstein, G. *Differential drawing size associated with unilateral brain damage.* Paper presented at the tenth annual meeting of the International Neuropsychological Society, Pittsburgh, February, 1982.

Lashley, K. S. The mechanisms of vision. XVI. The functioning of small remnants of the visual cortex. *Journal of Comparative Neurology,* 1939, *70,* 45-67.

Laurence, S., & Stein, D. B. Recovery after brain damage and the concept of localization of function. In S. Finger (Ed.), *Recovery from brain damage: research and theory.* New York: Plenum Press, 1978.

Lawrence, D. G., & Kuypers, H. G. J. M. The functional organization of the motor system in the monkey, II. The effects of lesions of the descending brain-stem pathways, *Brain,* 1968, *91,* 15-136.

Lebrun, Y., & Hoops, R. *Intelligence and aphasia.* Amsterdam: Sets & Zeitlinger, B. V., 1974.

Leech, R. W., & Shuman, R. M. *Neuropathology. A summary for students.* Philadelphia: Harper & Row, 1982.

Leipmann, H. Die linke Hemisphäre und das Handeln. In *Drei Aufsätze aus dem Apraxiegebiet.* Berlin: Springer, 1908.

Lenneberg, E. *Biological foundations of language.* New York: John Wiley and Sons, 1967.

Lesser, R. Verbal and non-verbal memory components in the Token Test. *Neuropsychologia,* 1976, *14,* 79-85.

Levin, H. S., & Grossman, R. G. Behavioral sequelae of closed head injury. *Archives of Neurology,* 1978, *35,* 720-727.

Levin, H. S., Grossman, R. G., Rose, J. E., & Teasdale, G. Long-term neuropsychological outcome of closed head injury. *Journal of Neurosurgery,* 1979, *50,* 412-422.

Levin, H. S., Myers, C. A., Grossman, R. G., & Sarwar, M. Ventricular enlargement after closed head injury. *Archives of Neurology,* 1981, *38,* 623-629.

Levin, H. S., O'Donnell, V. M., & Grossman, R. G. The Galveston Orientation and Amnesia Test. A Practical scale to assess cognition

305

after head injury. *Journal of Nervous and Mental Diseases*, 1979, *167*, 675-684.

Levy-Agresti, J., & Sperry, R. W. Differential perceptual capacities in major and minor hemispheres. *Proceedings of the National Academy of Science*, 1968, *61*, 1151.

Levy, J. Lateral specialization of the brain: behavioral manifestations and possible evolutionary basis. In J. A. Kiger, Jr. (Ed.), *The biology of behavior*. Corvallis, Oregon: Oregon State University Press, 1972.

Lewis R., & Kupke, T. *The Lafayette Clinic repeatable neuropsychological test battery: Its development and research applications*. Paper presented at the annual meeting of the Southeastern Psychological Association, Hollywood, Fla., May, 1977.

Lezak, M. D. Living with the characterologically altered brain injured patient. *Journal of Clinical Psychiatry*, 1978a, *39*, 592-598.

Lezak, M. D. Subtle sequelae of brain damage: perplexity, distractibility, and fatigue. *American Journal of Physical Medicine*, 1978b, *57*, 9-15.

Lezak, M. D. Recovery of memory and learning functions following traumatic brain injury. *Cortex*, 1979, *15*, 63-70.

Lezak, M. D. Coping with head injury in the family. In G. A. Broe & R. L. Tate (Eds.), *Brain impairment: Proceedings of the Fifth Annual Brain Impairment Conference*. Sydney: Postgraduate committee in Medicine of the University of Sydney, 1982a

Lezak, M. D. The problem of assessing executive functions. *International Journal of Psychology*, 1982b, *17*, 281-297.

Lezak, M. D. *Neuropsychological assessment*. New York: Oxford University Press, 1983.

Lezak, M. D., Cosgrove, J. N., O'Brien, K., & Wooster, N. *Relationship between personality disorder, social disturbance, and physical disability following traumatic brain injury*. Paper presented at the eighth annual meeting of the International Neuropsychological Society, San Francisco, 1980.

Lezak, M. D., Howieson, D. B., & McGavin, J. *Temoral sequencing of the remote events task with Korsakoff patients*. Paper presented at the eleventh annual meeting of the International Neuropsychological Society, Mexico City, February, 1983.

Lezak, M. D., & Newman, S. P. *Verbosity and right hemisphere damage*. Paper presented at the second European conference of the International Neuropsychological Society, Noordvijkerhout, Holland, 1979.

Lhermitte, F., & Signoret, J-L. Analyse neuropsychologique et différenciation des syndromes amnésiques. *Revue Neurologique*, 1972, *126*, 164-178.

Lhermitte, F., & Signoret, J-L. The amnesic syndromes and the hippocampal-mammillary system. In M. R. Rosenzweig & E. L. Bennett (Eds.), *Neural mechanisms of learning and memory*. Cambridge,

Mass.: Massachusetts Institute of Technology Press, 1976.

Lichtman, M. *REAL: Reading/Everyday Activities in Life*. New York: CAL Press, 1972.

Likert, R., & Quasha, W. H. *The revised Minnesota Paper Form Board Test Manual*. New York: Psychological Corporation, 1970.

Lindsey, B. A., & Coppinger, N. W. Age-related deficits in simple capabilities and their consequences for Trail Making performance. *Journal of Clinical Psychology*, 1969, *25*, 156-159.

Lishman, W. A. *Organic psychiatry*. Oxford: Blackwell Scientific Publications, 1978.

Lishman, W. A. Cerebral disorder in alcoholism syndromes of impairment. *Brain*, 1981, *104*, 1-20.

Long, C. J., & Brown, D. A. *Analysis of temporal cortex dysfunction by neuropsychological techniques*. Paper presented at the American Psychological Association Convention, New York, 1979.

Lubin, B. Adjective check lists for measurement of depression. *Archives of General Psychiatry*, 1965, *12*, 57-62.

Luria, A. R. Neuropsychological analysis of focal brain lesions. In B. B. Wolman (Ed.), *Handbook of Clinical psychology*. New York: McGraw-Hill, 1965.

Luria, A. R. *Higher cortical functions in man*. (B. Haigh, trans.). New York: Basic Books, 1966.

Luria, A. R. The frontal lobe and the regulation of behavior. In K. H. Pribram & A. R. Luria (Eds.), *Psychophysiology of the frontal lobes*. New York: Academic Press, 1973a.

Luria, A. R. *The working brain*. New York: Penguin Books, 1973b.

Luria, A. R., & Homskaya, E. D. Disturbances in the regulative role of speech with frontal lobe lesions. In J. M. Warren & K. Akert (Eds.), *The frontal granular cortex and behavior*. New York: McGraw-Hill, 1964.

Luria, A. R., & Hutton, J. T. A modern assessment of basic forms of aphasia. *Brain and Language*, 1977, *4*, 129-151.

Lyle, O. E., & Gottesman, I. I. Premorbid psychometric indicators of the gene for Huntington's disease. *Journal of Consulting and Clinical Psychology*, 1977, *45*, 1011-1022.

Mack, J. L. The MMPI and neurological dysfunction. In C. S. Newmark (Ed.), *MMPI: Current clinical and research trends*. New York: Praeger, 1979.

Mack, J. L., & Levine, R. N. The basis of visual constructional disability in patients with unilateral cerebral lesions. *Cortex*, 1981, *17*, 512-532.

MacQuarrie, T. W. *MacQuarrie Test for Mechanical Ability*. Monterey, Calif.: CTB/McGraw-Hill, 1925, 1953.

Malamud, N. Organic brain disease mistaken for psychiatric disorder.

In D. F. Benson and D. Blumer (Eds.), *Psychiatric Aspects of Neurological Disease*. New York: Grune and Stratton, 1975.

Mandleberg, I. A., & Brooks, D. N. Cognitive recovery after severe head injury: I. Serial testing on the WAIS. *Journal of Neurology, Neurosurgery, & Psychiatry*, 1975, *38*, 1121-1126.

Mandler, G. Organization and memory. *Psychology of Learning and Motivation*, 1967, *1*, 327-372.

Marin, O. S., & Gordon, B. Neuropsychologic aspects of aphasia. In H. R. Tyler & D. M. Dawson (Eds.), *Current neurology* (Vol. 2). Boston: Houghton-Mifflin, 1979.

Marsh G. G., & Hirsch, S. H. Effectiveness of two tests of visual retention. *Journal of Clinical Psychology*, 1982, *28*, 115-118.

Matthews, B. *Multiple sclerosis: The facts*. Oxford: Oxford University Press, 1978.

Matthews, C. G., & Haaland, , K. Y. The effect of symptom duration on cognitive and motor performance in Parkinsonism. *Neurology*, 1979, *29*, 951-956.

Matthews C. G., & Harley, J. P. Cognitive and motor-sensory performances in toxic and nontoxic epileptic subjects. *Neurology*, 1975, *25*, 184-188.

Matthews, C. G., & Kløve, H. *Instruction manual for the Adult Neuropsychology Test Battery*. Madison, Wisconsin: University of Wisconsin Medical School, 1964.

Mattis, S. Mental status examination for organic mental syndrome in the elderly patient. In L. Bellak & T. B. Karasu (Eds.), *Geriatric psychiatry*. New York: Grune & Stratton, 1976.

Mayeux, R., Stern, Y., Rosen, J., & Leventhal, J. Depression, intellectual impairment, and Parkinson disease. *Neurology*, 1981, *31*, 645-650.

McFie, J., *Assessment of organic intellectual impairment*. London: Academic Press, 1975.

McFie, J., Piercy, M. F., & Zangwill, O. I. Visual-agnosia associated with lesions of the right cerebral hemisphere. *Brain*, 1950, *73*, 167-190.

McFie, J. & Zangwill, O. I. Visual constructive disabilities associated with lesion of the left cerebral hemisphere. *Brain*, 1960, *83*, 243-260.

McKinlay, W. W., Brooks, D. N., Bond, M. R., et al. The short term outcome of severe blunt head injury as reported by relatives of the injured persons. *Journal of Neurology, Neurosurgery, and Psychiatry*, 1981, *44*, 527-533.

McSweeney, A. J., Grant, I., Heaton, R. K., et al. Life quality of patients with chronic obstructive pulmonary disease. *Archives of Internal Medicine*, 1982, *142*, 473-478.

Meadows, J. C. The anatomical basis of prosopagnosia. *Journal of Neurology, Neurosurgery, and Psychiatry*, 1974a, *37*, 489-501.

Meadows, J. C. Disturbed perception of colours associated with localized cerebral lesions. *Journal of Neurology, Neurosurgery, and Psychia-*

try, 1974b, *97*, 315-632.

Meer, B., & Baker, J. A. The Stockton Geriatric Rating Scale. *Journal of Gerontology*, 1966, *21*, 392-403.

Meier, M. J. The regional localization hypothesis and personality changes associated with focal cerebral lesions and ablations. In J. N. Butcher (Ed.), *MMPI: research developments and clinical applications*. New York: McGraw-Hill, 1969.

Meier, M. J. *Neuropsychological predictors of motor recovery after cerebral infarction*. Paper presented at the American Psychological Association Convention. New York, September, 1974.

Mercer, B., Wapner, W., Gardner, H., & Benson, D. F. A study of confabulation. *Archives of Neurology*, 1977, *34*, 429-433.

Messerli, P., Seron, X., & Tissot, R. Quelques aspects des troubles de la programmation dans le syndrome frontal. *Archives Suisse de Neurologie, Neurochirurgia, et de Psychiatrie*, 1979, *125*, 23-25.

Meyer V., & Falconer, M. A. Defects of learning ability with massive lesions of the temporal lobe. *Journal of Mental Science*, 1960, *106*, 472-477.

Miceli, G., Caltagirone, C., & Gainotti, G. Gangliosides in the treatment of mental deterioration. A double-blind comparison with placebo. *Acta Psychiatrica Scandinavica*, 1977, *55*, 102-110.

Miceli, G., Caltagirone, C., Gainotti, G., Masullo, C., & Silveri, M. C. Neuropsychological correlates of localized cerebral lesions in nonaphasic brain-damaged patients. *Journal of Clinical Neuropsychology*, 1981, *3*, 53-63.

Miller E., & Hague, F. Some characteristics of verbal behavior in presenile dementia. *Psychological Medicine*, 1975, *5*, 255-259.

Millham, J., Chilcutt, J., & Atkinson, B. *Criterion validity of the AAMD Adaptive Behavior Scale*. Symposium presented at the American Psychological Association Convention, Washington, D. C., 1976.

Millichap, J. G. Drugs in management of minimal brain dysfunction. *Annals of the New York Academy of Sciences*, 1973, *204*, 321-334.

Mills, L., & Burkhart, G. *Memory for prose material in neurological patients: a comparison of two scoring systems*. Research Bulletin #510. London, Canada: Department of Psychology, University of Western Ontario, July, 1980.

Milner, B. Lateral effects in audition. In V. B. Mountcastle (Ed.), *Interhemispheric relations and cerebral dominance*. Baltimore: John Hopkins University Press, 1962.

Milner, B. Some effects of frontal lobectomy in man. In J. M. Warren & K. Akert (Eds.). *The frontal granular cortex and Behavior*. New York: McGraw-Hill Book Co., 1964.

Milner, B. Visually-guided maze learning in man: effects of bilateral hippocampal, bilateral frontal, and unilateral cerebral lesions. *Neuropsychologia*, 1965, *3*, 317-338.

Milner, B. Brain mechanisms suggested by studies of temporal lobes. In C. H. Millikan & F. L. Darlely (Eds.), *Brain mechanisms underlying speech and language*. New York: Grune & Stratton, 1967.

Milner, B. Visual recognition and recall after right temporal-lobe excision in man. *Neuropsychologia*, 1968, *6*, 191-209.

Milner, B. Residual intellectual and memory deficits after head injury. In A. E. Walker, W. F. Caveness, & M. Critchley (Eds.), *The late effects of head injury*. Springfield, Ill.: C. C. Thomas, 1969.

Milner, B. Memory and the medial temporal regions of the brain. In K. H. Pribram and D. E. Broadbent (Eds.), *Biological basis of Memory*. New York: Academic Press, 1970.

Milner, B. Interhemispheric differences in the localization of psychological processes in man. *British Medical Bulletin*, 1971, *27*, 272-277.

Milner, B. Disorders of learning and memory after temporal lobe lesions in man. *Clinical Neurosurgery*, 1972, *19*, 421-446.

Milner, B. Hemispheric specialization: scope and limits. In F. O. Schmitt and F. G. Worden (Eds.). *The neurosciences: Third study program*. Cambridge, Mass.: MIT Press, 1974.

Milner, B. Psychological aspects of focal epilepsy and its neurological management. *Advances in Neurology*, 1975, *8*, 299-321.

Milner, B. Hemispheric asymmetry in the control of gesture sequences. *Proceedings of XXI International Congress of Psychology*. Paris, 1976.

Monakow, C. von. Diaschisis. In K. H. Pribram (Ed.), *Brain and behavior 1. Mood, states and mind*. Baltimore: Penguin, 1969.

Money, J. A. *A standardized Road Map Test of Direction Sense. Manual*. San Rafael, Calif.: Academic Therapy Publications, 1976.

Mooney, C. M. Age in the development of closure ability in children. *Canadian Journal of Psychology*, 1957, *2*, 219-226.

Mooney, C. M., & Ferguson, G. A. A new closure test. *Canadian Journal of Psychology*, 1951, *5*, 129-133.

Moran, L. J., & Mefford, R. D., Jr. Repetitive psychometric measures. *Psychological Reports*, 1959, *5*, 269-275.

Morrow. R. S., & Mark, J. C. The correlation of intelligence and neurological findings on 22 patients autopsied for brain damage. *Journal of Consulting Psychology*, 1955 *19*, 283-289.

Mueller, J. E. Test anxiety and the encoding and retrieval of information. In I. G. Sarason (Ed.), *Test anxiety: theory, research, and applications*. Hillsdale, N. J.: Erlbaum Associates, 1979.

Munday, C. S. *Emotional characteristics associated with laterality of brain lesion*. Unpublished doctoral dissertation, California School of Professional Psychology, Berkeley, 1979.

Murstein, B. I., & Leipold, W. D. The role of learning of motor abilities in the Wechsler-Bellevue Digit Symbol test. *Educational Psychological Measurement*, 1961, *21*, 103-112.

Najenson, T. *Rehabilitation of the severely brain damaged adult — a comprehensive approach.* Invited address to the Medical College of Virginia's Fourth Annual Post-Graduate Course on the Rehabilitation of the Traumatic Brain-injured Adult, Williamsburg, Virginia, June, 1980.

Nebes, R. D. Direct examination of cognitive function in the right and left hemispheres, In M. Kinsbourne (Ed.), *Asymmetrical function of the brain.* Cambridge, England: Cambridge University Press, 1978.

Nelson, H. E. A modified card sorting test sensitive to frontal lobe defects. *Cortex,* 1976, *12,* 313-324.

Nelson, H. E., & O'Connell, A. Dementia: the estimation of premorbid intelligence levels using the New Adult Reading Test. *Cortex,* 1978, *14,* 234-244.

Nemec, R. E. Effects of controlled background interference on test performance by right and left hemiplegics. *Journal of Consulting .and Clinical Psychology,* 1978, *46,* 294-297.

Neugarten, B. L., Havighurst, R. J., & Tobin, S. S. The measurement of life satisfaction. *Journal of Gerontology,* 1961, *16,* 134-143.

Newcombe, F. *Missile wounds of the brain.* London: Oxford University Press, 1969.

Nihira, K., Foster., R., Shellhaas, M., & Leland, H. *AAMD Adaptive Behavior Scale, 1974 Revision.* Washington, D. C.: American Association on Mental Deficiency, 1975.

O'Brien, M. T., & Lezak, M. D. *Long-term improvements in intellectual function following brain injury.* Paper presented at the fourth European conference of the International Neuropsychological Society, Bergen, Norway, July, 1981.

Obler, L. K., & Albert, M. L. *Language and communication in the elderly.* Lexington, Mass.: Lexington Books, 1980.

O'Brian, K., & Lezak, M. D. *Long-term improvements in intellectual function following brain injury.* Paper presented at the fourth European conference of the International Neuropsychological Society, Bergen, Norway, July, 1981.

Oddy, M., & Humphrey, M. Social recovery during the year following severe head injury. *Journal of Neurology, Neurosurgery, and Psychiatry,* 1980, *43,* 798-802.

Oddy, M., Humphrey, M., & Uttley, D. Subjective impairment and social recovery after closed head injury. *Journal of Neurology, Neurosurgery, and Psychiatry,* 1978b, *41,* 611-616.

Ojemann, G. Subcortical language mechanisms. In H. Avakian-Whitaker & A. Whitaker (Eds.), *Studies in neurolinguistics.* New York: academic Press, 1975.

Okawa, M., Maeda, S., Nukui, H., & Kawafuchi, J. Psychiatric symptoms in ruptured anterior communicating aneurysms: social prognosis. *Acta Psychiatrica Scandinavica*, 1980, *61*, 306-312.

Ommaya, A. K. head injury in the adult. In H. F. Conn (Ed.), *Current therapy*. Philadelphia: W. B. Saunder, 1972.

Ommaya, A. K., Fass, F., & Yarnell, P. Whiplash injury and brain damage. *Journal of the American Medical Association*, 1968, *204*, 285-289.

Ommaya, A. K., Grubb, R. L., & Naumann, R. A. Coup and contre-coup injury: observations on the mechanics of visible brain injuries in the rhesus monkey. *Journal of Neurosurgery*, 1971, *35*, 503-516.

Oscar-Berman, M. Neuropsychological consequences of long-term chronic alcoholism. *American Scientist*, 1980, *68*, 410-419.

Osgood, C. E., & Miron, M. S. *Approaches to the study of aphasia*. Urbana, Ill.: University of Illinois Press, 1963.

Osterrieth, P. A. Le test de copie d'une figure complexe. *Archives de Psychologie*, 1944, *30*, 206-356.

Overall, J. E., & Gorham, D. R. The Brief Psychiatric Rating Scale. *Psychological Reports*, 1962, *10*, 799-812.

Pankratz, L. Symptom validity testing and symptom retraining: procedures for the assessment and treatment of functional sensory deficits. *Journal of Consulting and Clinical Psychology*, 1979, *47*, 409-410.

Pankratz, L., Fausti, S. A., & Peed, S. A. A forced-choice technique to evaluate deafness in the hysterical or malingering patient. *Journal of Consulting and Clinical Psychology*, 1975, *43*, 421-422.

Panting, A., & Merry, P. H. The long-term rehabilitation of severe head injuries with particular reference to the need for social and medical support for the patient's family. *Rehabilitation*, 1972, *38*, 33-37.

Papez, J. W. A proposed mechanism of emotion. *Archives of Neurology and Psychiatry*, 1937, *38*, 724-744.

Parker, J. W. The validity of some current tests for organicity. *Journal of Consulting Psychology*, 1957, *21*, 425-428.

Parsons, O. A. Neuropsychological deficits in alcoholics: facts and fancies. *Alcoholism: Clinical and Experimental Research*, 1977, *1*, 51-56.

Parsons, O. A., & Farr, S. P. The neuropsychology of alcohol and drug use. In S. B. Filskov & T. J. Boll (Eds.), *Handbook of clinical neuropychology*. New York: Wiley-Interscience, 1981.

Parsons, O. A., Vega, A. Jr., & Burn, J. Differential psychological effects of lateralized brain damage. *Journal of Consulting and Clincal Psychology*, 1969, *33*, 551-557.

Paterson A., & Zangwill, O. L. Disorders of visual space perception associated with lesions of the right cerebral hemisphere. *Brain*, 1944, *67*, 331-358.

Payne, A. W. Disorders of thinking. In C. G. Costellor (Ed.), *Symptoms of psychopathology*. New York: Wiley, 1970.

Payne, R. W., & Hewlett, J. H. G. Thought disorder in psychotic patients. In H. J. Eysenck (Ed.), *Experiments in personality (Vol. 2, Psychodiagnostics and psychodynamics)*. New York: The Humanities Press, 1960.

Penfield, W., & Jasper, H. H. *Epilepsy and the functional anatomy of the human brain*. Boston; Little-Brown, 1954.

Penfield, W., & Roberts, L. *Speech and brain mechanisms*. Princeton, N. J.: Princeton University Press, 1959.

Perret, E. The left frontal lobe of man and the suppression of habitual responses in verbal categorical behavior. *Neuropsychologia*, 1974, *12*, 323-330.

Peyser, J. M., Edwards, K. R., & Posner, C. M. Psychological profiles in patients with multiple sclerosis. *Archives of Neurology*, 1980, *37*, 437-440.

Pfeiffer, E. SPMSQ: Short Portable Mental Status Questionnaire. *Journal of the American Geriatric Society*, 1975, *23*, 433-441.

Piaget, J. *Biology and knowledge*. Chicago: The University of Chicago Press, 1971.

Piercy, M. The effects of cerebral lesions on intellectual functions: a review of current research trends. *British Journal of Psychiatry*, 1964, *110*, 310-352.

Piercy, M., Hécaen, H., & de Ajuriaguerra, J. Constructional apraxia associated with unilateral cerebral lesions — left and right cases compared. *Brain*, 1960, *83*, 222-242.

Pincus, J. H., & Tucker, G. J. *Behavioral neurology*. 2nd ed.). New York: Oxford University Press, 1978.

Piotrowski, Z. The Rorschach inkblot method in organic disturbances of the central nervous system. *Journal of Nervous and Mental Disease*, 1937, *86*, 525-537.

Pirozzolo, F. J., Hansch, E. C., Mortimer, J. A., et al. Dementia in Parkinson disease: a neuropsychological analysis. *Brain and Cognition*, 1982, *1*, 71-83.

Plum F., & Caronn, J. J. Can one predict outcome of medical coma? In Ciba Foundation Symposium 34 (New Series) *Symposium on the outcome of severe damage to the central nervous system*. Amsterdam: Elsevier, 1975.

Plutchick, R., Conte, H., Lieberman, M., et al. Reliability and validity of a scale for assessing the functioning of geriatric patients. *Journal of the American Geriatric Society*, 1970, *18*, 491-500.

Plutchick, R., Conte, H., Lieberman, M. Development of a scale (GIES) for assessment of cognitive and perceptual functioning in geriatric patients. *Journal of the American Geriatric Society*, 1971, *19*, 614-623.

Pontius, A. A., & Yudowitz, B. S. Frontal lobe system dysfunction in some criminal actions as shown in the Narratives Test. *Journal of Nervous and Mental Disease*, 1980, *168*, 111-117.

Poon, L. W., Fozard, J. L., Cermak, L. S., et al. (Eds.), *New directions in memory and aging*. Hillsdale, N. J.: Lawrence Erlbaum Associates, 1980.

Porch, B. E. *Porch Index of communicative ability*. Palo alto, Calif.: Consulting Psychologist Press, 1967.

Porch, B. E., Friden, T., & Porec, J. *Objective differentiation of aphasic vs. non-organic patients.* Paper presented at the fifth annual meeting of the International Neuropsychological Society, Santa Fe, 1977.

Porteus, S. D. *The Maze Test and clinical psychology*. Palo Alto, Calif.: Pacific Books, 1959.

Porteus, S. D. *Porteus Maze Test. Fifty years' application*. Palo Alto, Calif.: Pacific Books, 1965.

Prigatano, G. P., & Pribram, K. H. Perception and memory of facial affect following brain injury. *Journal of Perceptual and Motor Skills*, 1982, *54*, 859-869.

Prisko, L. *Short-term memory in focal cerebral damage*. Unpublished Ph. D. thesis, McGill University, 1963.

Purdue Research Foundation. *Examiner's manual for the Purdue Pegboard*. Chicago: Science Research Associates, 1948.

Purisch, A. D., Golden, C. J., & Hammeke, T. A. Discrimination of schizophrenic and brain-injured patients by a standardized version of Luria's neuropsychological tests. *Journal of Consulting Clinical Psychology*, 1978, *46*, 1266-1273.

Pyke, S., & Agnew, N. McK. Digit Span performance as a function of noxious stimulation. *Journal of Consulting Psychology*, 1963, *27*, 281.

Raghaven, S. *A comparison of the performance of right and left hemiplegics on verbal and nonverbal body image tasks.* Master's Thesis. Northampton, Mass.: Smith College, 1961.

Ramier, A. -M., & Hécaen, H. Rôle respectif des atteintes frontales et de la latéralisation lésionnelle dans les déficits de la "fluence verbale." *Revue Neurologique*, Paris 1970, *123*, 17-22.

Randt, C. T., Brown, E. R., & Osborne, D. J., Jr. *A memory test for longitudinal measurement of mild to moderate deficits* (Rev.). Unpublished manuscript, Department of Neurology, New York Medical Center, 1980.

Rao, S. M., Hammeke, T. A., Huang, J. Y. S., et al. *Memory disturbance in chronic, progressive multiple sclerosis.* Paper presented at the tenth annual meeting of the International Neuropsychological Society, Pittsburgh, February, 1982.

Rappaport, M., Hall, K., Hopkins, K., Bellez, T., & Cope, N. Disability rating scale for severe head trauma patients: Coma to community. *Archives of Physical Medicine Rehabilitation*, 1982, *63*, 118-123.

Ratcliff, G. Disturbances of spatial orientation associated with cerebral lesions. In M. Potegal (Ed.), *Spatial abilities*. New York: Academic Press, 1972.

Raven, J. C. *Guide to the Standard Progressive Matrices*. New York: Psychological Corp.; London: H. K. Lewis, 1960.

Raven, J. C. *Guide to Using the Coloured Progressive Matrices*. New York: Psychological Corp.; London: H. K. Lewis, 1965.

Reitan, R. M. Investigation of the validity of Halstead's measure of biological intelligence. *A. M. A. Archives of Neurology and Psychiatry*, 1955, *73*, 28-35.

Reitan, R. M. Validity of the Trail Making Test as an indication of organic brain damage, *Perceptual and Motor Skills*, 1958, *8*, 271-276.

Reitan, R. M. Problems and prospects in studying the psychological correlates of brain lesions. *Cortex*, 1966a, *2*, 127-154.

Reitan, R. M. Psychological changes associated with aging and cerebral damage. *Mayo Clinic Proceedings*, 1967, *42*, 653-673.

Reitan, R. M., & Davison, L. A. *Clinical neuropsychology: current status and applications*. New York: Hemisphere, 1974.

Reitan, R. M., & Kløve, H. *Hypothesis supported by clinical evidence that are under current investigation*. Unpulished manuscript, 1959.

Reitan, R. M., & Wolfson, D. *Neuroanatomy and neuropathology: a clinical guide for neuropsychologists*. Tucson, Arizona: Neuropsychology Press, 1985.

Rey, A. L'examen psychologique dans les cas d'encéphalopathie traumatique. *Archives de Psychologie*, 1941, *28*, No. 112, 286-340.

Rey, A. *L'examen clinique en psychologie*. Paris: Presses Universitaires de France, 1964.

Riddoch, G. Dissociation of visual perceptions due to occipital injuries, with special reference to appreciation of movement. *Brain*, 1917, *40*, 15-47.

Riege, W. H., & Williams, M. V. *Modality and age comparisons in nonverbal memory*. Paper presented at the American Psychological Association Convention, Montreal, September, 1980.

Rosenzweig, M. R., & Leiman, A. L. Brain functions. *Annual Review of Psychology*, 1968, *19*, 55-98.

Roth, M. The psychiatric disorders of later life. *Psychiatric Annals*, 1976, *6*, 417-445.

Roth, M. Diagnosis of senile and related forms of dementia. In R. Katzman, R. D. Terry, & K. L. Bick (Eds.), *Alzheimer's disease: senile dementia and related disorders (Aging, Vol. 7)*. New York: Raven Press, 1978.

Rubens, A. The role of changes within the central nervous system during recovery from aphasia. In M. Sullivan & M. Kommens (Eds.), *Rationale for adult aphasia therapy.* Omaha: University of Nebraska Press, 1977.

Ruesch, J., & Moore, B. E. The measurement of intellectual functions in the acute stage of head injury. *Archives of Neurological Psychiatry*, 1943, *50*, 165-170.

Russell, E. W. *The effect of acute lateralized brain damage on Halstead's biological intelligence factors.* Paper presented at the American Psychological Association Convention, Honolulu, August, 1972.

Russell, E. W. A multiple scoring method for the assesment of complex memory functions. *Journal of Consulting and Clinical Psychology*, 1975, *43*, 800-809.

Russell, E. W. MMPI profiles of brain-damaged and schizophrenic subjects. *Journal of Clinical Psychology*, 1977, *33*, 190-193.

Russell, E. W., Neuringer, C., & Goldstein, G. *Assessment of brain damage. A neuropsychological key approach.* New York: Wiley-Interscience, 1970.

Ryan, C., & Butters, N. Further evidence for a continuum-of-impairment encompassing alcoholic Korsakoff patients and chronic alcoholics. *Alcoholism: Clinical and Experimental Research*, 1980a, *4*, 190-198.

Ryan, C., & Butters, N. Learning and memory impairments in young and old alcoholics: evidence for the premature-aging hypothesis. *Alcoholism : Clinical and Experimental Research*, 1980b, *4*, 288-293.

Ryan, C., & Butters, N. Cognitive effects in alcohol abuse. In B. Kissin & H. Begleiter (Eds.), *Cognitive effects in alcohol abuse.* New York: Plenum Press, 1982.

Ryan, C., Butters, N., Montgomery, K., Adinolfi, A., & DiDario, B. Memory deficits in chronic alcoholics: continuities between the "intact" alcoholic and the alcoholic Korsakoff patient. In H. Begleiter & B. Kissin (Eds.), *Biological effects of alcohol.* New York: Plenum Press, 1980.

Sanchez-Craig, M. Drinking pattern as a determinant of alcoholics' performance on the Trail-Making Test. *Journal of Studies on Alcohol*, 1980, *41*, 1083-1089.

Sarno, M. T. *The functional communication Profile: Manual of directions.* New York: Institute of Rehabilitation Medicine, New York University Medical Center, 1969.

Saunders, D. R. A factor analysis of the Information and the Arithmetic items of the WAIS. *Psychological Reports*, 1960a, *6*, 367-383.

Saunders, D. R. A factor analysis of the Picture Completion items of the WAIS. *Journal of Clinical Psychology*, 1960b, *16*, 146-149.

Schachter, D. L., & Crovitz, H. F. Memory function after closed head injury. A review of the quantitative research. *Cortex*, 1977, *13*, 150-

176.

Schaie, K. W. Rigidity-flexibility and intelligence: a cross-sectional study of the adult life span from 20 to 70 years. *Psychological Monographs*, 1958, *72* (9, Whole No. 462).

Schenkenberg, T., Bradford, D. C., & Ajax, E. E. Line bisection and unilateral visual neglect in patients with neurologic impairment. *Neurology*, 1980, *30*, 509-517.

Scherer, I. W., Klett, C. J., & Winne, J. F. Psychological changes over a five year period following bilateral frontal lobotomy. *Journal of Consulting Psychology*, 1957, *21*, 291-298.

Schonen, S. de Déficit mnésique d'origine organique et niveaux d'organisation des taches à mémoriser. *L'Anneé Psychologique*, 1968, *68*, 97-114.

Schuell, H. *Differential diagnosis of aphasia with the Minnesota Test.* Minneapolis: University of Minnesota Press, (2nd ed., revised), 1972.

Schulhoff, C., & Goodglass, H. Dichotic listening: side of brain injury and cerebral dominance. *Neuropsychologia*, 1969, *7*, 149-160.

Schulman, J. C., Kaspar, J. C., & Thorne, F. M. *Brain damage and behavior.* Springfield, Ill.: C. C. Thomas, 1965.

Schwartz, A. S., Marchok, P. L., & Flynn, R. E. A sensitive test for tactile extinction: results in patients with parietal and frontal lobe disease. *Journal of Neurology, Neurosurgery, and Psychiatry*, 1977, *40*, 228-233.

Scranton, J., Fogel, M. L., & Erdman, W. J. Evaluation of functional levels of patients during and following rehabilitation. *Archives of Physical Medicine Rehabilitation*, 1970, *51*, 1-21.

Seashore, C. E., Lewis, D., & Saetveit, D. L. *Seashore measures of musical talents (Rev. ed.).* New York: Psychological Corp., 1960.

Semmes, J., Weinstein, S., Ghent, L., & Teuber, H. -L. *Somatosensory changes after penetrating brain wounds in man.* Cambridge, Mass.: Harvard Univ. Press, 1960.

Semmes, J., Weinstein, S., Ghent, L., & Teuber, H. -L. Correlates of impaired orientation in personal and extra-personal space, *Brain*, 1963, *86*, 747-772.

Seron, X. Analyse neuropsychologique des lésions préfrontales chez l'homme. *L'Année Psychologique*, 1978, *78*, 183-202.

Shader, R. I., Harmatz, J. S., & Salzman, C. A new scale for clinical assessment in geriatric populations: Sandoz Clinical Assessment — Geriatric (SCAG). *Journal of the American Geriatrics Society*, 1974, *22*, 107-113.

Shallice, T. & Evans, M. E. The involvement of the frontal lobes in cognitive estimation. *Cortex*, 1978, *14*, 294-303.

Shankweiler, D. Effects of temporal lobe damage on perception of dichotically presented melodies. *Journal of comparative and Physio-*

logical Psychology, 1966, *62,* 115.

Shaywitz, B. A., Cohen, D. J., & Bowers, M. B., Jr. CSF monoamine metabolites in children with minimal brain dysfunction: Evidence for alteration of brain dopamine. *Journal of Pediatrics,* 1977, *90,* 67-71.

Sheer, D. E. Psychometric studies. In N. D. C. Lewis, C. Landis, & H. E. King (Eds.), *Studies in topectomy.* New York: Grune & Stratton, 1956.

Sherrington, C. S. *The integrative action of the nervous system.* New Haven, Yale University Press, 1906.

Shipley, W. C. A self-administered scale for measuring intellectual impairment and deterioration. *Journal of Psychology,* 1940, *9,* 371-377.

Shipley, W. C. *Institute of Living Scale.* Los Angeles: Western Psychological Services, 1946.

Sklar, M. Relation of psychological and language test scores and autopsy findings in aphasia. *Journal of Speech and Hearing Research,* 1963, *6,* 84-90.

Smith, A. Intellectual functions in patients with lateralized frontal tumors. *Journal of Neurology, Neurosurgery, and Psychiatry,* 1966, *29,* 52-59.

Smith, A. The serial sevens subtraction test. *Archives of Neurology,* 1967, *17,* 78-80.

Smith, A. *Symbol Digit Modalities Test Manual.* Los Angeles: Western Psychological Services, 1973.

Smith, A. Neurological testing in neurological disorders. In W. J. Friedlander (Ed.), *Advances in neurology* (Vol. 7). New York: Raven Press, 1975.

Smith, A. Practices and principles of neuropsychology. *International Journal of Neuroscience,* 1979, *9,* 233-238.

Smith, A. Principles underlying human brain functions in neuropsychological sequelae of different neuropathological processes. In S. B. Filskov & T. J. Boll (Eds.), *Handbook of clinical neuropsychology.* New York: Wiley-Interscience, 1980.

Snow, W. G. *The Rey-Osterrieth Complex Figure Test as a measure of visual recall.* Paper presented at the seventh annual meeting of the International Neuropsychological Society, New York, 1979.

Spence, J. T. Patterns of performance on WAIS Similarities in schizophrenic, brain-damaged, and normal subjects. *Psychological Reports,* 1963, *13,* 431-436.

Spitz, H. H. Note on immediate memory for digits: invariance over the years. *Psychological Bulletin,* 1972, *78,* 183-185.

Spreen, O., & Benton, A. L. Comparative studies of some psychological tests for cerebral damage. *Journal of Nervous and Mental Disease,* 1965, *140,* 323-333.

Spreen, O., & Benton, A. L. *Neurosensory Center comprehensive examination for aphasia.* Victoria, Canada: University of Victoria, 1969.

Squire, L. R., & Slater, P. C. Forgetting in very long-term memory as assessed by an improved questionnaire taxonomy. *Journal of Experimental Psychology: Human Language and memory*, 1975, *104*, 50-54.

Staples, D., & Lincoln, N. B. Intellectual impairment in multiple sclerosis and its relation to functional abilities. *Rheumatology and Rehabilitation*, 1979, *18*, 153-160.

Stevens, J. R. Psychiatric implications of psychomotor epilepsy. *Archives of General Psychiatry*, 1966, *14*, 461-471.

Stone, C. P., Girdner, J., & Albrecht, R. An alternate form of the Wechsler memory Scale. *Journal of Psychology*, 1946, *22*, 199-206.

Street, R. F. *A Gestalt Completion Test.* Contributions to Education, No 481. New York: Bureau of Publications, Teachers College, Columbia University, 1931.

Strich, S. J. Shearing of nerve fibers as a cause of brain damage due to head injury. *Lancet*, 1961, *ii*, 446-448.

Stroop, J. R. Studies of interference in serial verbal reactions. *Journal of Experimental Psychology*, 1935, *18*,   643-662.

Strub, R. L., & Black, F. W. *The mental status examination in neurology.* Philadelphia: F. A. Davis, 1977.

Strub, R. L., & Black, F. W. *Organic brain syndromes.* Philadelphia: F. A. Davis, 1981.

Suinn, R. M. *The predictive validity of projective measures.* Springfield, Ill.: C. C. Thoms, 1969.

Surridge, D. An investigation into some psychiatric aspects of multiple sclerosis. *British Journal of Psychiatry*, 1969, *115*, 749-764.

Talland, G. A. *Deranged memory.* New York: Academic Press, 1965a.

Talland, G. A. Three estimates of the word span and their stability over the adult years. *Journal of Experimental Psychology*, 1965b, *17*, 301-307.

Talland, G. A. Some observations on the psychological mechanisms impaired in the amnesic syndrome. *International Journal of Neurology*, 1968, *7*, 21-30.

Talland, G. A., & Ekdahl, M. Psychological studies of Korsakoff's psychosis: IV. The rate and mode of forgetting narrative material. *Journal of Nervous and Mental Disease*, 1959, *129*, 391-404.

Talland, G. A., & Schwab, R. S. Performance with multiple sets in Parkingson's disease. *Neuropsychologia*, 1964, *2*, 45-53.

Tarter, R. E. Psychological deficit in chronic alcoholics: a review. *International Journal of Addiction*, 1975, *10*, 327-368.

Tarter, R. E. Neuropsychological investigations of alcoholism. In G. Goldstein & C. Neuringer (Eds.), *Empirical studies of alcoholism.*

Cambridge, Mass.: Ballinger, 1976.

Tarter, R. E., & Jones, B. M. Absence of intellectual deterioration in chronic alcoholics. *Journal of Clinical Psychology*, 1971, *27*, 453-454.

Taylor, E. M. *The appraisal of children with cerebral deficits.* Cambridge, Mass.: Harvard University Press, 1959.

Taylor, L. B. Localization of cerebral lesions by psychological testing. *Clinical Neurosurgery*, 1969, *16*, 269-287.

Taylor, L. B. Psychological assessment of neurosurgical patients. In T. Rasmussen and R. Marino, (Eds.). *Functional Neurosurgery.* New York: Raven Press, 1979.

Taylor, M. A., Greenspan, B., & Abrams, R. Lateralized neuropsychological dysfunction in affective disorder and schizophrenia. *American Journal of Psychiatry*, 1979, *136*, 1031-1034.

Teasdale, G., & Jennett, B. Assessment of coma and impaired consciousness. *Lancet*, 1974, *ii*, 81-84.

Terman, L. M., & Merrill, M. A. *Stanford-Binet Intelligence Scale. Manual for the Third Revision, Form L-M.* Boston: Houghton Mifflin, 1973.

Terry, R. D. Structural changes in senile dememtia of the Alzheimer type. In L. Amaducci, A N. Davison, & P. Antuono (Eds.), *Aging of the brain and dementia.* New York: Raven Press, 1980.

Teuber, H. -L. Some alterations in behavior after cerebral lesions in man. In A. D. Bass (Ed.), *Evolution of nervous control.* Washington, D. C.: American Association for the Advancement of Science, 1959.

Teuber, H. -L. The riddle of frontal lobe function in man. In J. M. Warren and K. Akert, (Eds.). *The frontal granular cortex and behavior.* New York: McGraw-Hill Book Co., 1964.

Teuber, H. -L., & Weinstein, S. Performance on a formboard task after penetrating brain injury. *Journal of Psychology*, 1954, *38*, 177-190.

Thomas, J. C., Fozard, J. L., & Waugh, N. C. Age-related differences in naming latency. *American Journal of Psychology*, 1977, *90*, 499-509.

Thurstone, L. L. *Factorial study of perception.* Chicago: University of Chicago Press, 1944.

Thurstone, L. L., & Thurstone, T. G. *Primary Mental Abilities (Rev.).* Chicago: Science Research Associates, 1962.

Thurstone, L. L., & Jeffrey, T. E. *Closure Flexibility (Concealed Figures).* Chicago: Industrial Relations Center, University of Chicago, 1956.

Tissot, R., Lhermitte, F., & Ducarne, B. Etat intellectual des aphasiques. *L'Encéphale*, 1963, *52*, 286-320.

Torack, R. M. *The pathologic physiology of dementia.* New York: Springer-Verlag, 1978.

Tourette Syndrome Association, 41-02 Bell Blvd, Bayside, New York 11361.

Tourtellotte, W. W., & Shorr, R. J. Cerebral spinal fluid. In J. R.

Youmans (Ed.), *Neurological surgery*. Philadelphia: W. B. Saunders, 1982.

Tow, P. M. *Personality changes following frontal leucotomy*. London: Oxford University Press, 1955.

Tucker, D. M., Watson, R. T., & Heilman, K. M. Discrimination and evocation of affectively intoned speech in patients with right parietal disease. *Neurology*, 1977, *27*, 947-950.

Tweedy, J. R., Lapinski, R. H., Hines, T., et al. *Cognitive correlates of arteriosclerotic and depressive symptoms in a series of suspected Alzheimer patients*. Paper presented at the tenth annual meeting of the International Neuropsychological Association, Pittsburgh, February, 1982.

Twitchell, T. E. The restoration of motor functions following hemiplegia in man. *Brain*, 1951, *74*, 443-480.

Tyler, H. R. Disorders of visual scanning with frontal lobe lesions. In S. Locke (Ed.), *Modern Neurology*. London: Churchill, 1969.

Tzavaras, A., Hécaen, H., & Le Bras, H. Le probléme de la spécificité du déficit de la reconnaissance du visage humain lors des lesions hémisphériques unilaterales. *Neuropsychologia*, 1970, *8*, 403-416.

Van Zomeren, A. H., & Deelman, B. G. Long-term recovery of visual reaction time after closed head injury. *Journal of Neurology, Neurosurgery, and Psychiatry*, 1978, *41*, 452-457.

Varney, N. R. Colour association and "color amnesia" in aphasia. *Journal of Neurology, Neurosurgery, & Psychiatry*, 1982.

Vaughn, H. G., Jr., & Costa, L. D. Performance of patients with lateralized cerebral lesions. II. Sensory and motor tests. *Journal of Mental Disease*, 1962, *134*, 237-243.

Verhoff, A. E., Kaplan, E., Albert, M. L., et al. *Aging and dementia in the Framingham Heart Study population: preliminary prevalence data and qualitative analysis of visual reproductions*. Paper presented at the seventh annual meeting of the International Neuropsychological Society, New York, 1979.

Vernea, J. Considerations on certain tests of unilateral spatial neglect. In G. V. Stanley & K. W. Walsh (Eds.), Brain impairment. *Proceedings of the 1977 Brain Impairment Workshop*. Parkville, Victoria, Australia: Neuropsychology Group, Dept. of Psychology, University of Melbourne, 1978.

Vigouroux, R. P., Baurand, C., Naquet, R., A series of patients with cranio-cerebral injuries studies neurologically, psychometrically, electroenecephalographically, and socially. *International symposium on head injuries*. Edinburgh: Churchill Livingstone, 1971.

Visser, R. S. H. *Manual of the Complex Figure Test*. Amsterdam: Swets & Zeitlinger, B. V., 1973.

Vivian, T. N., Goldstein, G., & Shelly, C. Reaction time and motor speed in chronic alcoholics. *Perceptual and Motor Skills*, 1973, *36*, 136-138.

Vowels, L. M. Memory impairment in multiple sclerosis. In M. Malloy, G. V. Stanley & K. W. Walsh (Eds.), *Brain Impairment: Proceedings of the 1978 Brain Impairment Workshop*. Melbourne: University of Melbourne, 1979.

Wada, J & Rassmussen, T. Intra-carotid injection of sodium amytal for the lateralization of cerebral speech dominance. *Journal of Neurosurgery*, 1960, *17*, 266-282.

Walker, J. A., Posner, M. I., & Rafal, R. D. *Separation of effects on cognition versus motor performance due to the basal ganglia dysfunction of Parkinsonian patients*. Paper presented at the tenth annual meeting of the International Neuropsychological Society, Pittsburgh, February, 1982.

Walsh, K. W. *Neuropsychology*. New York: Churchill Livingston/ Longman, 1978

Walton, J. N. *Brain's diseases of the nervous system (8th ed.)*. London: Oxford University Press, 1977.

Walton D., & Black, D. A. The validity of a psychological test of brain damage. *British Journal of Medical Psychology*, 1957, *30*, 270-279.

Wapner, W., Hamby, S., & Gardner, H. The role of the right hemisphere in the apprehension of complex linguistic materials. *Brain and Language*, 1981, *41*, 15-33.

Warringron, E. K., & James, M. Disorders of visual perception in patients with localized cerebral lesions. *Neuropsychologia*, 1967a, *5*, 253-266.

Warrington, E. K., & James, M. An experimental investigation of facial recognition in patients with unilateral cerebral lesions. *Cortex*, 1967b, *3*, 317-326.

Warrington, E. K., & Rabin, P. Perceptual matching in patients with cerebral lesions. *Neuropsychologia*, 1970, *8*, 475-487.

Warrington, E. K., & Taylor, A. M. The contribution of the right parietal lobe to object recognition. *Cortex*, 1973, *9*, 152-164.

Warrington, E. K., & Weiskrantz, L. An analysis of short-term and long-term memory defects in man. In J. A. Deutsch (Ed.), *The physiological basis of memory*. New York: Academic Press, 1973.

Warrington, E. K., & Weiskrantz, L. Further analysis of the prior learning effect in amnesic patients. *Neuropsychologia*, 1978, *16*, 169-177.

Warrington, E. K., James, M., & Kinsbourne, M. Drawing disability in relation to laterality of cerebral lesion. *Brain*, 1966, *89*, 53-82.

Watson, C. G., Thomas, R. W., Anderson, D., & Felling, J. Differentiation of organics from schizophrenics at two chronicity levels by use of the Reitan-Halstead organic test battery. *Journal of Consulting Clinical Psychology*, 1968, *32*, 679-684.

Waxman, S. G., & Geschwind, N. Hypergraphia in temporal lobe epilepsy, *Neurology*, 1974, *24*, 629-636.

Wechsler, D. A Standardized memory scale for clinical use. *Journal of Psychology*, 1945, *19*, 87-95.

Weddell, R., Oddy, M., & Jenkins, D. Social adjustment after rehabilitation: a two year follow-up of patients with severe head injury. *Psychological Medicine*, 1980, *10*, 257-263.

Weigl, E. On the psychology of so-called processes of abstraction. *Journal of Abnormal & Social Psychology*, 1941, *36*, 3-33.

Weinberg, J., Diller, L., Gerstman, L., & Schulman, P. Digit span in right and left hemiplegics. *Journal of Clinical Psychology*, 1972, *28*, 361.

Weinberg, J., Diller, L., Laken, P., & Hodges, G. *Perceptual problems in right brain damage: the case for treatment.* Paper presented at the fourth annual meeting of the International Neuropsychological Society, Toronto, Canada, 1976.

Weingartner, H. Verbal learning in patients with temporal lobe lesions. *Journal of Verbal Learning and Verbal Behavior*, 1968, *7*, 520-526.

Weinstein, S. Deficits concomitant with aphasia or lesions of either cerebral hemisphere. *Cortex*, 1964, *1*, 154-169.

Weinstein, S., Semmes, J., Ghent, L., & Teuber, H.-L. Spatial orientation in man after cerebral injury: II. Analysis according to concomitant defects. *Journal of Psychology*, 1956, *42*, 249-263.

Weiskrantz, L., Warrington, E. K., & Saunders, M. D. Visual capacity in the hemianopic field following a restricted occipital ablation. *Brain*, 1974, *97*, 709-728.

Weissman, M. M. The assessment of social adjustment. *Archives of General Psychiatry*, 1975, *32*, 357-365.

Welford, A. T. Motor performance. In J. E. Birren & K. W. Schaie (Eds.), *Handbook of the psychology of aging.* New York: Van Nostrand, 1977.

Wells, C. E. Chronic brain disease: an overview. *American Journal of Psychiatry*, 1978, *135*, 1-12.

Wells, C. E. Chronic brain disease: an update on alcoholism, Parkinson's disease, and dementia. *Hospital and Community Psychiatry*, 1982, *33*, 111-126.

Wells F.L., & Ruesch, J. *Mental examiner's handbook* (Rev. ed.). New York: Psychological Corp., 1969.

Welsh, G. S., & Dahlstrom, W. G. (Eds.), *Basic readings on the MMPI in psychology and medicine.* Minneapolis: University of Minnesota Press, 1956.

Wepman, J. M., & Jones, L. V. *Studies in aphasia: An approach in testing.* Chicago University of Chicago Education-Industry Service, 1961.

Wepman, J. M., & Jones, L. V. Aphasia: diagnostic description and therapy. In W. S. Fields & W. A. Spencer (Eds.), *Stroke rehabilita-*

tion. St. Louis: W. H. Green, 1967.

Wepman, J. M., & Turaids, D. *Spatial Orientation Memory Test. Manual of Directions.* Palm Springs, Calif.: Language Research Associates, 1975.

Wertz, R. T. Review of Word Fluency Measure (WF). In F. L. Darley (Ed.), *Evaluation of appraisal techniques in speech and language pathology.* Reading, Mass.: Addison-Wesley, 1979.

Whitty, C. W. M., & Zangwill, O. L. Traumatic amnesia. In C. W. M. Whitty and O. L. Zangwill, (Eds.). *Amnesia.* London: Butterworths, 1966.

Wickens, D. D. Encoding categories of words: an empirical approach to meaning. *Psychological Review,* 1970, *77,* 1-15.

Williams, M. *Mental testing in clinical practice.* Oxford: Pergamon, 1965.

Williams, M. Geriatric patients. In P. Mittler (Ed.), *The psychological assessment of mental and physical handicaps.* London: Methuen, 1970.

Wilson, R. S., Bacon, L. D., Kasznick, A. W., & Fox, J. H. The episodic-semantic memory distinction and paired associate learning. *Journal of Consulting and Clinical Psychology,* 1982, *50,* 154-155.

Wilson, R. S., Rosenbaum, G., & Brown, G. The problem of premorbid intelligence in neuropsychological assessment. *Journal of Clinical Neuropsychology,* 1979, *1,* 49-54.

Wood, D. R., Reimherr, F. W., Wender. P. H., & Johnson, G. E. Diagnosis and treatment of minimal brain dysfunction in adults. *Archives of General Psychiatry,* 1976, *33,* 1453-1460.

Wood, F. B., Ebert, V., & Kinsbourne, M. The episodic-semantic memory distinction in memory and amnesia: clinical and experimental observations. In L. Cermak (Ed.), *Memory and amnesia.* Hillsdale, N. J.: Lawrence Erlbaum Associates, 1982.

Woodcock, R. L. *The Psycho-Educational Battery.* Boston: Teaching Resources, 1977.

Yacorzynski, G. K. Organic mental disorders. In B. B. Wolman (Ed.), *Handbook of clinical psychology.* New York: McGraw-Hill, 1965.

Yager, J. Intellectual impairment in uremic patients. *American Journal of Psychiatry,* 1973, *130,* 1159-1160.

Yntema, D. B., & Trask, F. P. Recall as a search process. *Journal of Verbal Learning and Verbal Behavior,* 1963, *2,* 65-74.

Zaidel, D., & Sperry, R. W. Some long term motor effects of cerebral commissurotomy in man. *Neuropsychologia,* 1977, *15,* 193-204.

Zangwill, O. L. Psychological deficits associated with frontal lobe lesions. *International Journal of Neurology,* 1966, *5,* 395-402.

Zubrick, S., & Smith, A. Minnesota Test for Differential Diagnosis of

Aphasia (MTDDA) (Review). In F. L. Darley (Ed.), *Evaluation of appraisal techniques in speech and language pathology*. Reading, Mass.: Addison-Wesley, 1979.

Zung, W. K. A self-rating depression scale. *Archives of General Psychiatry*, 1965, *12*, 63-70.

Zung, W. K. Factors influencing the self-rating depression scale. *Archives of General Psychiatry*, 1967, *16*, 543-547.